1995 MRKT
HKGS PRPRT

D0708151

THE ILLUSTRATED

DICTIONARY OF
NATURAL HEALTH

THE ILLUSTRATED
DICTIONARY OF
NATURAL HEALTH

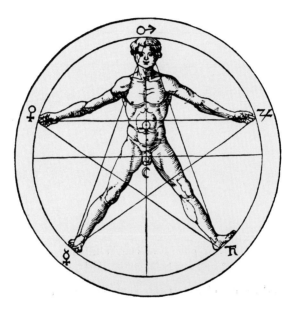

Compiled by
NEVILL & SUSAN DRURY

DAVID & CHARLES
Newton Abbot   London

NOTE TO READERS

This book is a work of reference only and should not be regarded as a source for individual treatments. Readers should consult qualified naturopaths, doctors and therapists for treating specific complaints since in many cases such complaints are multi-factorial.

First published in Great Britain
by David & Charles 1988

© Nevill and Susan Drury Publishing Pty Ltd 1988

British Library Cataloguing in Publication Data

Illustrated dictionary of natural health.
1. Medicine. Natural remedies
I. Drury, Nevill. II. Drury, Susan
615.5′35

ISBN 0-7153-9313-8

All rights reserved. No part of this publication
may be reproduced, stored in a retrieval system, or
transmitted, in any form or by any means, electronic,
mechanical, photocopying, recording or otherwise,
without the prior permission of David & Charles
Publishers plc.

Printed in Hong Kong by Mandarin Offset
for David & Charles Publishers plc
Brunel House
Newton Abbot   Devon

CONTENTS

PREFACE

During the last decade the general interest in alternative health therapies has increased enormously. There are several possible reasons for this. Among them is the undoubted mystique of the East, which has provided the West with the principles of yoga, meditation, tai chi and acupuncture as well as knowledge of a variety of important medicinal herbs and health foods, including ginseng and the various soyfoods used in macrobiotics. Then there is what can only be considered as the changing public perception of Western medicine itself — a mood towards self-reliance which tends to work against the aloof, authority-figure image presented by the traditional doctor. People these days want to know more about the treatments they take, participate in their own cures, feel more involved in the process of eliminating disease. The old notion of prescribing pills and allowing the illness to gradually subside is still prevalent, but more and more people are rejecting the very idea of treating disease with synthetic medicines that could have unforeseen side effects. Finally, there is a related perception that orthodox medicine has spent far too much time concerned with curative treatment, rather than with prevention. After all, if we are concerned about our health, a wholesome, nutritious diet coupled with regular exercise and a facility for reducing negative stress factors impinging on our lives — all of these are of undoubted importance. Yet, until very recently, modern medicine has had very little to say about nutrition, relaxation, or the psychosomatic aspects of disease. There has been little emphasis placed on individual or community-based health support systems, or on the idea of taking increasing responsibility for our own health, for these, to some extent, would erode the authority base of the doctor.

Nevertheless, as we have said, the times seem to be changing. More and more people are now looking for types of alternative health care with which they can become involved. And yet in terms of general reference works available to the public there has been no all-encompassing dictionary available in the English language, so far as we are aware, which has presented the terms and expressions used in alternative health therapies. This dictionary endeavours to fill that gap. And yet it does not ignore the frames of reference established by modern dietetics and Western medicine. Included are details of the nutrients required for a healthy diet and also numerous references to various systems, organs and functions of the body. Major diseases are also included, because in many cases natural therapies propose drug-free methods of treatment which deserve consideration. It is worth remembering that herbal remedies preceded the rise of the modern pharmaceutical companies, and many of the active constituents of modern medical drug treatments occur naturally in plants. So there is much 'traditional' knowledge that is still valid.

There is no doubt, of course, that the rise of alternative therapies has brought with it much that could be considered faddish, vogueish and scientifically unproven. This is a fair criticism, but references to health therapies of this type are also included here in an effort to be as broad as possible in the scope of the work. A dictionary, after all, is nothing other than a work of reference. However, inclusion of any given therapy should not be taken as an endorsement of its scientific validity, but simply as an indication that today some people are finding that modality to be of use in their day-to-day lives.

It is our belief that what has been called 'alternative medicine' in the past will increasingly come to be called 'complementary medicine' in the future. There is no doubting the miracles of modern Western medicine, especially in containing contagious diseases with antibiotics, but there is also much that can be added to conventional medical wisdom in terms of preventive diet, stress management and 'quality of life' considerations. The best aspects of alternative medicine, it seems to us, will survive and become increasingly important as adjuncts to modern health care. Chiropractic, osteopathy, the Alexander Technique, clinical hypnotherapy and acupuncture are well on the way to being accepted into orthodoxy, and more therapies will undoubtedly follow.

Meanwhile, we sincerely hope that *The Illustrated Dictionary of Natural Health* will make a modest contribution to delineating the seemingly vast range of alternative treatments now available. For the modern era, as always, has spawned an extraordinary diversity of approaches and techniques.

Nevill Drury
Susan Drury
1988

PART 1

HEALING PLANTS

A

ACACIA, gum arabic *(Acacia senegal)*

Several varieties of trees and shrubs occur within the genus *Acacia*. The gum from African species such as *Acacia senegal*, which exudes from the stem, can be dissolved in water; it has a soothing effect on irritated mucous membranes. It is an important ingredient in medicinal compounds used to treat coughs, sore throats, catarrh and also diarrhoea and dysentery. The gum from Australian species, known as wattle, is not as effective as that from certain African species, so an infusion made from bark is generally used instead. It should be noted that some species are poisonous. Acacia flowers can be used in perfumes and potpourris. When the Paiute Indians found their eyes inflamed by dust or other irritants they are said to have found relief by sleeping with 4 acacia seeds under each eyelid.

ACETUM

A solution of aromatic substances in vinegar.

ACONITE, monkshood, wolf's bane *(Aconitum napellus)*

A hardy, glossy-leafed plant with a tuberous root and dark blue flowers. Known since ancient times as a deadly poison, it was often used on arrow heads and also to kill rats and other pests. It can be used for medicinal purposes but only with extreme

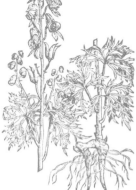

Aconite

caution as it acts as a depressant on the cardiac, respiratory and circulatory systems and causes strange hallucinations. Small doses can be used to combat fever and acute throat and lung infections. Applied externally it will ease the pain of complaints such as arthritis, rheumatism and neuralgia. Aconite mixed into an ointment with henbane and stramonium was rubbed on witches' broomsticks to give them the sensation of flying.

ADDER'S TONGUE *(Ophioglossum vulgatum)*

A single-leafed green plant traditionally used in infusion to treat wounds and skin problems but not widely used today.

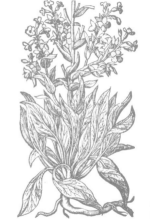

Adder's tongue

ADJUVANT

Any herb which can be added to a mixture to increase the effect of the main ingredient.

AGRIMONY, cockleburr, stickwort, sticklewort *(Agrimonia eupatoria)*

A long-leafed green plant with a tall, central, hairy stalk on which grow small yellow flowers. The plant grows wild in Europe, Asia and Africa and was used in the Middle Ages in the form of a solution to wash wounds and draw out splinters. When drunk as a herbal tea it is still said to be helpful for gastrointestinal problems and also for skin disorders, coughs and rheumatism.

ALDER, COMMON (*Alnus glutinosa*)

A tree with reddish catkins which turn a greenish yellow. The dried bark and leaves can be made into a tea which is said to be good for sore throats and dyspepsia. The fresh leaves were traditionally used to soothe inflamed skin and also to ward off fleas. A solution made from the inner bark boiled in vinegar and rubbed on the skin is said to kill lice, cure scabies and dry up any sores.

ALEXIPHARMIC

A medicine which neutralises a poison.

ALFALFA, buffalo herb, lucerne (*Medicago sativa*)

A perennial plant originally from China, today grown as fodder. It was named by the Arabs 'the Father of all Foods' because it contains such an unusually high number of vital nutrients including all the known vitamins, eight important digestive enzymes and also calcium, magnesium, phosphorus and potassium. The sprouts are a popular high-protein ingredient in salads and, if eaten regularly, are reported to help rebuild decayed teeth. Alfalfa tea helps to balance the acid production in the stomach and is taken to improve the appetite and aid digestion, to relieve urinary and bowel problems, and to help cure peptic ulcers. It is also helpful for people suffering from food allergies as it helps to break down protein residues which they find difficult to digest. Alfalfa tea is even said to be of some assistance in helping alcoholics and drug addicts to break their habits.

ALGIN

A natural substance derived from seaweeds in the form of alginic acid. Said to relieve heartburn, it is usually taken as sodium alginate tablets which are chewed and then washed down with a glass of milk. Their effectiveness is improved if crunched dolomite or magnesium oxide is added to the milk.

ALKALOID

A substance with alkaline properties which affect the circulatory and nervous systems. Often bitter and poisonous, alkaloids act as analgesics, tranquillisers, local anaesthetics and hallucinogens.

ALLSPICE, pimento, Jamaica pepper, clove pepper (*Pimenta officinalis*)

The dried, unripe berry from an evergreen tree native to the West Indies and Central and South America. Widely used in potpourris, and in cooking because it tastes like a combination of cinnamon, cloves and nutmeg, the berry is also used in ointments because of its anaesthetic effect. The oil from the crushed berries is used in medicines to relieve flatulence, indigestion and diarrhoea, and is also said to help cure headaches and toothaches. Made into a plaster, it can be helpful for rheumatism and neuralgia.

ALOE

Any of over 200 succulent plants of the genus *Aloe*, which is related to the lily. Aloes are grown in warm climates, particularly in Africa and the Americas, and have been used medicinally for over 2000 years. The bitter-tasting juice is a purgative which can be used for gastro-intestinal complaints, especially colitis, and is said to be helpful for peptic ulcers. When applied directly to the skin it has considerable healing powers.

The best known variety today is aloe vera, *Aloe barbadensis*, which is widely used in natural cosmetics. Cleopatra is said to have attributed her radiant skin and hair to her use of aloe gel. Modern beauticians assert that aloe vera is a unique substance which actually draws moisture from the air and so keeps the skin fresh and young-looking and softens ageing lines. It is also said to be an excellent hair conditioner. Aloe vera is a particularly effective first-aid plant. To give quick relief to burns, cuts, insect bites, bruises, sunburn or any skin irritation, simply break off a leaf and rub it over the skin. The gel which oozes out is a mild antiseptic and will seal the wound and allow it to heal naturally. Skin ulcerations resulting from X-ray burns have been greatly reduced by aloe vera. It is also said to soften corns and cure some fungal skin infections.

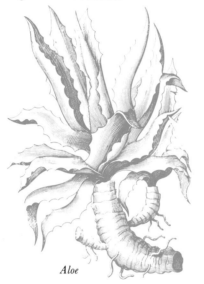

Aloe

ALTERATIVE

A somewhat imprecise term referring to any substance which will change and improve an unhealthy condition of the body and restore it to health. Alteratives are often used together with stimulants. Examples of alteratives are cod liver oil, sulphur, iodine, garlic, ginseng, sarsaparilla, sassafras and burdock root.

AMARANTH, lady bleeding
(Amaranthus hypochondriacus)

A flowering herb, the healing properties of which were known to the ancient Greeks who regarded it as a symbol of immortality and used it to decorate images of their gods and tombs. It has

astringent properties and is used in decoction to treat diarrhoea, dysentery, bleeding from the bowels, excessive menstruation and leucorrhoea. It is also helpful as a mouthwash for ulcerated throat and mouth infections. If woven into a wreath, it was reputed to make the wearer invisible and it has also been used in potions designed to curb the affections.

ANAESTHETIC

A substance which causes loss of sensation in the whole body or part of the body. The best known natural example is cocaine, a white, crystalline substance obtained from the leaves of the coca plant, *Erythroxylon coca*. It is sometimes used medicinally for minor surgery on the nasal passages. Clove oil, wintergreen, birch bark and mandrake also have anaesthetic properties.

ANALGESIC

A substance which relieves pain without causing loss of consciousness. One of the best known analgesics, aspirin, which is now made synthetically, also occurs naturally in some plants. Until 1874 all commercial aspirin was produced from the oils of sweetbirch bark or wintergreen leaves. Several other plants have natural analgesic properties; among them are valerian, St John's wort, mullein, cloves and chamomile.

ANAPHRODISIAC

An agent which decreases sexual desire or performance. Natural substances said to have this effect include ice, tobacco, cocaine, opium, camphor, lettuce and belladonna.

ANGELICA *(Angelica archangelica)*

A tall, large-leafed plant grown in cool shady areas, said to have been so named in the Middle Ages because of an angel who said that it would cure the plague. It has traditionally been highly regarded by herbalists as a general protection against infections. The sweet, pleasant-tasting plant is still included in many herbal tea blends for its soothing effect on the nerves and its qualities as a general tonic. Angelica tea (made either from the dried root or the whole plant) is also still used to relieve flatulence and indigestion. The root can be boiled in paraffin wax and made into an ointment for rheumatism or for minor skin problems, particularly itching. Large doses of angelica may have an adverse effect on blood pressure and respiration, and should be avoided particularly by diabetics as they may cause an increase of sugar in the urine.

ANISE, aniseed (Pimpinella anisum)

An aromatic herb whose small, licorice-flavoured seeds are widely used in cooking and herbal medicine. In Roman times a spicy aniseed cake was eaten after a large banquet to aid digestion. Aniseed tea is still drunk to dispel flatulence and alleviate cramps, nausea, diarrhoea and infant colic. It stimulates milk production in nursing mothers and is said to bring on menstruation. Aniseed is also helpful for respiratory ailments such as colds, flu and asthma and is used to flavour cough syrups. The seeds can be chewed to cure insomnia and hiccups and to sweeten the breath, or made into a calming drink for children. The oil from the seeds also acts as an insect repellent.

ANODYNE

A substance which lessens or stops pain. The best known painkiller is aspirin — see Analgesic.

ANTACID

A substance which neutralises the excess acid in the stomach and so relieves indigestion and its associated discomforts. Magnesium, charcoal and chalk (calcium carbonate) are common antacid remedies. Algin, a seaweed derivative, is becoming increasingly popular as an antacid — as are alfalfa, chamomile and meadowsweet.

ANTHELMINTICS

Agents used to destroy or expel intestinal worms. Also known as vermicides and vermifuges respectively. Plants used for this purpose include wormwood, horseradish, garlic, thyme, hydrangea, lily-of-the-valley, uva-ursi, aloes, wormseed, tansy, butternut.

ANTIASTHMATIC — see
Antispasmodic

ANTIBACTERIAL — see
Antiseptic

ANTIBIOTIC

A substance which arrests the growth of micro-organisms. The insectivorous plant, sundew, contains a natural antibiotic which, in its pure form, is effective against streptococcus, staphylococcus and pneumonococcus. Iceland moss is said to hinder the growth of the bacillus which causes tuberculosis.

ANTICOAGULANT

A substance which prevents or reduces blood clotting. The fragrant white chemical coumarin, which smells like vanilla, is a natural anticoagulant found in the herbs woodruff and melilot (sweet clover) and also in tonka beans. It is also produced synthetically from coal tar.

ANTI-EMETIC

A substance that relieves nausea and vomiting. Examples include spearmint, cloves, Iceland moss and raspberry.

ANTIFUNGAL

A substance used to treat fungal infections. Blackberry and sorrel are 2 common plants which can be used in this way.

ANTIHISTAMINE

A drug used in the treatment of allergies to neutralise the effect of histamines. Vitamin C is a natural antihistamine and some people find relief from allergic sneezing by eating orange peel which has been soaked in apple cider vinegar, drained, then cooked with honey and stored in the fridge.

ANTIHYDROTIC

A substance which reduces perspiration by decreasing the action of the sweat glands. Effective examples are belladonna and strychnine.

ANTI-INFLAMMATORY

A substance which reduces inflammation. Examples are ground ivy, mallow, melilot, white clover and comfrey.

ANTILITHIC

A substance which helps to dissolve urinary stones. Some examples are beans, bearberry, woodruff, knotweed and plum.

ANTIPERIODIC

A substance which prevents the periodic return of the seizures associated with certain feverish diseases such as malaria, or lessens the severity of these seizures. Examples are eucalyptus, iodine, cinchona bark, rue, senna, quebracho, salicin and arsenic.

ANTIPHLOGISTIC

A substance which reduces inflammation. Examples include chamomile, tormentil, goldthread, arnica, mallow, melilot and white clover.

ANTIPYRETIC

An agent which reduces high fevers either by causing the body to lose heat rapidly such as in perspiration, or by reducing circulation or slowing tissue change. Effective antipyretics are cold baths, drinks and ice packs, camphor, aspirin, quinine, wintergreen, strawberry and dandelion.

ANTIRHEUMATIC

A substance which reduces rheumatic pain. Examples include couch grass, nettle, violet, comfrey, wintergreen and celery.

ANTISCORBUTIC

A rich source of vitamin C which acts as a remedy for scurvy. Some examples are rosehips, capsicum, watercress, sorrel and citrus fruits.

ANTISEPTIC

An agent which stops the growth of micro-organisms on living tissue. There are many plants which have natural antiseptic properties. Some of these are anise oil, bay laurel, cassia, gum benzoin, oxalis, comfrey, coffee, hydrogen peroxide, clove oil, garlic, eucalyptus, golden seal, lily-of-the-valley, rosemary, thyme, peppermint, sandalwood, tobacco, witch hazel and wormwood.

ANTISPASMODIC

Any substance which stops or reduces muscular spasms or convulsions. Examples include cohosh, catnip, hemlock, thyme, mistletoe, valerian, fennel and melilot.

ANTITHROMBIC

A substance said to help prevent clotting and thrombosis. Melilot is believed to have these qualities.

ANTITUSSIVE

A substance which relieves coughing. Examples include coltsfoot, horseradish, comfrey, horehound, licorice and mullein.

APERIENT

A gentle purgative which acts as a mild stimulant for the bowels. Examples include asparagus, dandelion, cucumber, calendula and burdock.

APHRODISIAC

A substance which stimulates sexual desire and function. There is much disagreement over the effectiveness of aphrodisiacs. Amongst those considered worthwhile by many people are yohimbe, saw palmetto, muira-pauma and marijuana.

Baths containing plants such as civet, vervain and orris root are often recommended as aphrodisiacs, as are those sprinkled with orange and rose buds, jasmine and acacia flowers, rosemary and myrtle. Other people have more faith in a romantic dinner which includes foods widely believed to act as aphrodisiacs, such as oysters, artichokes, anchovies, asparagus, onions, garlic, cucumber, bananas or dates.

APPETISER

A substance which stimulates the appetite. Some examples: alfalfa, mint, watercress, parsley, rosemary and chamomile.

APPLE CIDER VINEGAR

A folk medicine traditionally used in Vermont, USA. Its effectiveness was researched by a country doctor, D. C. Jarvis, who in 1958 used his findings as a basis for his best selling book *Folk Medicine*. He found apple cider vinegar was an effective remedy for a variety of ailments including headaches, fatigue, sore throats, high blood pressure and gastric upsets, and that it was particularly useful as a cure for arthritis because it contains a high level of the mineral salt potassium. His recommended dose was 1 teaspoon in a glass of water taken after each meal. It is said to be even more beneficial when sweetened with unprocessed honey.

ARNICA, leopard's bane (*Arnica montana*)

A poisonous plant which has healing powers when applied externally in a diluted form. A professionally prepared tincture can be helpful for sprains, bruises, boils and abrasions, though it must be used cautiously as it can cause inflammation of the skin. It has been claimed to restore hair growth when applied to the scalp.

AROMATIC

A spicy, fragrant-smelling plant often used to mask unpleasant or nauseating substances. In small doses aromatics usually stimulate the mucous membranes of the gastro-intestinal tract and expel wind. They should not be used in large doses or where there is any inflammation of the stomach or intestines. Examples include cinnamon, nutmeg, ginger, allspice, basil, orange, angostura, caraway, wintergreen, summer savory and musk seed.

ARROWROOT (*Maranta arundinacea*)

A root plant from the West Indies and the Americas, so named because it was used by American Indians to heal wounds from poisoned arrows. It is now widely used as a starchy food and is especially valuable for infants and invalids because it is so easy to digest. Made into a paste and boiled with milk or water, it is an excellent natural remedy for diarrhoea.

ASAFOETIDA, devil's dung, stinking gum (*Ferula asafoetida*)

Strong smelling gum from a kind of giant fennel. It is a popular seasoning in Indian food and is used in some Asian perfumes and potpourris. A piece of the gum hung around the neck is believed, in some countries, to protect the wearer from disease. Used in a more orthodox way, it is made into a pill to relieve croup and colic in children and as a stimulant, an expectorant and a remedy for hysteria and spasmodic nervous diseases.

ASTRINGENT

A substance which contracts the tissues of the body and so lessens the discharge of mucus, blood or other fluid. Often used to refer to cosmetic substances which clean the skin and contract the pores, leaving a tight, refreshing feeling. Examples of astringents are witch hazel, geranium, rose, bistort root and white oak bark.

AUSTRALIAN BINDWEED (*Convolvulus erubescens*)

A trailing plant with hairy leaves and funnel-shaped flowers used by the Aborigines of New South Wales in decoction as a remedy for indigestion, gastric disturbances and diarrhoea.

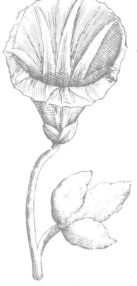

Bindweed, Australian

B

BALM, lemon balm, sweet balm, bee balm (*Melissa officinalis*)

A lemon-scented herb found in most herb gardens and used extensively in cooking and in bath additives and herb pillows because of its soothing qualities. Its medicinal qualities have been known since ancient times. The fresh leaves are made into a refreshing tea, especially valuable in hot weather, which is often used to induce perspiration and bring down a mild fever. Balm tea aids digestion and relieves many stomach complaints and has been traditionally thought to contribute to a long and active life. It is used for a wide variety of nervous complaints such as headaches, insomnia and nausea, and to regulate menstruation and alleviate symptoms of pregnancy and menopause. Mixed with honey, balm tea soothes sore throats. Balm leaves are an effective mouth-freshener, and can also relieve toothache and soothe insect bites.

BALSAM

A healing, soothing substance — usually an ointment.

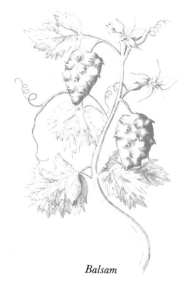

Balsam

the digestive system, stimulating the appetite and relieving flatulence, stomach cramps and diarrhoea. It has also been used in childbirth to hasten the expulsion of the afterbirth. The fresh leaves help to draw the poison from insect bites, and the dried leaves can be made into snuff which is often helpful for headaches and other cold symptoms.

substance obtained , particularly the *balsamea*. It is often n healing ointments but may aken orally.

ARBERRY, jaundice berry, pperidge, sowberry *(Berberis vulgaris)*

ornamental shrub with yellow flowers I red berries. It may be prescribed as erbal tincture in very small doses to at liver conditions, particularly jaune, gall bladder conditions and gastric oblems. The bark of the root is said to aid digestion, to make a good mouthwash for throat infections, and to dilate the blood vessels and lower blood pressure. The raw berries can be eaten to control the symptoms of typhus fever or rubbed onto the gums to relieve pyorrhoea. Both the root and berries have laxative properties.

BARLEY, pearl barley, Scotch barley *(Hordeum vulgare)*

A widely cultivated cereal important for its nutritional qualities and especially rich in vitamins B and E. Given as barley water or malt, it is generally recommended for convalescents. Barley water soothes inflamed mucous membranes and is especially helpful for diarrhoea and stomach pains, and in relieving the pain of cystitis. It is also sometimes applied to external sores. The root produces hordenine which is similar to ephedrine and can be used to treat asthma and bronchitis.

BASIL, sweet basil *(Ocimum basilicum)*

A fragrant green herb, regarded as sacred in ancient India, today used widely in cooking. The fresh leaves are more effective than the dry and can be made into a refreshing tea which clears the head and acts as a general stimulant. It acts on

BAY, sweet bay, bay laurel *(Laurus nobilis)*

An evergreen shrub with great historical and mythological significance; once thought to give protection against evil. It has been used to cure a wide variety of ailments but is now used mainly in cooking. Modern herbalists still use the oil from the leaves and berries (applied externally) to treat rheumatism and sometimes sprains and bruises. It was once a popular remedy for earaches, itchiness and stomach complaints. The fresh leaves will keep away fleas and generally freshen the atmosphere in a house. American Indians have used them for headaches and to clear the breathing passages.

BEACH BEAN, fire bean *(Canavalia rosea)*

A pink-flowered trailing plant found on sand dunes in warm areas of Australia. An infusion of the roots was used by the Aborigines to cure colds and was applied externally for rheumatism and other aches and pains.

BEANS, French bean, kidney bean, green bean, string bean, navy bean *(Phaseolus vulgaris)*

A common garden vegetable which comes in a great many varieties and is usually eaten for its nutritive qualities. Bean pods, when eaten in large quantities, lower the blood sugar level and can be helpful in treating diabetes. They also have a diuretic action, so bean pod tea is helpful for kidney, bladder and urinary tract disorders. As a homeopathic tincture, beans are used to treat rheumatism. Bean meal can be applied directly to the skin to treat acne, eczema and itching skin.

BEARBERRY, mountain
cranberry, bear's grape, arberry, kinnikinnik *(Arctostaphylos uva-ursi)*

A small evergreen shrub with red berries which grows wild in highland areas of Europe, North America and Asia. Usually taken as an infusion, it is well known for its effectiveness in treating all kinds of urinary tract disorders, diseases of the bladder and kidneys and particularly cystitis. It has also been used for bronchitis and, when combined with blueberry, for treating diabetes. Some people find it helpful for treating bed-wetting. Bearberry should not be used for prolonged periods as it can produce chronic poisoning.

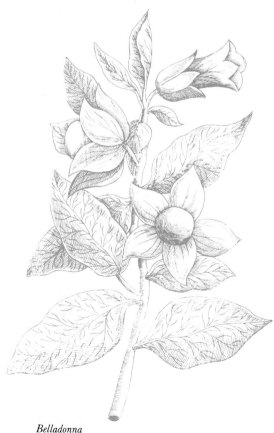

Belladonna

BELLADONNA, deadly
nightshade, bane wort, black cherry *(Atropa belladonna)*

A highly poisonous plant which grows wild in Europe. It is very dangerous to handle and should be prescribed only by qualified persons. The raw root and leaves are sometimes used medicinally in very small doses as a sedative and a pain reliever, and to relieve spasms in diseases like whooping cough. It can be used externally to relieve gout and rheumatism and to treat ulcers and boils, and also to dilate the pupils of the eyes. It was this last property which gave the plant its name, literally 'beautiful woman': its berries were used as a cosmetic by Italian ladies who wished to draw attention to their eyes.

BENZOIN, benjamin *(Styrax benzoin)*

A balsamic resin obtained from Indonesian trees of the genus *Styrax*. It is an antiseptic and is used mainly as a stimulating expectorant to clear the lungs in cases of chronic bronchitis. Mixed with glycerine, it is very effective for sore nipples on nursing mothers, for soothing chapped hands, and even for removing freckles. It is also used to treat fungal skin irritations, chronic laryngitis, diarrhoea and disorders of the genito-urinary tracts. One of the more bizarre uses of this fragrant gum, often used in incense and in fumigants, is as the scent-essence in a seance to call forth the spirits of the dead.

BERGAMOT, bee balm,
horsemint *(Monarda didyma)* wild bergamot *(Monarda fistulosa)*

There are two varieties of this wild herb, both native to North America. Both are used in cooking but also have medicinal qualities. Bergamot tea is an old Indian remedy for colds, sore throats and chest complaints. When mixed with milk, it is said to induce sleep. The leaves make a refreshing addition to bath water and for use on sprains, cuts and sores. Betony tea has been recommended as a sedative to alleviate asthma and hayfever and also as a general tonic for children who are not growing healthily; it is said to be effective against worms. The root should never be used as it tastes terrible and causes vomiting.

BILBERRY, blueberry, buckleberry, whortleberry, huckleberry, whimberry *(Vaccinium myrtillus)*

A wild shrub whose blue-black berries are enjoyed as a nutritious fruit containing vitamin C, bioflavonoids, copper and iron. The dried berries can be made into a tea which will improve blood circulation and is especially helpful for old people or those who have undergone surgery. They are sometimes used by homeopaths to treat diabetes and can also be used for coughs, gastric upsets and skin problems including burns and ulcers. The fresh berries make a good mouthwash and are especially helpful for inflamed gums and catarrh.

BISTORT, adderwort, dragonwort, snakeweed, Easter giant, patience dock *(Polygonum bistorta)*

A low-growing herb found in damp areas of Europe and North America. The root is rich in tannin and is a very strong astringent. It is prepared as a decoction and used for diarrhoea, dysentery, incontinence, haemorrhages and mucous discharges. It can also be used for haemorrhoids, as a mouthwash for sore throats or gums, and as a powder applied to a wound to stop bleeding.

BITTER

A substance which stimulates the appetite and digestion by acting on the mucous membranes of the mouth and stomach to stimulate the gastric juices. Examples include black alder, angelica, privet and dandelion.

BLACKBERRY, bramble *(Rubus fructicosus)* American blackberry *(Rubus villosus)*

This plant is best known for its edible fruit, but the roots and leaves are also used medicinally for their astringent and tonic qualities. Made into a tea, they are an excellent home remedy for diarrhoea and can also be helpful for chronic appendicitis, dysentery and leucorrhoea. The leaves can be chewed to cure bleeding gums, or bruised and placed directly onto haemorrhoids to relieve discomfort.

BLACK COHOSH, snakeroot,
squawroot, cimicifuga (*Cimicifuga racemosa*)

A perennial plant widely used by the North American Indians as an antidote to snakebite. It relieves painful menstruation and is used in natural childbirth to stimulate contractions of the uterus. Usually drunk as a tea, it can help rheumatism, asthma and bronchitis, headaches, high blood pressure and diarrhoea, and is an effective remedy for hysteria. It acts as a sedative on the nervous system but is a cardiac stimulant. Black cohosh must be used with care as large doses are poisonous. The leaves make a good insect repellent.

BLESSED THISTLE, milk
thistle, holy thistle (*Carduus benedictus/ Cnicus benedictus*)

An annual plant with large purple flowers which grows wild in wastelands, particularly in southern Europe. Widely used by ancient Romans both medicinally and as a food, this plant has bitter tasting leaves which are used by some herbalists to improve the appetite and to cure dyspepsia. It may cause vomiting if taken in too large a dose. The seeds are sometimes used for jaundice and for gall bladder and liver problems.

BLUE COHOSH, blue ginseng,
yellow ginseng, squawroot, beechdrops (*Caulophyllum thalictroides*)

A tall North American perennial with yellow flowers and single dark blue berries. The root is used in a tea for menstrual problems, especially cramps, and to speed contractions of the uterus and alleviate pain in childbirth. It can also be

used for children's colic and for rheumatism, or made into a poultice for skin sores and rashes. The berries are poisonous and often very irritating to the skin.

BOLDO (*Peumus boldus*)

A small shrub from Chile with dark leaves that smell strongly of lemon, and unpleasant-tasting, greenish-yellow fruit. The leaves are blended with other herbs into teas and can help people lose any excess weight which is due to sluggish, inefficient digestion. Boldo acts on the digestive system, stimulating gastric acid production, and on the liver, gall bladder and pancreas. It is also an antiseptic.

BORAGE, burrage (*Borago officinalis*)

A well-known herb with bright blue edible flowers, originally from the Mediterranean area. The leaves and flowers are used in salads and drinks, and also have medicinal qualities. The dried leaves, often combined with basil, make a stimulating and refreshing tea often used as a general tonic, particularly during convalescence, and recommended as a mid-morning drink for busy people. Borage also has an anti-inflammatory action and is helpful for reducing fevers and treating colds, bronchitis and other respiratory complaints, as well as rheumatism. The fresh leaves can be used in an eyewash and also made into a poultice to reduce inflammations and help varicose veins. The seeds and leaves are sometimes taken by nursing mothers to increase their milk supply. Some people develop skin rashes on contact with the fresh leaves.

BRYONY (*Bryonia dioica*)

A wild climbing plant from Europe and North America, bryony is extremely poisonous and should only be used according to instructions from thoroughly trained practitioners. It is used by homeopaths to treat whooping cough and some chest problems, and as a tincture to cure chilblains and stop them recurring.

BUCKBEAN, bogbean, water
trefoil, marsh clover, water shamrock
(Menyanthes trifoliata)

An aquatic plant from marshy areas in the northern hemisphere, buckbean is known as an old cure for scurvy. Its dried leaves can be made into a tea to relieve fever, migraine, indigestion, liver diseases and rheumatism. Applied externally it helps glandular swellings, sores and skin diseases such as herpes.

BURDOCK, cockleburr, burrseed
(Arctium lappa)

A large-leafed weed from Europe and North America with irritating burrs which stick to clothes. The root, leaves and seeds are used in healing. Used as a decoction it is said to be a particularly effective blood purifier and acts on the kidneys to increase their effectiveness. It can also be used for gout, jaundice, and liver and stomach problems. Applied externally it is helpful for sores, acne, eczema, boils and swellings of many kinds. The fresh, bruised leaves are a useful home remedy for poison oak or poison ivy stings, for bruises and sprains, and to bring down fever by increasing perspiration.

C

CACAO BUTTER

An oil extracted from the seeds of the chocolate tree (*Theobroma cacao*) for use in manufacturing skin-protection creams and oils. It has a demulcent action and is yellow-white in colour.

CACTUS *(Cactus grandiflorus)*

The stem and root can be made into a tea which acts as a cardiac stimulant similar to digitalis, and is also helpful for bladder and kidney problems.

CAJEPUT OIL, cajuput

An oil distilled from the leaves of a swamp tea-tree, *Melaleuca leucadendron*, found mainly in Australia and parts of South-East Asia. It is a powerful antiseptic, useful for cuts, scratches and insect bites, and will relieve the pain of bruises, strained muscles and rheumatism. It is very good for toothache and headache, and to relieve colic and flatulence. Just the smell of a few drops of the oil will revive a person who is feeling faint. The Aborigines of northern Queensland drank a decoction of young leaves for colds, flu and headaches.

CALAMINT, mountain balm
(Calamintha officinalis)

A European weed with pale blue flowers and a minty smell. Considered by the early English herbalist, Nicholas Culpeper, to be good for an enormous number of illnesses ranging from persistent coughs to leprosy, and said to be a natural contraceptive. It is now used mainly as an expectorant and is made into a cough syrup by adding sugar to an infusion. The dried leaves can be made into a mint tea which is good for the heart, helps colic and is a general tonic. The fresh leaves can be made into a poultice and used on bruises or for rheumatism.

CALAMUS, sweet flag, myrtle
grass *(Acorus calamus/Calamus aromaticus)*

A very pleasant-smelling, reed-like plant which grows beside water. Its dried rhizome has been used medicinally for thousands of years and is also used in flavouring and in perfumes. The ancient Greeks found it an excellent remedy for eye troubles and in parts of Turkey the candied root is still chewed to soothe coughs and build up the body's resistance to other diseases. Calamus can be made into an infusion or chewed raw, but it is rather bitter. It is a useful tonic and stimulant, and is helpful for indigestion and flatulence. It is sometimes chewed by smokers who are trying to give up the habit. The oil from the pressed root is used in inhalations.

CALENDULA, marigold
(Calendula officinalis)

A well-known garden plant with bright orange or yellow flowers. Only the variety with deep orange flowers has medicinal value. The juice, either freshly pressed from the flowers or made into a tincture, is good for sprains, pulled muscles, bruises, boils, cuts and sores, and is applied externally. The fresh juice is said to get rid of warts and also to relieve the pain of insect stings. The flowers can also be made into an infusion and drunk to relieve fevers, stomach complaints, vomiting, diarrhoea, boils and menstrual problems. A snuff to get rid of mucus from the nose is sometimes made from the dried flowers.

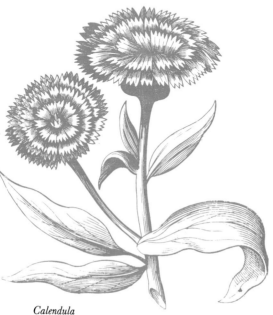

Calendula

CALMATIVE

A substance with a mildly sedative effect such as chamomile, bergamot or valerian.

CAMPHOR, camphor laurel, gum camphor *(Cinnamomum camphora)*

A translucent, crystalline mass obtained by passing steam through the wood of a large tree *Cinnamomum camphora*, which is native to eastern Asia and now growing wild in Australia. It is poisonous in large doses but can be used in small quantities as a sedative, to reduce fevers and as an antispasmodic helpful for conditions like whooping cough, epilepsy and vomiting. It has also been used for rheumatism, gout and diarrhoea. Applied externally it can heal bruises and sprains. It was used by the Arabs to lessen sexual desire and in parts of Asia to preserve the bodies of the dead. It also happens to be a very effective insect repellent.

CAPSULE

A container made of gelatin used to administer nauseous liquids or solids and to make them easier to swallow.

CARAWAY, caraway seed *(Carum carvi)*

A feathery-leafed cultivated plant whose seeds have been used in cooking and medicine for over 5000 years. Its pleasant flavour makes it a popular ingredient in medicines, especially for children, and it is sometimes used to settle the stomach after a dose of nauseous medicine. The seeds can be chewed after a meal to cure indigestion or flatulence, and to sweeten the breath. They can also be crushed into a powder and taken in hot milk to ward off a cold, and are said to be useful for menstrual problems and to increase the milk supply of nursing mothers. The oil from the seeds makes a good painkiller for toothache when put on a cotton pad placed directly onto the tooth. The seeds can also be crushed into a poultice for sprains and bruises. Caraway seeds were traditionally considered an essential ingredient in love potions as they were said to keep lovers faithful.

CARDAMOM (*Elettaria cardamomum*)

A perennial shrub of the same family as ginger, grown in hot climates, particularly in Malabar and Sri Lanka. The aromatic seeds are used in cooking, particularly in curries and spiced cakes, and also to flavour medicines. They were chewed by the ancient Egyptians to whiten their teeth but are more often used today for indigestion. An infusion of cardamom seeds stimulates the appetite and helps prevent flatulence.

CARDIAC

Any substance which acts on the heart. It may be a cardiac stimulant such as alcohol, lily-of-the-valley or digitalis, or a cardiac depressant like aconite or pulsatilla.

CARMINATIVE

An agent used to expel gas from the stomach and intestines and to relieve flatulence and pains. Some effective carminatives are aniseed, allspice, peppermint, ginger, eucalyptus, fennel, nutmeg, caraway, orange, coriander and pepper.

CARRAGEEN

An emulsifier used in cosmetic lotions and creams. Derived from Irish moss, it has an aroma reminiscent of seaweed — *see Irish moss*.

CASSIA

Any shrub or tree belonging to the genus *Cassia* which is characterised by tropical or subtropical plants with bright yellow flowers and long, many-seeded pods. A well-known example is *Cassia fistula*, known as pudding stick, the pulped pods of which can be used as a mild laxative. The cathartic drug senna is obtained from the dried leaves of some species of cassia. *Cassia alata*, known as ringworm shrub or seven golden candlesticks, is mainly used to treat itchy skin complaints such as eczema and ringworm. The freshly crushed leaves can be rubbed directly onto the affected area or made into a wash or an ointment. In India the leaves were scattered over elephants to prevent them from shaking off their loads, probably because they eased skin irritations caused by the loads.

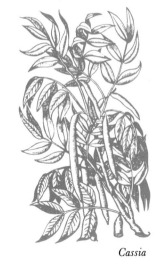

Cassia

CASSIA, Chinese cinnamon, cassia bark (*Cinnamomum cassia*)

An aromatic plant similar to the better known Ceylon cinnamon (usually called 'cinnamon'). The bark is used as a tonic, a carminative and an aid to digestion. It is also used in potpourris and in incense and sometimes as a substitute for Ceylon cinnamon. Oil from the plant is marketed in the United States as 'oil of cinnamon' and in Britain as 'oil of cassia'.

CASTOR OIL, Palma Christi, Mexico seed (*Ricinus communis*)

An unpleasant-tasting oil from the crushed seeds of the castor oil plant, once considered essential to keep children healthy. The oil is a simple, non-irritating purgative useful for constipation and colic in small children. It can also be used externally for ringworm, itchiness and warts, and has been used by women in the Canary Islands to increase their milk supply.

CATHARTIC, purgative, laxative

An agent used to hasten the evacuation of the bowel. Some gentle laxatives which merely increase peristaltic action are coffee, manna, cassia, tamarind and lemon. Purgatives which loosen the contents of the bowels include aloe, castor oil, rhubarb and senna. Some purgatives have a rather drastic effect and cause pain and spasms; among these are croton oil, scammony and mandrake.

CATNIP, catmint, catnep (*Nepeta cataria*)

A perennial shrub traditionally thought to excite cats, though not all cats seem to be affected by it. The leaves are made into an infusion which usually produces a tranquillising effect and so is often recommended for sick children. It brings down body temperature by promoting perspiration, is helpful for relieving pains and colic, and usually causes sleepiness. It can be injected into the bowel to relieve severe colic and is also used to relieve the discomfort of piles. Catnip is also said to increase a woman's fertility.

CAUSTIC VINE (*Sarcostemma australe*)

A tangled vine found in most of the warmer parts of Australia. Its stems exude a milky sap which can be applied directly to bleeding wounds, sores and ulcers.

CELANDINE, greater celandine, garden celandine (*Chelidonium majus*)

A common garden plant in Europe which also grows wild. It has yellow flowers and a reddish-brown root. The plant contains a bitter orange-yellow juice which turns red when exposed to air; this juice is an effective remedy for corns and warts and for itching skin diseases like eczema and ringworm. Mixed with brimstone it will fade spots on the skin. The plant can be made into an ointment for sore eyes and the root can be chewed to relieve toothache. An infusion can be taken internally to produce sweating and for liver and gall bladder complaints, but should be used in moderation as it can cause poisoning.

CELANDINE, lesser celandine, pilewort (*Ranunculus ficaria*)

A yellow flowering plant similar to a buttercup. It has astringent properties which make it a very good treatment for piles or haemorrhoids. The plant can be made into an ointment and applied directly to the piles, or made into an infusion of about 30 g (1 oz) in 600 ml (1 pint) of boiling water and drunk in doses of a small glassful at a time.

CENTAURY, fever wort, European centaury (*Centaurium erythraea*)

A red-flowered herb from Europe used as a general tonic and once considered to be almost a panacea. (It was so named because it was said to have healed the injured foot of the centaur, Chiron.) The whole plant or just the leaves can be made into an infusion which will stimulate all parts of the digestive system and cure biliousness. It is also said to kill worms, to relieve rheumatism, sore throats and feverishness, and to bring on menstruation. Combined with dandelion root it is used for jaundice. Applied externally it is said to fade freckles and skin blemishes.

CERATE

A preparation of oils, often with added herbs, that is made by being mixed with wax. It is used externally.

CEREBRAL DEPRESSANT

A sedative substance which decreases the vital activity of the brain. Examples are morphine, opium and black cohosh.

CEREBRAL EXCITANT

A stimulant; any substance which increases the vital activity of the brain. Examples are caffeine, camphor, musk and valerian.

CHAMOMILE, camomile, true chamomile, wild chamomile, German chamomile (Matricaria chamomilla) English, Roman or lawn chamomile (Anthemis nobilis)

Some herbalists say that only the German or true chamomile has medicinal value while others do not differentiate between the two varieties of this well-known herb. Chamomile tea, made from the small flower heads, has been a popular herbal remedy for centuries. Its soothing, relaxing qualities and its pleasant flavour make it an excellent drink for fretful, overtired or feverish children, and it is also useful to relax adults suffering from tension headaches, indigestion, sleeplessness or menstrual difficulties.

Chamomile is also helpful for relieving abdominal pains, rheumatism, cystitis and asthma, and will increase perspiration and elimination. It can be applied directly to ease the pain of bruises and sprains, haemorrhoids, boils and abscesses, eczema, earache and toothache. Added to bathwater it will relieve sunburn, leave the skin smooth and soft,

and soothe tired and aching muscles. Severe muscle pain or rheumatism can be treated effectively by rubbing the body with chamomile oil, then taking a sauna.

In addition, chamomile makes an excellent rinse to lighten and condition blonde hair, and is used in many face creams to soften and rejuvenate the skin. It makes an excellent eyewash to brighten the eyes and, if used regularly, will cure a stye in the eye. Some people use it as a refreshing mouthwash and it has even been reported to help alcoholics who are suffering from the dt's. A chamomile plant in the garden will keep away harmful insects.

CHERRY BARK (Prunus virginiana)

The young bark of the cherry tree, often used to give a sweet cherry flavour to cough medicine. It is also helpful for curing diarrhoea, bronchitis and indigestion.

CHERVIL (Anthriscus cerefolium)

A feathery green herb tasting rather like aniseed and used widely in cooking. It has been known since Roman times as a blood purifier, and is taken to help the kidneys and digestive system and to give the user a clear, healthy complexion. It is taken by infusion in Europe to treat high blood pressure and is also thought to be helpful in preventing anaemia in teenage girls. Chervil is a stimulant and expectorant, and is good for treating coughs. Applied externally it is helpful for swellings and bruises and for eczema.

CHESTNUT, sweet chestnut (Castanea sativa) horse chestnut (Aesculus hippocastanum)

A large tree with edible brown fruit. The leaves of the sweet chestnut can be made into an astringent, expectorant tea useful for coughs. An infusion of the bark of the horse chestnut is used to treat fevers and a tincture of the fruit can relieve haemorrhoids.

CHICKWEED, starweed, tongue grass, satin flower (*Stellaria media*)

Originally from Europe, chickweed is now known worldwide as a troublesome garden weed. It can be eaten as a vegetable, boiled lightly in water, or used raw as a cress; it has considerable nutritional value, being rich in vitamins A, B and C, and in several minerals. It is also helpful for constipation and as a soothing demulcent for inflammations of the lungs and digestive system. Applied externally it is good for sores, skin irritations, eczema, bruises, haemorrhoids, rheumatism and chilblains. It is quite a mild herb and safe to use in large quantities.

CHICORY — *see Succory*

CHOLAGOGUE

A substance which stimulates the flow of bile from the liver. Examples include aloe, dandelion, golden seal, rhubarb and wood betony.

CHOLERETIC

A substance which stimulates the liver to produce bile. Examples are dandelion and sage.

CINCHONA BARK, Peruvian bark, Jesuit's bark (*Cinchona* species)

The bark of any of the several varieties of cinchona tree, originally grown in the Andes, now cultivated in India and Java. Cinchona bark contains 24 alkaloids, the most important of which is quinine, an astringent, bitter antiseptic substance which is a specific treatment for malaria. Quinine is also useful for other intermittent fevers, neuralgia and dyspepsia, and as a general tonic. It can be given during labour to stimulate contractions of the uterus.

CINNAMON, Ceylon cinnamon (*Cinnamomum zeylanicum*)

Traditionally a highly valued spice, once more valued than gold. It was used by the ancient Egyptians in witchcraft and for embalming, and later it became a very important part of the Portuguese and Dutch spice trade. The dried bark is used in cooking and also for medicinal purposes. Made into a tea or simmered in milk, it is an excellent remedy for indigestion, diarrhoea, nausea and flatulence. Cinnamon is also sold as an oil, distilled from the bark and leaves, and useful for all sorts of digestive complaints as well as for cramps and pains, especially toothache. It is a general stimulant, warming the body and toning the nervous system. When used in incense it is said to arouse sexual feelings in females. Cinnamon is particularly useful to quell morning sickness in early pregnancy and is also said to be effective in stopping bleeding from the uterus.

CINQUEFOIL, five finger grass, silverweed (*Potentilla* species)

Any of the creeping grassy plants of the genus *Potentilla*. Their astringent properties make them useful for sore throats. They are also helpful for cramps and diarrhoea.

CLARY, clear eye, clary sage (*Salvia sclarea*)

A small European herb the seeds of which were made into an eyewash in the Middle Ages. The leaves are pleasantly aromatic and can be used as a flavouring or eaten as a vegetable fried in batter. Clary is most often used today for digestive upsets and for its soothing and antispasmodic properties. The oil is a highly aromatic fixative and is used in perfumes.

CLEAVERS, goosegrass, catchweed, clivers, clevers *(Galium aparine)*

A European herb now found over much of the world as a weed with a prickly stem and seed capsules which attach themselves to passers-by. It is a relaxing diuretic and laxative, and is an important herb for kidney and bladder complaints, particularly cystitis, which is often treated by an infusion of cleavers and marshmallow. It is also taken internally to treat skin complaints such as eczema and psoriasis. Cleavers acts on the lymphatic system, reducing the size of enlarged nodes, and is thought by some to prevent the growth of tumours. It can also be used to treat fevers and to lower blood pressure. Externally it can be applied as an ointment to wounds and burns. The seeds can be roasted and used as a coffee substitute.

CLOVES *(Eugenia caryophyllata)*

The dried unopened flower buds of a South-East Asian tree, first brought to Europe by the Arabs and Venetians. Cloves are highly aromatic and widely used in spicy cooking. They were once important as a natural food preservative and were also used in embalming. They are still used sometimes to make a local anaesthetic and particularly to relieve toothache. Cloves may be included in ointments for rheumatism. The oil acts on the digestive system relieving flatulence, colic, vomiting and bad breath, and also acts as a general stimulant. Pregnant women often find that cloves, combined with cinnamon and spearmint, will relieve morning sickness. Cloves are often added to other herb teas to settle an upset stomach. Clove oil is used commercially in toothpaste, mouthwashes and germicides because of its antiseptic qualities. It is used widely in soaps, perfumes and incense, and is sometimes said to be an aphrodisiac. A pomander of cloves makes an excellent insect repellent and is particularly useful in protecting stored clothes.

COAGULANT

An agent which helps clotting, particularly of blood. Examples are alum, lady's mantle, plantain and equisetum.

COCCULUS, moonseed *(Cocculus indicus)*

A plant used as a homeopathic treatment for travel sickness. It is related to the buttercup and was recommended by the homeopathic physician, Dr Margery Blackie, to Her Majesty Queen Elizabeth II as a remedy for travel sickness. Cocculus is also taken as a remedy for nausea in pregnancy.

COCKY APPLE *(Planchonia careya)*

A small tree, found in dry areas of northern Australia, with leaves which turn bright red before they fall and flowers which open only at night. The bark can be made into a decoction and used to bathe sores and wounds and to relieve itching rashes. The leaves are an old bush remedy for ulcers.

COLTSFOOT, coughwood, foalswort, horsehoof *(Tussilago farfara)*

A hardy weed from Europe which is used widely in cough mixtures. The dried leaves can be made into a herbal tobacco which is smoked for chest complaints such as bronchitis, asthma, persistent coughing or breathlessness. It can also be made into a tea which acts as an expectorant and loosens mucus so that it can be coughed up. Some people recommend its use by smokers to counteract some of the bad effects such as accumulation of coal tar in the lungs. Because it also has demulcent qualities it will soothe irritated mucous membranes in either the respiratory or digestive systems. Externally coltsfoot leaves can be made into a poultice to heal sores, wounds, burns, insect bites and any skin inflammations and swellings.

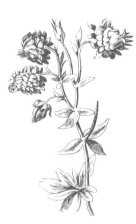

Columbine

COLUMBINE *(Aquilegia vulgaris)*

An attractive flowering plant often cultivated in gardens. It was formerly used in lotions for sore throats and mouth ulcers, and as a remedy for diarrhoea; it was even said to hasten the delivery of a child. It is slightly poisonous so is not used much by modern herbalists except externally, when its astringent properties make it helpful to relieve rheumatic pains. The seeds can be crushed and rubbed onto the scalp to repel head lice.

COMFREY, knitbone, slippery root, boneset *(Symphytum officinale)*

A fleshy-leafed plant from Europe, known since the Middle Ages for its healing properties and as a vegetable. The leaves or root, made into a poultice or an ointment, have traditionally been used to heal injuries, particularly broken bones, sprains, torn muscles, bruises, boils and other wounds. Recent research has shown that this healing power is due to the presence of allantoin and choline, 2 substances which stimulate circulation and reproduction of red blood cells. The whole plant is made into a hot poultice to soothe aches and pains such as rheumatism and also for varicose veins. Comfrey is an astringent and has a very high mucilage content. It is often made into a soothing, demulcent tea for digestive problems, especially ulcers and colitis and respiratory complaints like bronchitis, chest congestion and persistent coughs. A decoction of the root can be used for internal bleeding and is often recommended after surgery to promote cell regeneration and minimise scar tissue. The leaves are also used cosmetically to remove wrinkles and rejuvenate ageing skin. They can be used either fresh or as an ointment. Comfrey is poisonous if used in large doses over a long period of time.

COMPRESS

A thick piece of wet cloth, either hot or cold, which is applied to some part of the body, usually to ease pain, inflammation or swelling, though a cold compress can also be used to reduce fever. A compress is usually changed frequently.

CORIANDER *(Coriandrum sativum)*

A well-known aromatic culinary herb used in spices and curries. The seeds have generally beneficial effects on the digestive system, stimulate the appetite and relieve colic and flatulence. Coriander can be used to flavour other medicines and as a general tonic. The crushed seeds can be breathed in to cure dizziness and were once considered to have aphrodisiac qualities.

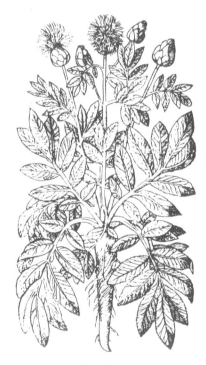

Cornflower

CORNFLOWER, hurtsickle, blue bottle *(Centaurea cyanus)*

Once a wild plant thought to have many medicinal qualities, it is now mainly grown for its attractive blue flowers. The flowers are still sometimes made into a eyewash and into a tea which is drunk as a general stimulant and tonic, and considered helpful for dyspepsia.

CORN SILK *(Zea mays)*

The protective covering around corn cobs, inside the leaves — actually the pistil of the corn plant. It can be made into a tea which is a useful demulcent and diuretic used for urinary problems, especially cystitis, and for bed-wetting, when mixed with agrimony. It can also be helpful for respiratory problems.

CORYDALIS *(Corydalis cava)*

A small reddish-flowered plant from Europe with a very high alkaloid content. Its effect is antispasmodic and it is particularly good for palsy, trembling hands and Parkinson's disease, and even for general over-excitement. It has been used to expel worms from the intestines.

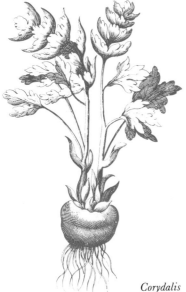

Corydalis

COTTON *(Gossypium herbaceum)*

This Mediterranean plant is cultivated commercially in many parts of the world. The bark of the root can be used like ergot to contract the uterus either during childbirth or to cause abortion. The mucilaginous seeds can be made into a cough remedy.

COUCH GRASS, twitchgrass, dog's grass *(Agropyron repens)*

A common weed generally regarded as a nuisance in gardens, it has been known since the time of the ancient Greeks as an effective diuretic useful for treating disorders of the kidneys and bladder, particularly cystitis. Couch grass tea can be very helpful for elderly people to tone up the sphincter muscle of the bladder, but should be used with caution. It can also help gout and rheumatism. Cats and dogs eat couch grass when they are sick. Couch grass root can be made into a soothing drink and is popular in France.

COUNTERIRRRITANT

A substance used to cause inflammation on the surface of the skin so as to relieve a deeper inflammation — *see also Irritant.*

COWSLIP, paigle, paegle *(Primula veris)*

A yellow-flowering plant related to the primrose. The fragrant flowers can be made into wine or eaten fresh with cream or as a decoration on cakes. Made into an ointment they can fade skin blemishes, freckles and wrinkles, and will sooth sunburn. Taken as a sedative tea they will cure insomnia, dizziness, headaches and stomach cramps. A decoction of the root is said to be helpful for bronchitis and for pains in the back.

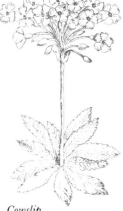

Cowslip

CRAMP BARK, guelder rose,
high cranberry *(Viburnum opulus)*

An attractive shrub with white flowers often grown in gardens. The bark is antispasmodic and is useful for colic, period pains, muscle pains, spasms, asthma, convulsions, fits and other nervous disorders. It is particularly helpful for pains in the uterus and ovaries. Cramp bark is usually combined with other plants such as ginger, angelica and chamomile. It is regarded as safe for children and can be helpful in stopping bedwetting.

CRANESBILL, spotted
cranesbill, alumroot, American cranesbill, storksbill, dove's foot *(Geranium maculatum)*

A common North American woodland plant with blue flowers, widely used by the American Indians. Its root has strong astringent properties; it is helpful when applied to sores, wounds and swellings of all kinds, and will stop bleeding. It can be made into an eyewash or a mouthwash useful for children with thrush, sore throats or mouth ulcers. It is also used for piles and for leucorrhoea. Taken internally it is helpful for diarrhoea and for internal bleeding. It is also used in deodorants.

CREOSOTE BUSH,
greasewood *(Larrea divaricata)* chaparral *(Larrea tridentata)*

The leaves and stems of this bush are widely used by the American Indians as a general tonic and panacea. As a tea it is helpful for digestive and respiratory problems as well as rheumatism, venereal disease and menstrual cramps. Some people believe it can cause remissions of cancers and shrinkage of tumours because of an ingredient called NDGA (nordihydroguiaretic acid). The plant has antiseptic qualities and the dried powdered leaves can be used for sores, wounds and snakebites, or made into a poultice to relieve rheumatism, sprains and all muscular pains. It makes an excellent disinfectant which can be used to remove body odours and to get rid of any scalp diseases. A resin is commercially extracted from the plant and used to prevent fats and butter from becoming rancid. The leaf residue is then used as a high-protein food for livestock.

CROSSWORT *(Galium cruciata)*

A yellow-flowered plant, common in Europe, which can be made into an ointment for cuts and abrasions.

CUBEB, java pepper *(Piper cubeba)*

The unripe berries from the cubeb vine of South-East Asia. They look like black pepper but when crushed turn red and give off a strong smell of sulphuric acid. The resultant oil has stimulant and diuretic properties. It is helpful for indigestion and urinary problems. Cubeb has a stimulating effect on the mucous membranes and is helpful for all sorts of respiratory complaints. It can be made into a tea for coughs, bronchitis and catarrh, or taken in capsules, made into lozenges or used in herbal cigarettes.

CUCUMBER *(Cucumis sativus)*

Usually eaten as a low-calorie salad vegetable, cucumber has aperient and diuretic qualities, so is good for chronic constipation and for bladder and kidney problems as it helps dissolve uric acid. The seeds will expel tapeworms from the body. Cucumber can also be used as a skin cleanser to soften and whiten the skin, fade freckles and soothe sunburn, bed sores and other skin inflammations. Made into an ointment, it can be used to get rid of wrinkles.

CUMIN *(Cuminum cyminum)*

A common culinary spice used especially in curries. It aids digestion and helps dispel flatulence, but is not widely used medicinally; it is often used by veterinary scientists, however.

CURRANT, black currant *(Ribes nigrum)*
red currant *(Ribes rubrum)*

A well-known plant usually grown for its fruit which is very high in vitamin C and bioflavonoids. The leaves can be made into a soothing tea for sore throats, hoarseness and children's coughs, and also used as a diuretic for kidney problems, rheumatism and gout. The berries can also be made into a mouthwash for bleeding gums and other mouth sores, or used as a basis for medicated throat lozenges.

Red currant berries can also be made into a mouthwash or can be used to stimulate the appetite and help digestion. They can be made into a particularly refreshing drink which some people use as a substitute for alcohol.

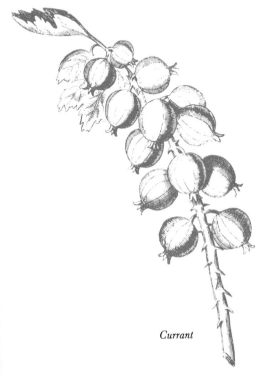

Currant

CYCLAMEN — *see Sowbread*

D

DAISY, ox-eye daisy, marguerite, white weed, white daisy, golden daisy *(Chrysanthemum leucanthemum)*

The large, white, yellow-centred daisy is often grown in gardens, but is also found wild. It can be used as a general tonic with diuretic and antispasmodic properties, and for coughs and respiratory complaints. The fresh leaves and flowers are sometimes used to treat warts. The daisy has similar qualities to chamomile, the latter being the more frequently used herb.

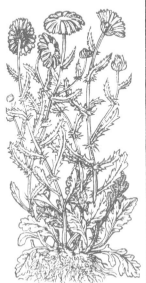

Daisy

DAISY CRESS *(Spilanthes paniculata)*

A common plant with long-stemmed conical flowers. It contains the chemical spilanthol which acts as a local anaesthetic. In many parts of Asia and Australia the roots and sometimes the leaves are chewed to relieve toothache. In India the flowerheads are also used for headaches, sore throats and gums, and even to correct stammering in children. Spilanthol is also a very effective insecticide.

DAMIANA *(Turnera diffusa)*

A medium-sized shrub found in Mexico and Texas. Its leaves and stem are prepared as a tea which is a general tonic and antidepressant, and is said to be an effective aphrodisiac.

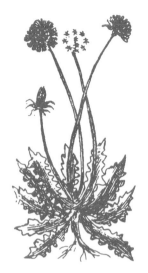

Dandelion

DANDELION, lion's tooth, piss-a-bed (*Taraxacum officinale*)

A common garden weed which contains many important nutrients including vitamins A, B, and C, mineral salts of potassium, calcium, manganese, sodium and sulphur, and also choline. The young leaves can be eaten as a wholesome salad vegetable, the flowers made into a blood-purifying wine, and the root roasted and used as a coffee substitute. Dandelion tea has considerable medicinal qualities. Its diuretic properties make it especially useful for all diseases of the liver, kidneys, gall bladder and urinary tract, so it is often used for jaundice, hepatitis, cirrhosis, gallstones, rheumatism, gout and fluid retention. It stimulates the appetite and aids digestion. The juice from the stem is said to remove warts and corns. According to gypsy lore, to dream of dandelions is a bad sign which suggests some impending disaster. However, it is believed that if you blow the down in the right direction you can send fond thoughts to your lover.

DECOCTION

A liquid made by simmering a medicinal plant in water, usually in a ratio of 1 part plant to 20 parts water. Roots, bark or seeds are often made into decoctions. They should be cut or crushed into small pieces, soaked for 10 minutes, then simmered in a covered, non-metal container for about 15 minutes, left to steep for another 10 minutes, then finally drained. It is usual to drink a cupful of the decoction 3 times a day before meals, but doses do vary according to the herb and the complaint.

DECONGESTANT

A substance used to relieve congestion, particularly in the upper respiratory tract. Examples are eucalyptus, ephedra, sage and thyme.

DEER'S TONGUE, vanilla leaf, hart's tongue (*Liatris odoratissimum*)

A plant grown on the west coast of North America. The dried leaves are used in sachets and potpourris, and to flavour tobacco. They can be used medicinally as a stimulant, diuretic and general tonic.

DEMULCENT

A substance taken internally to soothe inflamed tissues, particularly mucous membranes, and to protect them from further irritation. Demulcent plants are said to have a high mucilage content. Examples are burdock, comfrey, coltsfoot, licorice and arrowroot.

DEODORANT

A substance which masks or destroys unpleasant odours. Some plants with this quality are witch hazel, eucalyptus, lovage, willow and thyme.

DEPURATIVE

A substance which cleanses and purifies the system, especially the blood. Some examples are dandelion, cowslip, red clover, wild strawberry and nettle.

DEVIL'S BIT (*Scabiosa succisa*)

A purple-flowering plant which grows wild in the fields in Britain. It was so named, according to the English herbalist Nicholas Culpeper, because the devil bit off a piece of its root, envying its usefulness to mankind. Once believed to have a wide range of healing powers (it was even said to be effective against the plague), it is now used mainly to reduce fevers and cure old sores and internal inflammations by causing the toxins to be excreted through the skin. It is also used for coughs.

DIAPHORETIC

A substance which increases perspiration, often used to treat fevers. Very powerful ones are called sudorifics. Effective diaphoretics are burdock, catnip, angelica, thyme, lemon balm and spearmint.

DIGESTIVE

A substance which helps to digest food — *see Carminative and Stomachic.*

DILL *(Anethum graveolens)*

A feathery-leafed herb related to fennel and caraway, and widely used in cooking, particularly to flavour salads, soups, cheese and eggs. The seeds can be crushed and made into a tea which aids digestion, cures flatulence and indigestion, and is particularly good for children as it can be drunk cold. A teaspoon of dill tea is a good way to prevent colic in babies, and has also been said to increase milk production in nursing mothers. The seeds boiled in wine and breathed deeply are claimed to be a cure for hiccups.

DISINFECTANT — *see Antiseptic*

DIURETIC

A substance which increases the flow of urine and helps cleanse the bloodstream and excretory system. Examples are dandelion, alfalfa, caffeine, marshmallow, parsley, plantain and, of course, water.

DOCK — *see Sorrel*

DODDER, dodder of thyme *(Cuscuta epithymum)*

A parasitic plant of the convolvulus family, with pinkish-white flowers but no leaves, found in grassy areas. The bitter-tasting plant can be prepared as an infusion, which is a mild laxative and also helpful for diseases of the kidneys, the urinary tract and particularly of the liver.

DOG ROSE, brier hip, brier rose *(Rosa canina)*

A wild climbing rose; its fruit, known as rosehips, are very high in ascorbic acid or vitamin C. It is usually made into rosehip syrup, which is often given to babies and young children. Rosehips are a general tonic and aid to digestion, and are particularly recommended for kidney and bladder problems when their diuretic effect can be very helpful.

DOWN, cotton thistle, Scotch thistle *(Onopordum acanthium)*

A prickly thistle with a purple-flowering head. The juice was traditionally used to cure some cancers and has been used with some success by modern herbalists to reduce tumours and ulcers.

DRAGON'S BLOOD *(Daemonorops draco)*

A resinous coating around the ripe, cherry-sized fruits of the dragon tree, native to Indonesia. The resin has astringent qualities and is used to heal wounds and skin disorders. It is also thought to be an aphrodisiac and is used in incantations to bring back a wayward lover. Its red colour makes it useful in colouring varnishes and lacquers.

DYER'S GREENWEED,
dyer's broom, waxen woad *(Genista tinctoria)*

A perennial herbaceous shrub from Europe and north-eastern America. It stimulates the central nervous system and raises the blood pressure. Because it is a mild diuretic and cathartic, it is recommended for fluid retention, gout and rheumatism. The tincture can be applied externally for herpes.

DYSENTERY PLANT
(Grewia retusifolia)

The leaves of this plant are a well-known bush remedy for diarrhoea, used by both the Australian Aborigines and the early white settlers. They can either be chewed or made into a decoction.

E

ECHINACEA, cornflower, black
sampson *(Echinacea augustifolia)*

A perennial herb from the prairies of North America. The odourless, bitter-tasting rhizome is antiseptic and has remarkable qualities as a blood purifier and natural antitoxin. It is prepared as a decoction and taken either internally or externally for blood poisoning and septic infections of all kinds, boils, eczema, abscessed teeth, acne, snakebites and even cancer. It will also reduce fevers and help digestion, and has been used successfully for typhoid fever.

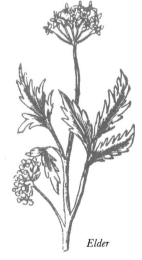

Elder

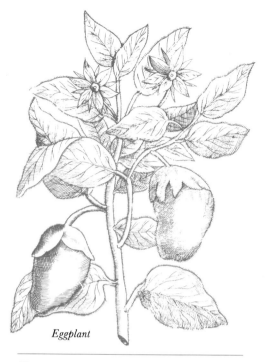

Eggplant

EGGPLANT, aubergine *(Solanum melongena)*

The purplish-black fruit of a leafy plant originally from India, now cultivated widely for use as a vegetable. It is a very nutritious food containing protein, carbohydrates, minerals and vitamins A, B and C, and is sometimes referred to as 'poor man's meat'. Eggplant is said to be helpful in regulating cholesterol levels, and can also be made into an ointment and used externally to relieve haemorrhoids.

ELDER, black elder *(Sambucus nigra)*

A tall, straggling shrub with white flowers and black berries which are used in jams and syrups or made into wine, but should not be eaten raw. The berries are rich in mineral salts and vitamins, particularly vitamins B and C. The plant is used widely in herbal medicine. The flowers can be made into a relaxing tea which acts as a general tonic, helps digestion, induces sleep, increases perspiration and is a traditional remedy for colds and flu. A tea made from the young leaves is a diuretic useful for diabetics, and can be used for urinary problems, fluid retention and rheumatism. Elder flower water is used externally as an eyewash, a bath additive and a skin toner. It is said to remove wrinkles, smooth roughened skin, soothe sunburn, fade freckles and clear up minor skin infections. Held in the mouth for a few minutes, it will often relieve toothache. The leaves can be made into a soothing ointment for bruises, sprains and chilblains. The berries can be made into a black dye which some American Indians used on their hair. The hard, close-grained wood is often used for musical instruments but, according to Danish legend, brings bad luck if it is made into furniture.

ELECAMPANE, elfdock,
scabwort, wild sunflower, horseheal
(Inula helenium)

A yellow-flowering plant from Europe and Asia, used particularly frequently in Chinese herbal medicine as a general tonic and digestive aid which expels gas and has laxative qualities. It is also used for respiratory problems, especially coughs and bronchitis, and will expel intestinal worms. Externally it is helpful for itchy skin conditions. Its root is one of the richest natural sources of insulin or diabetic sugar. When it is burnt the smoke will repel insects.

ELM, common elm, field elm *(Ulmus campestris)*

A large European tree, the bark of which can be used as an astringent decoction for itching skin diseases such as herpes or ringworm. It is also soothing and diuretic. The American species often known as slippery elm, *Ulmus fulva*, has similar properties but in a stronger form, so the American tree is much more important in modern herbalism. Its powdered bark can be obtained commercially and is used to soothe most irritations resulting from inflammations of the mucous membranes, such as sore throats, bronchitis and inflammatory bowel diseases. Because it contains considerable nutrients, it is injected into the bowel in

severe cases of diarrhoea and dysentery. It can also be used externally as a poultice to soothe wounds and skin irritations.

EMBELIA *(Embelia ribes)*

An Indian plant with a single reddish-brown fruit about the size of a peppercorn. The crushed fruit dissolved in milk and taken with any purgative is an effective way to expel tapeworms. Embelia is a diuretic and a digestive aid which is often used for dyspepsia; it is also used for rheumatism.

EMETIC

A substance which causes vomiting. Local emetics act on the gastric nerves alone. Among these are alum, mustard, salt and large quantities of warm water. Systemic emetics act through the medium of the circulation and include ipecac, senega and squill.

EMMENAGOGUE

A substance which stimulates menstruation. Examples include ergot, thyme, rosemary, nasturtium seeds and watercress.

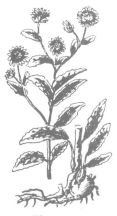

Elecampane

EMOLLIENT

A substance which soothes, softens and protects the skin. Examples include aloe vera, chickweed, marshmallow, comfrey and oatmeal.

EPHEDRA, mormon plant, desert
tea, brigham weed, teamsters tea
(Ephedra species)

A broom-like shrub found in arid areas of the northern hemisphere. It was widely consumed by the American Indians as a pleasant-tasting tea which was also thought to be a general tonic. It can be used as a blood purifier and a diuretic; it is especially helpful for flushing out the kidneys, but should not be used by people suffering from high blood pressure or heart disease. The roots can be used to stop internal bleeding and cure venereal disease.

Ma huang, the Chinese species of ephedra (*Ephedra sinica*), has been used for over 5000 years to treat coughs, headaches, asthma, hayfever and some skin infections. It contains the alkaloid ephedrine, a powerful decongestant which is found only in small quantities in other species. It may be taken by mouth or by injection.

EQUISITUM — *see Horsetail*

ERGOT *(Claviceps purpurea)*

A fungus which grows on rye plants and other cereals. It causes certain muscles to contract, so is useful in stimulating contractions of the uterus in labour, in menstrual disorders, and in preventing haemorrhages. It is sometimes used to relieve migraine headaches by contracting the swollen blood vessels, and can also be helpful for diarrhoea, diabetes and night sweats. Ergot is a source of the hallucinogen LSD and is available only by medical prescription in the USA, though it is freely available in Europe.

ERRHINE

A substance that causes sneezing and promotes nasal discharges. Examples include cubeb, coltsfoot, ginger and lavender.

ERYNGO, eringo, sea holly *(Eryngium campestre)*

A prickly-leafed plant that grows in sandy coastal soils in Europe. Its large white root is used as a diuretic for urinary diseases, particularly urethritis and cystitis, and also for irritations of the uterus. It is also an expectorant and can be useful for coughs and respiratory complaints.

EUCALYPTOL

The essential oil distilled from eucalyptus leaves — *see Eucalyptus*.

EUCALYPTUS, blue gum *(Eucalyptus globulus)*

A native Australian tree now widely cultivated in southern parts of Europe and the USA. Its leaves and the oil *eucalyptol* which is distilled from them are highly aromatic and are a powerful antiseptic. Eucalyptus oil is an excellent inhalant used to clear the nasal passages in a heavy head cold. It is useful as an expectorant in all kinds of respiratory ailments, either made into lozenges for coughs and sore throats, smoked as a tobacco, or made into a tea for bronchitis and asthma. It is also good for treating intermittent fevers such as malaria and for colds and flu. It can be applied externally to disinfect cuts, sores and ulcers, or added to bathwater to get rid of offensive odours from skin infections.

EUPHORBIA, asthma weed, catshair *(Euphorbia hirta)*

A bitter-tasting herb grown in India and other tropical countries. The plant is prepared as an infusion and taken for quick relief during an asthma attack, as well as for coughs and respiratory complaints.

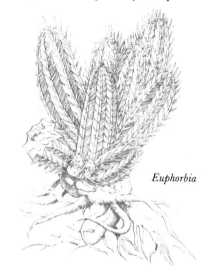

Euphorbia

EUPHORIANT

A substance which induces an abnormal feeling of vigour and buoyancy. Examples include nutmeg and cannabis.

EVENING PRIMROSE, tree primrose (*Oenothera biennis*)

A wild yellow-flowering plant from North America, cultivated in European gardens. The leaves and bark are astringent and mucilaginous. They can be used for coughs, asthma, gastrointestinal disorders and menstrual problems. Made into an ointment, they will soothe rashes and skin irritations. Evening primrose is a sedative sometimes used in cases of mental depression.

EVEWEED, double rocket (*Hesperis matronalis*)

A wild herb with large white and blue or pinkish-purple flowers. The whole plant can be dried and powdered, then taken mixed with water to prevent scurvy. In large doses it is an emetic (induces vomiting) and can be used instead of ipecac in cases of accidental poisoning.

EXPECTORANT

A substance which encourages the expulsion of mucus from the lungs and respiratory passages. Examples include licorice, horehound, garlic, coltsfoot and acacia.

EYEBRIGHT (*Euphrasia officinalis*)

A partially parasitic plant found in grassy areas. It is very widely used in infusion as an eye lotion, particularly for conjunctivitis. Its anti-inflammatory qualities make it an effective remedy for colds, sinusitis and catarrh. It can also be drunk as a general tonic.

F

FEBRIFUGE

A substance which reduces fever — *see Antipyretic*.

FENNEL (*Foeniculum vulgare*)

A tall feathery-leafed herb with bright yellow flowers and a smell like aniseed. There are several different varieties and all have been used since ancient times for both culinary and medicinal purposes. The Romans believed that fennel strengthened the eyesight, and fennel tea (made from the seeds) is still used by some people as a soothing eyewash which will fade yellowish patches on the whites of the eyes. It can also be used as a general skin freshener and wrinkle remover. Fennel tea relieves flatulence and is believed by some to have a slimming effect because it stimulates the pancreas and improves the metabolism of fats and sugars. For this reason it is sometimes recommended for diabetics. The seeds are sometimes added to rich fatty foods to aid their digestion. Fennel is rich in mineral salts, especially sulphur, potassium and sodium. Fennel tea is a diuretic and is also said to increase the milk supply of nursing mothers. It can be gargled to sooth coughing and hoarseness. The seeds can be chewed to sweeten the breath.

FENUGREEK, foenugreek, bird's foot, Greek hayseed (*Trigonella foenum-graecum*)

A hardy annual originally from the Mediterranean area and used since ancient times for culinary and medicinal purposes. The seeds are pungent-tasting and usually used in curries. Many people find the taste of fenugreek tea unpleasantly strong. However, it can be very helpful for reducing the symptoms of heavy colds and flu, particularly catarrh and blocked sinuses. It is sometimes prescribed as a digestive aid to help with the breakdown of fatty foods, and is said to be helpful in fighting minor infections and for acne. The seeds can also be made into a paste and applied to boils, wounds, corns and mouth ulcers, or made into an infusion to improve the condition of the skin and hair. Recent research has shown that fenugreek seeds contain diosgenin, which is an important ingredient in oral contraceptives.

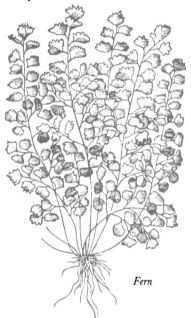

Fern

FERN, royal fern, buckhorn brake
(Osmunda regalis)
maidenhair fern *(Adiantum pedatum)*

A large fern with stiff, branched leaves, the royal fern grows wild and thrives on moist ground. The leaf fronds can be made into a useful ointment for sprains, bruises and rheumatism; this ointment can also be mixed with alcohol and used as a back rub. Pillows and mattresses stuffed with fern fronds are said to give relief to sufferers of rheumatism. The root can be made into a decoction to soothe coughs and act as a general tonic.

Maidenhair fern can be dried and made into an infusion which may be drunk to increase the milk supply of nurs-ing mothers or to soothe coughs and hoarseness. It is also said to be helpful for alcoholics. Maidenhair is used in hair conditioners and is said to prevent dandruff and hair thinning.

FEVERFEW, pyrethrum
(Chrysanthemum parthenium)

A perennial cultivated plant, also found growing wild, which has a number of small, white, daisy-like flowers with yellow centres. It was popular in the eighteenth century when its leaves were made into a tea drunk by women to cure a wide variety of nervous disorders such as 'hysteria', headaches and fever, as well as being used for colds, to bring on menstruation, and to hasten the expulsion of afterbirth. It has recently been recognised as a very effective remedy for headaches and migraine, and is still used by herbalists to reduce fever and regulate contractions during labour. A tincture of feverfew will relieve the pain of insect bites, and can be diluted and applied as an insect repellent.

FIG TREE, common fig *(Ficus carica)*

A deciduous tree originally from the Middle East and Mediterranean countries, the fruit of which are often dried. Eaten for their nutritional qualities as well as their sweet taste, figs are also a natural laxative and can be made into a syrup for children. A decoction of figs can be used as a demulcent to soothe inflamed mucous passages. Roasted fresh figs can be applied as a soothing poultice to boils, and the milky juice from the stem and leaves can be used to remove warts.

FIGWORT, throatwort
(Scrophularia nodosa)

A perennial plant with small purple flowers, found wild in Europe and North America. It can be taken in infusion as a diuretic and kidney tonic, and to purify the blood and regulate menstruation. It is particularly helpful for chronic skin complaints such as eczema and can be made into an ointment for minor wounds, boils, bruises, sprains and swellings. Homeopaths may recommend a tincture of figwort for conjunctivitis, mastitis or piles.

FIR, Norway spruce, spruce, Norway pine (*Picea abies*)

A tall evergreen tree from northern Europe. The young shoots can be made into an expectorant tea useful for coughs, flu and catarrh, and to promote perspiration. The steam from a vapour bath of these shoots can be inhaled to relieve bronchitis or they can be used as a soothing bath additive. The resin from these trees is made into oil of turpentine, which is antiseptic and rubefacient, and can be used in medicinal plasters. Oil of tar, which is made commercially from fir trees, is often used in ointments to soothe itching skin conditions like eczema.

The North American species, *Picea mariana* (often called black spruce), was an important source of vitamin C for the American Indians and early settlers who drank a decoction from the bark and needles.

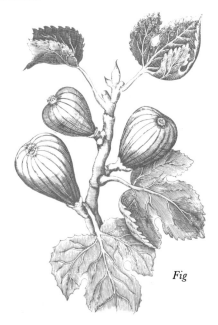

Fig

FIXATIVE

A substance which can be added to a mixture such as a perfume to prevent the more volatile ingredients evaporating too quickly.

FLAG, blue flag, wild iris, iris (*Iris versicolor*)

This is the iris most commonly used by herbalists. It grows wild in swamps of North America and the root can be used to prevent vomiting and to help liver, gall bladder and sinus problems. A tincture of blue flag is said to be useful for reducing an enlarged thyroid gland and the fresh, bruised leaves can be used to heal burns and sores.

FLAX, linseed (*Linum usitatissimum*)

A fibrous plant best known because its stems are made into linen and the oil from its seeds used in furniture polish and printer's ink. The seeds are also used medicinally. They can be crushed and made into a poultice to soothe swellings, rheumatism, haemorrhoids and other inflammations or applied to burns, or mixed with mustard and put on the chest to soothe bronchitis. They are often crushed and made into a soothing, lubricating tea used to relieve constipation, kidney or urinary infections, sore throats, coughs and catarrh.

FLEABANE, simson, Canadian fleabane (*Conyza canadensis*)

A weed from North America with broad, brown lower leaves and small white flowers. The whole herb can be made into an astringent diuretic infusion useful for kidney disease and diarrhoea. The oil from the leaves, taken a few drops at a time, perhaps with a lump of sugar, will stop bleeding from the lungs or colon.

FLEUR-DE-LYS, blue flag, garden iris, common iris (*Iris germanica*)

Originally found wild in the Mediterranean, now seen mostly in gardens. The root is used as an aromatic to flavour other medicines, and when fresh can be used as a purgative. *See also Flag.*

FLUELLEN — *see Speedwell*

FOMENTATION

The application of heat and moisture to reduce pain and inflammation.

FO-TI-TIENG (*Hydrocotyle asiatica*)

A Chinese herb, the leaves and seeds of which have been found to contain a substance sometimes called 'vitamin X' which has a rejuvenating effect on the brain, nerves and endocrine glands, and can be used to treat general debility. Li Chung Yun, a Chinese herbalist who is said to have lived 256 years, drank a daily tea of fo-ti-tieng and ginseng.

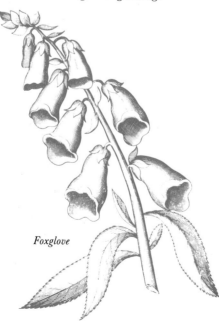

Foxglove

FOXGLOVE, digitalis (*Digitalis purpurea*)

A highly poisonous plant, often grown for its decorative flowers, but now also grown commercially for its leaves which yield the drug digitalis, used by orthodox doctors as a powerful cardiac stimulant that slows and strengthens the pulse. It is not generally recommended for use except under strict medical supervision, as it is a cumulative poison.

FRAGRANT VALERIAN — *see Valerian*

FRANKINCENSE, olibanum (*Boswellia carterii*)

A gum resin from a southern Arabian tree once widely used for embalming. It is still used in some parts of the East as an external application to cure boils and sores, as well as being taken internally for gonorrhoea.

FRINGE TREE, old man's beard, poison ash, snowflower (*Chionanthus virginicus*)

A small tree with fragrant, white flowers with fringe-like petals which grows wild in the USA. The bark of the root, prepared as a decoction, will reduce fever and is used as a tonic and diuretic to relieve kidney and liver disorders as well as acute dyspepsia. The bark can also be made into a poultice to soothe skin irritations.

FUCHSIA (*Zauschneria californica*)

Best known as a colourful flowering plant. Some North American Indians drank a decoction of its leaves and flowers for respiratory and urinary disorders. They also used its leaves either as a powder or a wash to heal cuts and sores.

G

GALACTOGOGUE

A plant which increases milk supply in nursing mothers. Some examples are carrots, aniseed, fennel, blessed thistle and vervain. A poultice of buckwheat is also said to be helpful.

GALANGA, catarrh root, galangal (*Alpinia officinarum*)

A pungent rhizome related to ginger, originally cultivated in China. Like ginger, it is used as an aromatic, appetiser and carminative. In the Middle Ages it was believed to be an aphrodisiac.

GALL OAK (*Quercus infectoria*)

A small oak tree native to Asia which produces acorns and round woody substances called galls. These are powdered and made into an astringent tincture for diarrhoea and dysentery, or into an ointment used on bleeding haemorrhoids. They can also be made into an infusion for leucorrhoea and as a mouthwash.

GAMBOGE, cambogia (*Garcinia hanburyi*)

The resinous gum from a South-East Asian tree. It is an extremely strong cathartic and diuretic, and is poisonous in large doses; it is used only in small doses in combination with other drugs. Gamboge is best known as a bright yellowish-orange commercial colouring pigment.

GARDEN VIOLET — *see* Violet

GARLIC (*Allium sativum*)

Originally from Asia, garlic has been widely cultivated for over 2000 years both for its culinary and medicinal uses. It is perhaps best known as a flavouring, but unfortunately its medicinal qualities are destroyed when it is cooked. Raw garlic is useful for a wide variety of disorders and many people eat it regularly as a general tonic. It has antibacterial qualities which make it an excellent preventive medicine to guard against colds, flu and even more deadly diseases such as typhoid and dysentery. It is particularly effective for respiratory disorders such as bronchitis, catarrh and persistent coughs and hay fever, as well as for digestive problems, especially of the liver and gall bladder, for high blood pressure and hardening of the arteries, and for headaches, faintness and nervous disorders. Garlic is believed by some to stop the growth of tumours. It will expel intestinal worms and, when eaten regularly, will cure acne. Its antiseptic qualities are so strong that raw garlic juice was used to prevent infection of wounds during World War I. Garlic oil is rich in vitamins A, B and C, and in sulphur, copper, manganese, iron and calcium. Used externally it will ease the pain of earache and toothache. The odour of garlic can be removed by chewing parsley or mint. Garlic plants in the garden will repel many insect pests, particularly aphids.

GELSEMIUM, yellow jasmine, yellow jessamine, woodbine (*Gelsemium sempervirens*)

A climbing plant with yellow flowers, found wild in parts of North and Central America, and cultivated elsewhere as an ornamental vine. It was once commonly used as a sedative and to treat migraine, neuralgia, sciatica and hypertension, but is no longer recommended as it is a poison which can easily be fatal.

GENTIAN *(Gentiana lutea)*

A European alpine plant with bright yellow flowers (the well-known *Gentiana acaulis* is blue). The bitter-tasting root has been used in healing since ancient times, particularly as a general tonic and to improve the appetite and digestion in cases such as anorexia and general debility. It will disperse blood clots, stimulate the production of blood corpuscles, and relieve fever. It has also been used for malaria and jaundice, and to discourage smoking. It should be taken at least 1 hour before eating or it will adversely affect digestion. Gentian should not be taken in early pregnancy or by anyone with high blood pressure.

GERANIUM — *see Herb Robert*

GERMANDER, wall germander *(Teucrium chamaedrys)*

A creeping European plant with leaves shaped like oak leaves which can be dried and used in infusion as a stimulating diuretic tonic with anti-inflammatory properties. It is useful for gout, rheumatism, fevers and to bring on menstruation, and is sometimes used for coughs and chest complaints as a substitute for horehound.

GERMICIDE — *see Antiseptic*

GINGER *(Zingiber officinale)*

Originally from South-East Asia, ginger is now cultivated commercially in most warmer parts of the world. The knotty rhizome has been used in cooking and medicine for thousands of years, and it is still an important drug in Chinese medicine. Ginger is a general tonic and stimulant, and is particularly helpful for stimulating the digestive system, easing flatulence, and preventing nausea. Its antispasmodic qualities make it useful for treating colic, cramps and period pain, and it will improve the circulation. Hot ginger tea may be taken to relieve colds and flu, and to cleanse the system by increasing perspiration; it will also sometimes induce menstruation. Externally, ginger can be used in a compress or ointment to relieve the pain of stiff joints. People suffering from skin complaints are not advised to take large doses of ginger.

GINSENG, RED, Korean red ginseng *(Panax ginseng)*

A plant cultivated in China and Korea for many centuries and popular as a general panacea. *Panax ginseng*, the Korean variety, was named by the Russian botanist C. A. Meyer in 1843. Recent research in Japan has identified 16 ginsenosides (ginseng glycosides, active constitutents) together with various anti-oxidants, phenolic compounds and acidic peptides. Of the 16 ginsenosides, Rb and Re have been shown to produce an insulin-like effect against diabetes, while the so-called phenolic compounds, including salicylic acid, vanillic acid, syringic acid and ferulic acid, have an apparent anti-ageing effect through the inhibition of lipid peroxide formation. They also help slow down tissue destruction and reduce cell membrane degeneration.

Ginseng seedlings are nurtured on a seedbed for 18 months and then transferred to a partially shaded bed for a further 5 years. The mature plants, when harvested, may be up to 50 centimetres in height. It is the root which has medicinal value. When taken from the earth it is creamy yellow and has a profusion of 'limbs' and filaments. The root is dried and steamed, making it pink in colour, and it may then be taken in the form of tea, as powder, in capsules or as nectar.

Scientific research into the properties of ginseng is still continuing, but ginseng has already been shown to have a number of remarkable medicinal and nutritive properties. It helps to stimulate protein synthesis, regenerate the liver, and reduce blood cholesterol level. It also suppresses proliferation of cancer cells, stimulates lipid metabolism, bolsters the immune system, and is useful in treating hepatitis B and anaemia.

GINSENG, WHITE,
American ginseng (*Panax quinquefolius*)

A variety of ginseng which is cultivated for only 4 to 5 years (red ginseng is grown for 6 to 7 years) and is not steamed (as is red ginseng). It appears to contain fewer metabolites than the more mature red form.

GLYCOSIDE

A plant drug with cardiac, antiseptic, aromatic, antithrombic, expectorant or laxative properties.

GOAT'S FOOT CONVOLVULUS, coast
morning glory (*Ipomoea pes-caprae*)

A common plant on coastal sand dunes with succulent leaves and large purple flowers. The leaves were used by Aborigines to treat skin inflammations, infection and haemorrhoids. Some tribes heated them before placing them on boils to bring them to a head. The juice was also taken internally as a diuretic and laxative, and a decoction of the whole plant was claimed by some to be a remedy for venereal disease.

GOLDENROD, European
goldenrod (*Solidago virgaurea*)

A tall herb with yellow flowers which can be used in infusion to treat arthritis, eczema, kidney problems, nausea, diarrhoea and excessive menstruation. The crushed leaves, fresh or dried, can be applied externally to cuts, sores and insect bites to assist healing.

GOLDEN SEAL, yellow root
(*Hydrastis canadensis*)

A small shade-loving plant which once grew wild in North America but has become almost unknown except as a cultivated plant. It was used by the American Indians as a tonic for gastric and liver disorders, as a laxative and douche, and to relieve morning sickness. It acts on the mucous membranes and is good for catarrh, sore mouths and gums, inflamed eyes and many skin diseases such as acne, eczema and ringworm. Combined with capsicum, it can be used as a remedy for chronic alcoholism.

GOLDTHREAD, mouth root
(*Coptis trifolia*)

A small plant found in mossy woods in North America. The root is made into a decoction which is a popular folk remedy for sores in the mouth, gums and throat, and around the eyes. It can also be used for dyspepsia.

GOTU KOLA (*Centella asiatica/ Hydrocotyle asiatica*)

An Indian plant alleged to have youth-giving properties similar to those of fo-ti-tieng and ginseng, and to act particularly on the brain to prevent its degeneration.

GRAPE (*Vitis vinifera*)

The grapevine is one of the oldest cultivated plants and is usually valued for its fruit and the wine which is made from them. However, the plant also has medicinal value. Grapes are laxative and diuretic and, being full of vitamins and minerals, are often recommended for convalescents. Grapes can also be used to treat low blood pressure, poor circulation, anaemia and skin blemishes. The liquid from the broken branches is a good diuretic and can also be used as an eyewash.

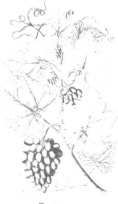

Grape

GREAT BURNET, Italian pimpernel (*Sanguisorba officinalis*)

A purple-flowered plant from damp areas of Europe and North America which can be used to coagulate blood and stop bleeding, and has also been recommended for inflamed varicose veins. Its astringent qualities make it useful in treating diarrhoea.

GREEN MAGMA

The juice extracted from young barley leaves, used for a variety of therapeutic purposes. These include use as a treatment for pancreatisis, and inflammation of the oral cavity, the stomach and the duodenum. According to Dr Kazuhito Kubota of the Science University, Tokyo, green magma juice contains a potent anti-inflammatory glycoprotein (a combination of sugar and protein) which possesses an anti-peptic-ulcer action. Research scientists at the University of California, San Diego, also claim that the juice stimulates repair of cellular DNA and that this effect extends to the body's somatic cells: this means potentially that green magma may slow the ageing process and promote longevity. However research into the properties of green magma is ongoing and scientific evaluation of the barley juice is at a preliminary stage.

GROUND ELDER, goat's foot, goutweed, bishop's elder (*Aegopodium podagraria*)

A garden weed cultivated in monastery gardens in the Middle Ages as a remedy for gout and used in some European countries as a green vegetable. It is a diuretic and sedative, and is still taken in infusion to ease the pain of rheumatism and arthritis. A hot fomentation of the root and leaves may be applied externally to an aching joint.

GROUND IVY, creeping Jenny, alehoof, creeping Charlie (*Nepeta hederacea*)

A creeping evergreen ground cover with small purplish flowers, found in moist soils. It was used in medieval Britain to brew beer, before the introduction of hops. Modern herbalists make the leaves into a tea for a diuretic tonic which stimulates the appetite and digestive system, and it is recommended for kidney complaints. It can also be used to bring on menstruation and to soothe inflammation of the mucous membranes, especially in colds, sore throats and chest complaints. The fresh juice can be inhaled to clear the head and relieve nasal congestion. Ground ivy can be mixed with chamomile flowers and made into a poultice for boils, or added to bathwater to relieve sciatica and gout. It is used in China to relieve fever and pain of many kinds.

GUAIACUM, lignum vitae (*Guaiacum officinale*)

The resin from a tree native to the West Indies and Central and South America. It is antiseptic and diuretic, and is used for gout, rheumatism, syphilis and skin complaints. Its expectorant qualities make it helpful for catarrh and, mixed with sarsaparilla, it is sometimes used in blood-purifying medicines. It is an antioxidant sometimes used in packaged and tinned food.

GUARANA, Brazilian cocoa (*Paullinia cupana*)

A tall shrub, found in Brazil and Venezuela, with seeds which contain about 4 times more caffeine than coffee beans. They are dried, crushed and made into a stimulating drink which prevents sleepiness and dulls the appetite. It can be used to cure headaches and hangovers, to bring on menstruation, and to give relief from arthritis.

H

HAEMOSTATIC

A substance which controls bleeding by contracting the blood vessels or tissues. Examples include nettle, shepherd's purse, wood sorrel, great burnet and plantain.

HALLUCINOGEN

A substance which causes hallucinations. Examples include cannabis, nutmeg, Scotch broom and peyote.

HAWTHORN, maybush, white thorn, quickthorn (*Crataegus oxyacantha/Crataegus monogyna*)

A small shrub-like tree native to Europe but now found growing wild in many temperate parts of the world. It has formed part of the famous British hedgerows for centuries and has many religious and magical associations. Its branches were believed to give protection against witchcraft but, if brought inside the house, to be harbingers of death. Hawthorn has many uses of a more orthodox nature. The berries are particularly effective in increasing the muscular action of the heart, and are used to treat angina, palpitations, arteriosclerosis, irregular pulse and other disorders of the heart or circulatory system. The blossoms too can be made into a mild heart tonic which can be taken daily as a preventive measure against heart disease. Hawthorn tea is sometimes used to cure insomnia and as a diuretic helpful for kidney diseases. In some areas hawthorn has been sprayed with poisonous herbicides, so care should be taken before collecting wild berries.

HEART'S EASE — *see Pansy*

HEATHER (*Calluna vulgaris*)

A hardy shrub found on poor soils in Europe. The flowers are sometimes taken in infusion for insomnia, or to strengthen the heart and cure coughs, stomach pains and rheumatism.

HELLEBORE, black hellebore, Christmas rose (*Helleborus niger*)

A white-flowered plant native to Europe but grown in gardens elsewhere. It has been used as a heart stimulant, a diuretic, and to treat depression, but is not generally recommended for domestic use as it is poisonous except in very small doses. Some modern homeopaths prepare a tincture from the fresh root to treat nervous disorders and epilepsy. The ancient Greeks used hellebore to cure madness and it was later used in witchcraft.

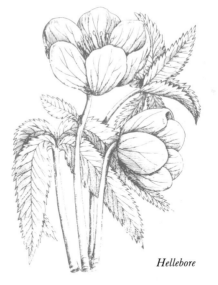

Hellebore

HELLEBORE, white hellebore, green hellebore, American hellebore, Indian poke (*Veratrum album*)

This variety is also poisonous, but is used in small doses as a cardiac depressant. Although not generally used by herbalists, alkaloids from the plant are used in orthodox medicine to treat hypertension. A homeopathic tincture is available to treat some liver disorders.

HEMLOCK, poison parsley
(Conium maculatum)

A common wild plant in Europe, best known as a deadly poison. It was used in ancient times as a way of executing criminals. Socrates was forced to drink a cup of hemlock juice and some people believe Jesus Christ was given hemlock together with vinegar and myrrh as he hung on the cross. Although it is not widely used today because of the obvious danger of overdose, small amounts were formerly used as a sedative, an anaesthetic and a pain reliever. It is still sometimes used externally to heal sores and also to relieve the pain of terminal cancer. A homeopathic tincture is sometimes prescribed for an enlarged prostate gland.

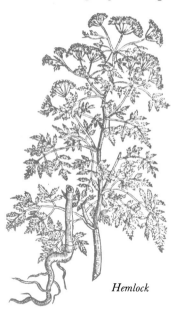

Hemlock

HEMLOCK SPRUCE,
Canada pitch tree *(Tsuga canadensis)*

A North American evergreen with bark and young twigs which can be made into a diuretic tea useful for kidney problems and as an astringent enema for diarrhoea. It can also be used as a mouthwash and an external wash for sores and ulcers. The powdered bark will prevent sweating and foot odour if sprinkled inside the shoes.

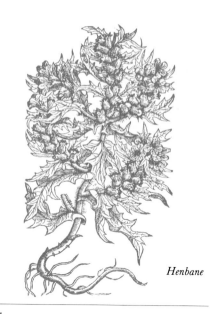

Henbane

HENBANE, hogbean, black henbane, devil's eye *(Hyoscyamus niger)*

A highly poisonous plant which grows wild, especially on waste ground in Europe and North America. It is a strong sedative and narcotic, and should be used only under close medical supervision. Henbane is an antispasmodic which has been used for treating nervous complaints, particularly Parkinson's disease. It is sometimes used externally in drops for earache and for rheumatism. Some pharmaceutical preparations for whooping cough and asthma contain small amounts of henbane.

HENNA *(Lawsonia inermis)*

A small North African shrub, the powdered leaves of which have been used as a hair and nail colouring since the time of the ancient Egyptians. The leaves also have astringent qualities and can be made into a mouth and throat gargle, a treatment for skin irritations and a drink to cure headaches.

HEPATIC

A drug which acts on the liver. Examples include asparagus, dandelion, parsley, sandalwood and rosemary.

HERB ROBERT, dragon's blood, geranium *(Geranium robertianum)*

A type of geranium with astringent and sedative properties. The leaves can be taken in infusion for diarrhoea, internal bleeding and peptic ulcers, as well as to lower the blood sugar level in diabetics. They can also be used as a mouthwash for sore throats and gum inflammations, or diluted and used as an eyewash. The fresh leaves can be crushed and applied directly to wounds, bruises and skin irritations to ease pain and aid healing.

HERBS

Herbs are part of an ancient tradition in Europe, the Middle East and Asia, and have been used both to enhance the flavour of food and as medicinal cures.

Herbal medicines were the major source of treatment for illness before the development of modern synthetic drugs, and it is fair to say that knowledge of herbal remedies developed by trial and error: it was gradually discovered that certain roots, plants and seeds had curative properties, and this knowledge was passed from one generation to the next.

In China a major book on medicinal herbs titled *Pen Tsao* was compiled in 3000 BC by Emperor Shen-ung. He praised the healing properties of ginseng, cinnamon, the bark of the mulberry tree and the roots of rhubarb. The ancient Egyptians valued olive oil, cloves, myrrh and castor oil, and developed a wide knowledge of 'essential oils' for curative and embalming purposes. Pliny's *Natural History* records that herbalism was also practised in ancient Greece and endorsed by the great physician Hippocrates.

Possibly because of its pagan associations and frequent references to the healing deities Apollo and Aesculapius, much of the herbal knowledge that filtered through to the Middle Ages from ancient Greece was discarded as non-Christian and linked to witchcraft and magic. In England, Nicholas Culpeper (1616–54) combined astrology, magic and herbalism in his book *The English Physician* (1653),

while the Swiss herbalist and alchemist Paracelsus (1493–1541) classified plants according to the colour symbolism of their flowers. Paracelsus also believed in the curative properties of metals like mercury and antimony and was, in this sense, a precursor both of modern scientists and naturopaths advocating mineral supplements in the diet.

In the nineteenth century, as scientific interest in classifying plants increased, there was once again a revival of interest in the medicinal power of herbs, especially in the United States. Samuel Thompson (1769–1843) angered doctors in New Hampshire by advocating the use of herbal medicines and not charging his patients for treatment, while in 1896 the herbalist Dr Benedict Lust opened the first health food store in that country.

Today herbs are used either singly (as 'simples') or in combination remedies. A common practice among herbalists these days is to use only non-toxic remedies, thereby following Hippocrates' dictum: *do no harm.* Herbal remedies are comparatively cheap and easy to prepare. As synthetic medicines become increasingly expensive and often produce unwanted side effects, it is not surprising that herbalism is once again reviving in popularity. *(For specific herbal treatments see plant listings.)*

Herb Robert

HIBISCUS, African mallow, karkade, Jamaica sorrel *(Hibiscus sabdariffa)*

An exotic tropical flower which can be dried and made into a thirst-quenching drink, karkade, which contains vitamin C, iron and copper. In Europe tea-bags containing a mixture of rosehip and hibiscus make a popular herbal drink characterised by a rich ruby-red colour.

HOLLY *(Ilex aquifolium)*

An evergreen shrub usually associated with Christmas. The red berries are poisonous but can be powdered and used to prevent bleeding. An infusion of leaves is a diuretic and will also produce sweating, as well as being used for colds, fevers, catarrh and rheumatism.

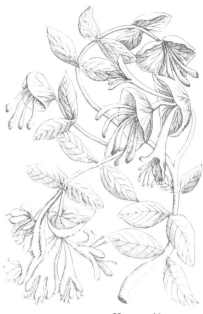

Honeysuckle

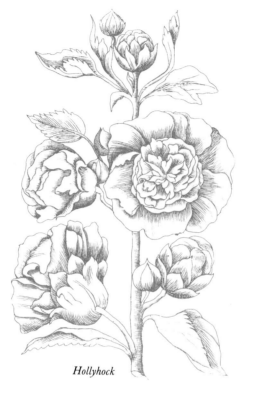

Hollyhock

HOLLYHOCK, blue malva
(Althaea rosea)

A tall colourful garden plant, the dried flowers of which can be made into a soothing infusion for coughs and bronchitis, and for inflammations of the mouth and throat. A vapour bath of the tea is sometimes recommended for earache. The flowers are used in some cosmetics as a skin softener.

HONEYSUCKLE *(Lonicera periclymenum)*

A well-known climbing shrub, the leaves of which, in infusion, can be used as a laxative. Its flowers can be made into a gargle for coughs, catarrh and sore throats. It is poisonous in large doses.

HOPS *(Humulus lupulus)*

The dried female flowers of a climbing plant native to Europe but introduced to many other parts of the world and famous for their part in brewing beer. Hop tea, often used in combination with other herbs, is a soothing drink especially recommended for those suffering from nervous indigestion, insomnia, tension headaches and general restlessness. It can also help alleviate period pain, neuralgia and spasmodic coughs, and can be used as a diuretic. Hops have antibacterial qualities and can be applied as a poultice to wounds, ulcers and itching skin irritations. A hop pillow, made from the dried flowers, is a well-known folk remedy for sleeplessness.

HOREHOUND, white
horehound, common horehound
(Marrubium vulgare)

A common pasture weed native to Europe and Asia but now widespread in many countries. It is a famous cough remedy which has been used since the time of the Egyptians, and is now used in commercial cough medicines and lozenges. Because of its very bitter taste, it is often combined with other herbs in a tea or else made into a syrup. It is a particularly good expectorant used for bronchitis, asthma and chest coughs, and is suitable to give to children. Taken as a hot tea it will induce perspiration and reduce fever, and in large doses it is a diuretic and laxative, sometimes prescribed for obesity. In small doses it is a tonic which will stimulate the appetite and increase the flow of bile. It can also be used to bring on suppressed menstruation. Horehound is an antiseptic which can be applied externally to cuts and skin irritations, and will also repel insects. It is one of the 5 bitter herbs traditionally eaten by Jewish people at Passover.

HORSERADISH, red cole, wild radish (*Cochlearia armoracia/Armoracia rusticana*)

A European plant usually grown for its pungent edible root. It also has medicinal qualities and can be used as an appetite stimulant and digestive aid, as well as a strong diuretic. It stimulates the circulation and, if taken regularly, is good for catarrh, coughs and sinus pains, and is thought to help build up resistance to colds. Horseradish must be taken raw to be effective; its taste can be made more palatable by mixing it with honey. Applied externally it is helpful for insect bites, sores, eczema, chilblains and rheumatism and, mixed with milk, to fade freckles and freshen the skin. Freshly grated horseradish can be inhaled to clear the head and relieve the symptoms of a heavy cold.

HORSETAIL, equisitum, shave grass, bottlebrush (*Equisitum arvense*)

A non-flowering, fern-like plant usually regarded as a troublesome weed in the northern hemisphere. There are over 20 different species in the genus *Equisitum*, some of which contain so much silica that they can be used for household cleaning. All species contain a high concentration of silicate compounds, as well as salts of magnesium and calcium which help the silica to be correctly absorbed. Equisitum tea is drunk as a remedy for respiratory complaints, even tuberculosis, and as a powerful diuretic which stimulates the kidneys and bladder and removes any gravel and stones. The tea stimulates the formation of blood corpuscles and promotes blood coagulation, so it is helpful for anaemia and internal bleeding, especially from stomach ulcers, and also for external bleeding. It makes a good wash for wounds, sores, mouth and gum inflammations, ulcers and nosebleeds. Its silica content can help skin complaints such as acne and eczema. It should not be used in large doses or for long periods.

HORSEWEED, Canada fleabane (*Erigeron canadensis*)

A North American weed with astringent leaves which can be taken in infusion for diarrhoea and haemorrhoids, and also act as a diuretic which can be helpful for bladder problems and rheumatism.

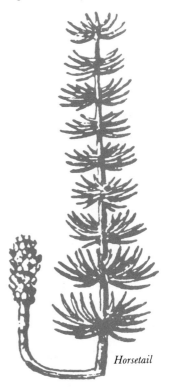

Horsetail

HOUND'S TONGUE, dog's tongue (*Cynoglossum officinale*)

A weed with large furry leaves which at one time were boiled in fat and applied to the scalp to prevent balding. Its astringent root can be used for diarrhoea and to reduce the pain and irritation of piles.

HOUSELEEK, Jupiter's beard (*Sempervivum tectorum*)

A European garden plant, the fresh leaves of which are astringent and cooling, and can be crushed and applied directly to ease the pain of headaches, burns, insect stings and haemorrhoids. The juice from the leaves, applied regularly, is said to soften corns and warts and to fade freckles.

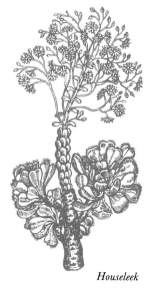

Houseleek

HYDROGUE

A purgative drug which produces a copious watery discharge from the bowels — *see Purgative and Cathartic*.

HYPNOTIC

A substance which induces sleep. Examples include tarragon, periwinkle, corydalis and valerian.

HYPOGLYCAEMIC

A substance which reduces blood sugar levels. Examples include burdock, chickweed, chicory and nettle.

HYSSOP (*Hyssopus officinalis*)

An aromatic herb of the mint family used in Mediterranean areas for medicinal purposes for over 2000 years, as well as being used as a deodorant herb in the cleansing of holy temples. The flowers can be made into hyssop tea, which can be used for sore throats, catarrh and irregular blood pressure. It helps the digestion, particularly of fatty foods, and can be helpful for skin irritations, burns, bruises, insect bites and as a wash for eye and throat infections. The crushed leaves can be placed directly onto wounds to prevent infection and promote healing.

I

ICELAND MOSS (*Cetraria islandica*)

A type of lichen found in country areas in the far northern parts of Europe, North America and Asia. It can be collected in summer, dried and made into a tea useful for coughs, hoarseness and bronchitis, and even for tuberculosis. It is also helpful for gastric and intestinal inflammations and can stimulate the flow of milk in nursing mothers. It is a nourishing food but must be boiled for a long time to make it palatable.

IMPERIAL MASTERWORT — *see Masterwort*

INDIAN CORN — *see Corn silk*

INFUSION

An extraction of the water-soluble properties of a substance by steeping it in water for about 15 minutes. The method is similar to making a pot of tea and is most suitable for leaves and flowers, though powdered seeds, bark or roots can also be used. Infusions are usually made with boiling water in a covered container so that the volatile oils are not lost through evaporation, but occasionally cold water can be used. The proportions are 25 g of herb to 500 ml of water (or 1 oz to 1 pint). The infusion is then strained and usually drunk warm, normally in a dose of 1 cupful 3 times a day, though a smaller dose is sometimes prescribed.

INSECTICIDE

A substance which kills or repels insects. Examples include wormwood, camphor, oil of mint, feverfew and bay laurel.

IODINE PLANT *(Ervatamia orientalis)*

A small tree from northern Australia used by the Aborigines and early settlers in the same way as iodine. When broken, the leaves exude latex which can be applied directly to wounds and sores.

IRISH MOSS, carrageen, pearl moss *(Chondrus crispus)*

A seaweed that grows on rocks off the coast of France and Ireland, and contains a gelatinous substance called 'carrageen' which is used as a suspending agent in pharmaceutical preparations. It soothes inflamed mucous membranes and is recommended for coughs, bronchitis, sore throats and intestinal irritations. It is also a nutritious food for convalescents and is sometimes used for kidney and urinary-tract disorders. Externally it is used in skin lotions and anti-wrinkle creams.

IRRITANT

A substance which causes inflammation or irritation of the skin. Examples include mustard, cayenne, hellebore and horseradish.

ISCADOR

A substance obtained from mistletoe which can be given in the form of injections to treat cancer. It is used at Lucas Klinik in Arlesheim, Switzerland, in combination with herbs and special foods.

IVY, English ivy, common ivy *(Hedera helix)*

A climbing evergreen vine with black berries which ripen in winter. These are poisonous and may also cause skin irritations if handled. The leaves can be boiled and used in a poultice for boils, ulcers, sores and other skin problems. A tincture made from the leaves can be used for whooping cough.

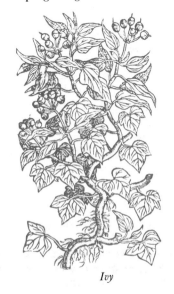

Ivy

J

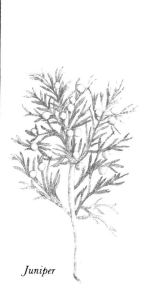

Juniper

JAMU

Indonesian herbal medicines derived from leaves, roots, barks and fruits, and used to treat a variety of health disorders. These include infirm muscles, superfluous body fluids, excess fat and kidney stones. Jamu remedies are also used by women to stimulate the uterus following childbirth, and generally as blood purifiers, diuretics and astringents.

JASMINE, jessamine (*Jasminum officinale*)

A white-flowered vine originally from India, now cultivated in gardens. The oil from the sweet-smelling flowers is said to be a relaxant and antidepressant, as well as an aphrodisiac. It can be added to bathwater or taken internally in a dose of 2 drops on a lump of sugar. It is used in aromatherapy massage to treat respiratory problems and menstrual pain. The flowers can also be made into a syrup for coughs and catarrh. The berries are poisonous but can be used in a homeopathic tincture to treat tetanus and convulsions. In India jasmine is used as a remedy for snakebite and the leaves are made into a eyewash. Jasmine oil is extremely expensive and many people believe the scent of the fresh flowers has the same relaxing and erotic qualities.

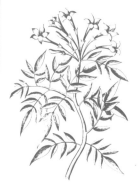

Jasmine

JIMSON WEED, thorn apple, devil's apple (*Datura stramonium*)

An extremely poisonous plant which is ritually used in some parts of the world to produce visions and hypnotic states, but may easily be fatal in inexperienced hands. It is also sometimes used medicinally as a tincture for spasmodic coughing, chronic laryngitis and Parkinson's disease. The leaves can be smoked in medicinal cigarettes for asthma and other respiratory complaints. An ointment from the seeds can be used for rheumatism.

JUNIPER (*Juniperus communis*)

A small evergreen tree which, since ancient times, has been believed to have magical properties. Its leaves have been used to freshen stale air and were believed to give protection against evil spirits as well as plagues. The black berries, which take 3 years to ripen, are well known for their use in distilling gin, and are also used as a culinary spice which stimulates the appetite and helps prevent flatulence and indigestion. The berries, which can be eaten raw or taken in infusion, have diuretic and antiseptic qualities and are useful for cystitis and kidney stones as well as for gastrointestinal infections, rheumatism and gout. Juniper oil, breathed in a vapour bath, is helpful for bronchitis and other lung infections.

K

KAMALA (*Mallotus philippinensis*)

A fruit from Asia with capsule hair which is taken internally to expel tapeworms or externally for skin diseases such as scabies.

KAVA KAVA (*Piper methysticum*)

A lilac-smelling plant from Hawaii which is a diuretic and can be used as a douche for vaginal disorders and as a local anaesthetic. It can also be made into a potent drink which produces mild hallucinations.

KEFIR

A drink made from cow's milk fermented with a mushroom grown in the Caucasus Mountains. It is used in parts of Asia to treat anaemia, stomach ailments and lung disorders.

KIDNEY VETCH, ladies' fingers, wound-wort *(Anthyllis vulneraria)*

A yellow-flowered European plant which can be used in infusion to wash wounds and also as a poultice. It is sometimes given to children as a tea to stop vomiting.

KINO

The juice from an Indian plant *Pterocarpus marsupium* which is used as a tincture in gargles and for diarrhoea.

KNAPWEED, greater knapweed *(Centaurea scabiosa)*

A red-flowered European plant, the roots and seeds of which can be made into a decoction useful for catarrh or into an ointment for cuts and bruises. Black knapweed *(Centaurea nigra)*, a smaller plant, is more useful for piles or as a gargle for a sore throat.

KNOTWEED, knotgrass

A general name used to refer to several species of common weeds belonging to the family Polygonaceae. They have creeping stems with knot-like stipules at the base of the leaves and tiny flowers which are often pink. They have astringent and diuretic properties and can be used for diarrhoea, respiratory problems and kidney stones. Externally they can be used on wounds, boils, haemorrhoids and varicose veins, as well as on flabby skin. One species, *Polygonum persicaria*, known as lady's thumb, has been used in European folk medicine as a cure for arthritis.

KOLA, kola nut, caffeine nut

The seeds of the tree *Cola nitida* and other similar species which are used as a chocolate-tasting, stimulating drink in parts of Africa. They were once an ingredient in Coca Cola and contain more caffeine than do coffee beans. They can be used as a cardiac tonic and for headaches and neuralgia, and will make it possible for the user to keep active for long periods without food or sleep.

KOUSSO *(Hagenia abyssinica)*

A plant from north-eastern Africa, the dried flowers of which can be used to expel tapeworms without having any other effects on the digestive system.

KUKICHA

A Japanese herbal tea. Alkaline in nature, it contains more calcium than cow's milk and twice as much vitamin C as orange juice. Kukicha helps to purify the blood and is suitable for people with a suspected heart condition.

KUZU, kudzu

A Japanese root extract used in a variety of herbal preparations, as a cream, as an ingredient in tea, and in combination with lotus root and umeboshi (Japanese salty plum). Kuzu roots yield an alkaline starch and the extract is regarded as strongly 'yang' in nature. Kuzu cream is used primarily to treat intestinal pains and stomach disorders. It may also be combined with lotus root powder to treat asthma, whooping cough and respiratory problems. Umesho-kuzu, the salty plum combination, is ideal for colds, dysentery and fever.

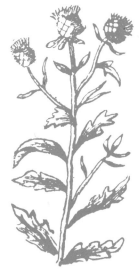

Knapweed

KYOLIC

Purified garlic extract, developed in Japan in the 1960s. Kyolic has been widely prescribed in that country as a treatment to lower cholesterol levels, reduce blood pressure and eliminate heavy metals like lead, mercury and copper from the body. It is also used for a variety of other complaints including sinus infections, bronchitis, asthma, haemorrhoids, toe fungus, athlete's foot and influenza. According to Dr Satosi Kitahara of Kunamoto University, who is a specialist toxicologist, kyolic also increases the fibrinolytic or anticlotting activity of blood platelets and fights the germs which cause pneumonia, tuberculosis, diphtheria, typhus and the common cold. *See also Garlic.*

L

LADY'S BEDSTRAW, cheese rennet *(Galium verum)*

A yellow-flowered herb with the unusual ability to curdle milk in the same way as rennet. It can be used in infusion as a diuretic blood purifier for urinary diseases and kidney stones. A decoction of the plant makes a soothing foot bath.

LADY'S MANTLE, lion's foot, bear's foot, nine hooks *(Alchemilla vulgaris)*

A low-growing herb with greenish flowers found in damp shady areas in cooler parts of the northern hemisphere. It is sometimes known as 'woman's best friend' and has been used for centuries for many kinds of female complaints. The herb is an astringent and is particularly good taken in infusion to control excessive

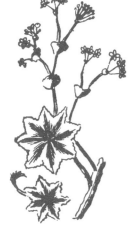

Lady's mantle

menstruation. It is sometimes taken just before childbirth, and to help coagulate the blood in any internal bleeding. The seventeenth-century herbalist, Nicholas Culpeper, recommended adding it to the bath water to help prevent miscarriage, and also suggested it was good for women with 'over-flagging breasts, causing them to grow less and hard'. As a tonic it can be taken to improve the appetite and strengthen the heart and blood vessels. Externally it is an astringent which makes an excellent vaginal douche and helps to heal wounds and sores of all kinds. The freshly pressed juice is said to be helpful for acne and also to fade freckles. A decoction of the root is good for diarrhoea.

LADY'S SMOCK, meadow bitterness, cuckoo flower *(Cardamine pratensis)*

A wild plant with pinkish-white flowers found in damp places. It has a pungent taste like watercress and can be used fresh in salads; it is thought to stimulate the appetite and help digestion. Lady's smock has tonic and expectorant qualities and is sometimes recommended for coughs. It contains a considerable amount of vitamin C and has been a traditional remedy for scurvy.

LAXATIVE

A mild purgative which relieves constipation and brings on evacuation of the bowels. Examples include rhubarb, dandelion, coffee, alfalfa, fennel and dock.

LEMON BALM — *see Balm*

LEMON VERBENA *(Lippia citriodora)*

A tropical plant introduced to Europe from Chile in the eighteenth century. It is a popular sedative tea in some European countries and is considered soothing for bronchitis and nasal congestion. The leaves can be used as a refreshing flavouring and the scent is often used in perfumes and cosmetics.

LINIMENT

A thin medicinal substance which may be rubbed onto the skin to ease sprains and bruises.

LIQUOR

A solution of medicinal substances in water. This differs from a tincture, which is a solution in alcohol.

LIQUORICE, licorice (*Glycyrrhiza glabra*)

A tall purple-flowered plant native to Mediterranean and northern Asian countries, the root of which has been used medicinally since the time of the ancient Egyptians. A literal translation of its name is 'sweet root'. It is a good expectorant widely used for coughs, bronchitis and other respiratory complaints, and its demulcent and anti-inflammatory qualities make it excellent for sore throats and laryngitis, and for stomach and intestinal ulcers. It is also a mild laxative. Cold liquorice tea mixed with linseed is a popular remedy for coughs and colds. Liquorice is particularly important in Chinese medicine because it increases the effectiveness of other drugs. It is also widely used to flavour bitter or unpleasant medicines. Liquorice should not be taken in large doses or for long periods as it can cause sodium retention and potassium loss, which may lead to high blood pressure, headaches, breathlessness and fluid retention. People with any condition such as diabetes, hypertension, pregnancy or kidney disorders should seek medical advice before taking liquorice.

LOTION

A liquid which is applied to the skin, usually for its cleansing, softening or astringent qualities.

LOTUS ROOT

A Japanese herb taken as a tea for asthma, whooping cough and other respiratory disorders. Lotus root tea is a powder extracted from the tuberous root of the lotus lily and, according to Japanese herbal tradition, a cup of the tea should be taken 3 times a day for effective results.

M

MACE (*Myristica fragrans*)

The nutmeg tree, native to the Moluccas and other islands of the East Indies, bears a large fleshy fruit (the nutmeg). The kernel of this fruit is wrapped in a bright red net-like substance called mace. When dried, it turns an orangey-brown and gives off a pungent aroma. Mace can be used as a carminative helpful for flatulence and vomiting, as a flavouring in cakes, and as a scent in soap and perfume. Together with nutmeg, it can be made into an ointment used as a counter-irritant in the treatment of arthritis. *See also Nutmeg.*

MADDER (*Rubia tinctorum*)

A herbaceous plant from the Mediterranean area used to make red dye and sometimes used for liver and urinary complaints, and to improve menstrual flow.

MAGNOLIA *(Magnolia glauca)*

An evergreen tree from the southern parts of the USA with large cream-coloured flowers. The bark can be made into a tea said to be good for fever, dyspepsia and some skin diseases. It has also been used to break the smoking habit.

MAIDENHAIR — *see Fern*

MALLEE RICE FLOWER *(Pimelea microcephala)*

A slender shrub from inland Australia with small heads of silky flowers. Some Aboriginal tribes plaited the bark and tied it around the neck to treat a cold or around an afflicted area to relieve pain. A decoction of the root bark was used for respiratory complaints or sore throats.

MALVA *(Malva rotundifolia)*

A roadside weed in North America said to contain a lot of vitamin A. It has been used for kidney troubles and as a demulcent for dysentery.

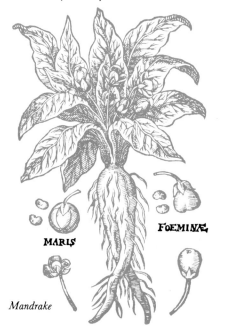

MARIS   FOEMINÆ

Mandrake

MANDRAKE, American mandrake, May apple *(Podophyllum peltatum)*
European mandrake, satan's apple *(Mandragora officinarum)*

The roots of this plant are poisonous and were used by some American Indians to commit suicide. However, they yield the drug podophyllin which is used in commercial wart-killing preparations and is being investigated in Switzerland as a possible cancer cure.

European mandrake is a poisonous Mediterranean plant with a large brown root divided into branches and sometimes resembling a human figure. It was thought in ancient times to have magical properties, and was also used as an anaesthetic for surgery and as a sleeping pill to relieve pain. The fresh plant is used today by homeopaths as a tincture for hayfever, coughs and asthma.

MAPLE TREE *(Acer* species)

There are many varieties of this tree, including the American sugar maple which is tapped for its sweet syrup, often regarded as a healthier substitute for sugar. The bark of the red maple and the sycamore maple is astringent and is used in decoction as a lotion for sore eyes.

MARIGOLD — *see Calendula*

MARJORAM, wild marjoram *(Origanum vulgare)*
sweet marjoram *(Origanum majorana)*

A small-leafed creeping plant with purple flowers. It grows wild in the Mediterranean and Asia, and was used by the ancient Romans as a medicinal and culinary herb, as well as being considered a symbol of peace and happiness. Used in cooking it has a stronger flavour than other varieties of marjoram, and is generally known as oregano. Made into an infusion, it can be taken as a general tonic which will increase perspiration, stimulate digestion and ease flatulence. It is a useful expectorant for easing coughs, and can also bring on menstruation and relieve cramp. An infusion of flowers is said to prevent sea sickness. Externally the oil can be used to relieve sore joints, arthritis, rheumatism and bruises, or placed directly onto an aching tooth. Added to bathwater it has a calming effect. The bruised leaves can be made into a herbal pillow for insomnia. Marjoram snuff is sometimes used to clear nasal congestion.

Sweet marjoram has similar attributes, but its flavour is not as strong so it is more commonly used in cooking. It is sometimes combined with chamomile and taken as a general tonic, and can be used in a weak tea to ease children's colic.

MARSHMALLOW (Althaea officinalis)

A decorative plant originally from marshy areas of China, now found wild and commercially cultivated. It was known to the ancient Greeks who considered it almost a panacea. Marshmallow is an excellent source of easily digested mucilage, and is famous for its soothing, demulcent qualities which help to heal any inflammation of the respiratory, digestive and urinary organs. The dried root is made into a tea, often combined with other herbs such as coltsfoot and horehound, and used for all chest complaints. The tea is also used for cystitis, diarrhoea and vomiting and, combined with other laxative herbs, can ease the discomfort of chronic constipation. The powdered root can be used to enrich and increase the milk flow in nursing mothers. Made into an ointment marshmallow root is soothing for burns, and in a poultice it will reduce the inflammation of boils, abscesses, bruises, eczema and blood poisoning. A decoction of the root can be gargled for sore throats, applied to inflammations in the mouth and gums, or diluted as an eyewash. Marshmallow can also be eaten in salads or cooked as a green vegetable.

MARSH TEA (Ledum palustre)

An evergreen shrub from cool moist areas, sometimes cultivated in gardens. It can be made into a stimulating infusion for the nerves and stomach, and to treat coughs. Externally it can be used for all kinds of skin problems.

MASTERWORT, imperial masterwort (Imperatoria ostruthium)

A European alpine plant now cultivated in gardens; its root can be made into an infusion or a decoction useful for asthma, catarrh and breathlessness. It is also taken to stimulate the appetite, relieve flatulent colic and migraine, and to bring on delayed menstruation. Externally it can be applied to skin irritations.

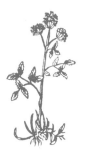

Masterwort

MASTIC

A transparent yellow resin from the Mediterranean shrub *Pistacia lentiscus*. It is occasionally used as a stimulant, diuretic and for bronchial problems. It can be softened and used as a temporary tooth filling, and is used commercially as a dental adhesive.

MATICO (Piper angustifolium)

A tall shrub from Peru, the dried leaves of which are used internally as a tonic, stimulant and for bronchitis and diarrhoea. Used externally they stop bleeding and make a good mouthwash. In Peru the plant is regarded as an aphrodisiac.

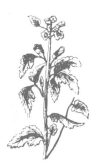

Marshmallow

MAUI WORMWOOD (Artemisia naviensis)

A type of sage brush grown on Maui, one of the Hawaiian Islands. It is used like sage for colds, sore throats and fevers, and as a tonic after childbirth.

MAYWEED, dog fennel, stinking chamomile (*Anthemis cotula*)

An unpleasant-smelling European weed which looks like chamomile. Its flowers can be made into a poultice for piles, or a weak infusion to stimulate menstruation and relieve migraine.

MEADOW SAFFRON, naked ladies, autum crocus (*Colchicum autumnale*)

A large bulb with lilac or purple crocus-like flowers. It is extremely poisonous but contains the alkaloid colchicine which is used medicinally for gout and arthritis. Anti-cancerous drugs derived from colchicine were among the first to be used successfully against leukaemia.

MEADOWSWEET, bridewort, lady of the meadow (*Filipendula ulmaria/ Spiraea ulmaria*)

A tall, fragrant, flowering herb common in damp European meadows. In 1839 it was discovered to contain salicylic acid, the substance from which aspirin was later synthesised. In fact the name 'aspirin' means literally 'from spiraea'. So meadowsweet is a natural substance with many of the same qualities as aspirin. It is particularly useful to relieve the pain of rheumatism, arthritis and gout, either taken in infusion or applied directly in an ointment or poultice. It is also helpful for feverish colds and flu, for gastric complaints (especially dyspepsia or 'acid stomach') and for vomiting in children, as well as being a specific remedy for peptic ulcers. As a diuretic it is useful for kidney complaints, cystitis and fluid retention, and its astringent qualities make it helpful for diarrhoea. It can be used externally to bathe wounds and reduce eye inflammation.

MEEMEEI, weeping pittosporum (*Pittosporum phylliraeoides*)

A slender, graceful tree with pale yellow flowers and yellow berries. It has been used by Aborigines throughout Australia as a medicinal plant, both internally and externally. A decoction can be used for colds, internal pains, sprains and eczema, and the warmed leaves made into a compress were used to encourage the flow of breast milk.

MELALEUCA — *see Tea-tree, Paperbark*

MELILOT, sweet clover, hay flower (*Melilotus officinalis*)

A strong-smelling type of clover once widely grown for cattle fodder, and also used in flavouring Gruyère cheese and tobacco, and to scent potpourris. Its carminative properties make it helpful for flatulence and digestive troubles, and it is used to improve the flavour of nauseous medicines. The whole plant, including the flowers, is made into an infusion which can be taken as a sedative for neuralgia and insomnia, or as a mild expectorant to relieve catarrh. The plant contains the anticoagulant coumarin, and can be taken to relieve inflammations of the eyes and to bring other inflammations to a head. Made into a poultice it can be helpful for headaches and arthritis, and has even been claimed to strengthen the memory.

MELLITA

A liquid medicine mixed with honey instead of syrup.

MESQUITE (*Prosopis juliflora*)

A Central American weed used by some Indians as a glue and a blue dye, and taken for indigestion, as a lotion to soothe sore eyes and to kill head lice.

MEXICAN DAMIANA
(Turnera aphrodisiaca)

A small shrub from Texas and northern Mexico, the leaves of which can be taken as a stimulant, general tonic or laxative. It is said to be an aphrodisiac.

MEZEREON, Mexican spurge, spurge laurel *(Daphne mezereum)*

A hardy deciduous European shrub with red berries, often grown in gardens. It is used by homeopaths for mental depression, skin problems and some respiratory and digestive ailments. The whole plant, particularly the berries, is very poisonous.

MILKWEED, silkweed *(Asclepias syriaca)*

A common North American plant which can be used in infusion for kidney and urinary complaints, and also for stomach ailments. The juice is said to remove warts.

MINT — *see Peppermint, Spearmint*

MISTLETOE, European mistletoe, all-heal, devil's fuge *(Viscum album)*
American mistletoe *(Phoradendron flavescens)*

An evergreen parasitic plant which for centuries has been thought by some to have mystical properties such as bringing good luck or protection against sorcery. It is an important plant in modern herbal and homeopathic medicine, and is used to strengthen the heart, reduce blood pressure and regulate menstruation. Combined with valerian root and vervain, it is used as a nerve tonic. A homeopathic tincture is used in treating cancer and the powdered leaves, in carefully measured doses, are used for epilepsy. In small doses it helps digestion,

but large doses can affect the heart. The berries can be very dangerous if eaten. Used externally, mistletoe can be made into a compress for varicose veins and for chilblains.

American mistletoe has quite a different effect. It increases blood pressure, stimulates contractions of the uterus, and has been used to stop bleeding after childbirth. However, it is dangerous to use except under medical supervision.

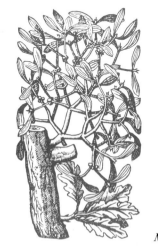

Mistletoe

MONARDA, horsemint *(Monarda punctata)*

A native plant from the USA which was used by the American Indians for fevers, inflammations, digestive problems, diarrhoea and rheumatism, and to relieve backache and stimulate the heart. The oil from the leaves induces sweating.

MONKSHOOD — *see Aconite*

MOONSEED — *see Cocculus*

MOTHERWORT, lion's tail *(Leonurus cardiaca)*

A tall strong-smelling plant with small pink flowers, found in gardens and waste places mostly in Europe. As its name suggests, it is useful for a variety of female complaints such as irregular or painful menstruation, and reduces problems such as palpitations during menopause. Taken in infusion it is a good general heart tonic and helps lower blood pressure. As an antispasmodic and sedative it is useful for anxiety, insomnia, convulsions and restless or delirious fevers. It is also helpful for stomach cramps, shortness of breath and rheumatism. Motherwort is collected in summer and dried before use. The fresh plant causes dermatitis in some people.

MOUNTAIN LAUREL
(Kalmia latifolia)

A highly poisonous evergreen shrub from cooler parts of North America. In very small doses it can be used as a sedative and to ease the pain of neuralgia. Externally it can be used for skin irritations.

MOUSE EAR (Hieracium pilosella)

A small plant found in dry parts of the USA. Taken in infusion it can be used for diarrhoea, liver problems and as a gargle for sore throats. As a powder it can be sniffed to stop nosebleed. Some people believe it will help cataracts if taken over a long period.

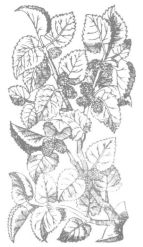

Mulberry

MUCILAGE

A jelly-like substance used to soothe irritations, particularly of the respiratory tract. It is found in plants such as cotton, elm, fenugreek fern and pansy.

MUGWORT, St John's plant
(Artemisa vulgaris)

A common aromatic wild herb once used to flavour beer. When used to season fatty meats it helps to prevent indigestion by its beneficial effect on bile production,

and it is recommended for diabetics. It can be used in infusion to regulate menstruation and for fevers, nervous disorders and rheumatism. As a bath additive it is helpful for rheumatism and tired, aching legs. Pilgrims once placed the herb in their shoes to give them strength to walk long distances. The fresh juice can be used as an antidote to opium, and will also relieve itching due to poison oak irritation. The American Indians used a decoction of the leaves for colds, fever and bronchitis, and as a poultice for wounds. A fresh leaf placed in 1 nostril is said to cure headache. Legend has it that a good night's sleep on a pillow stuffed with mugwort will produce dreams that reveal one's future.

MUIRA-PUAMA (Liriosma ovata)

A Brazilian plant with a root which can be used as an aphrodisiac and nerve stimulant.

MULBERRY (Morus nigra/ Morus rubra/Morus alba)

There are three kinds of mulberry tree bearing black, red or white fruit. The bark of the root, made into a decoction, is a traditional remedy for intestinal worms. The berries are laxative, as well as being rich in grape sugar which provides easily assimilated energy for convalescents. American Indians used the milky juice at the base of the red mulberry leaf to cure ringworm.

MULLEIN (Verbascum thapsus)

A tall yellow flower believed in its native Europe and Asia to have the power to ward off evil spirits and said to be the plant Ulysses took with him to protect himself against Circe. The leaves and flowers are made into an infusion which is excellent for respiratory complaints, particularly asthma, bronchitis and croup, and in combination with garlic and comfrey it is a specific treatment for tuberculosis. It acts as an expectorant and stimulant, and also relieves pain and has a sedative action. The dried leaves can be smoked as medicinal cigarettes or inhaled in a steam bath to clear sinus congestion and relieve asthma. They can also be gargled in infusion for laryngitis. An oil made from the flowers is good for piles, bruises and nappy rash, and is used in Europe for ear complaints. A poultice of leaves can help slow-healing sores, reduce swollen glands and help painful swollen or rheumatic joints. A strong infusion of leaves will slow any internal bleeding, and is also a useful diuretic, a kidney tonic and a remedy for diarrhoea. The crushed fresh flowers are said to remove warts.

MUSK BASIL (*Basilicum polystachyon*)

An aromatic herb with pale lilac flowers used by some Australian Aborigines to reduce fever. In Indonesia the crushed leaves were used externally to relieve strained muscles.

MUSK ROOT, sumbul (*Ferula sumbul*)

Found in Asia and Russia, this plant smells rather like musk. Its root can be used as a stimulant, an antispasmodic and a nerve tonic, and it is sometimes prescribed for asthma and nervous diseases. It is also used in cosmetics and perfumes.

MUSTARD

This widely cultivated yellow-flowered plant comes in several varieties, the most commonly grown being black mustard (*Brassica nigra*), which has black seeds, and white mustard (*Brassica alba*), which has pale seeds. Their properties are similar, though black mustard is stronger. Mustard is best known as a flavouring, but has also been used since the time of the ancient Greeks for medicinal pur-

poses. It is now used mainly externally, the seeds being made into a poultice used to relieve acute pain and lung congestion, particularly with regard to bronchitis. The poultice should not be left on too long as it may redden and inflame the skin. A mustard foot bath can be used for tired and aching feet. Many sufferers from rheumatism and muscular pain find relief in a mustard bath.

MU TEA

A Japanese herbal tea containing a number of ingredients balanced in their yin and yang attributes. Mu tea contains, among other things, cinnamon, cypress, cloves, liquorice, peach kernels, ginger root and Japanese ginseng. It is taken for wheezing coughs and respiratory disorders.

MYRRH (*Commiphora myrrha*)

An aromatic, gummy resin used by the Arabs and ancient Egyptians in embalming, as incense, in cosmetics and perfumes, and for medicine. It is antiseptic and astringent, and makes a good gargle for sore throats, sore teeth and gums, bad breath, coughs and asthma. It can also be used to wash wounds and as a douche. Myrrh is said to improve circulation and increase the number of white blood cells.

MYRTLE (*Myrtus communis*)

A small, fragrant, white-flowering tree used since ancient times for culinary and religious purposes. Its leaves were made into garlands for the winners of the Olympic Games, were used by Jews at the Feast of the Tabernacle, and were carried by English brides as a symbol of fertility. Today it is used medicinally as an infusion, to make a douche for leucorrhoea or an expectorant tea helpful for chest complaints. The oil is used in perfumes and potpourris.

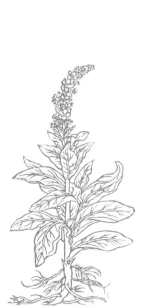

Mullein

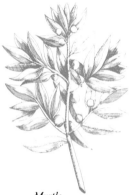

Myrtle

N

NARCOTIC

A drug which, in small doses, relieves pain and induces sleep, but in large doses causes convulsions, coma or even death. Examples include deadly nightshade, opium, wormwood and aconite.

NASTURTIUM, Indian cress (*Tropaeolum majus*)

A creeping garden plant with bright red, orange and yellow flowers, originally from Peru. Its flowers and leaves can be used in salads and teas. They have a strong peppery taste and a high vitamin C content. The seeds can be used as a substitute for capers. The plant has antiseptic and expectorant qualities, and is useful for respiratory congestion and as a tonic for the blood (it promotes the formation of blood cells) and the digestive system. It also helps clear the skin and eyes. The crushed seeds can be made into a poultice for boils.

NATIVE MINT BUSH (*Prostanthera rotundifolia*)

A common Australian bush with rounded leaves and purple flowers. The aromatic leaves can be used, like garden mint, in a tea to relieve flatulence, colic and nausea.

NATIVE PEAR, Austral doubah (*Leichhardtia australis*)

A climbing plant with clusters of star-shaped flowers and elongated olive-green fruits which, when dried, release masses of flat black seeds which were ground and used by some Aborigines in Western Australia as an oral contraceptive.

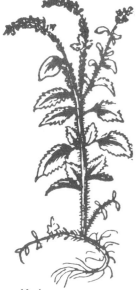

Nettle

NATIVE PEPPER (*Piper novae-hollandiae*)

A climbing rainforest plant, the leaves of which were chewed by Aborigines to relieve sore gums. The plant has been shown to stimulate the mucous membranes, making it useful in the treatment of gonorrhoea. Recent studies have shown it is effective in combating one form of lung cancer in mice.

NEPHRITIC

A substance which can be used to treat diseases of the kidneys. Examples include hepatica, horseradish, aloe, celery and sassafras.

NERVE ROOT, lady's slipper, moccasin flower (*Cypripedium pubescens*)

A North American plant with a characteristic moccasin-shaped flower of yellow lined with purple. Its root can be made into a tranquillising tea for headaches, insomnia and general anxiety, and also to relieve muscle cramps and spasms. Large doses may cause hallucinations.

NERVINE

A herb which has a calming or soothing effect on the nerves. Examples include hops, mistletoe, skullcap, passion flower, gentian and valerian, all of which can be used to make teas.

NETTLE, common nettle, stinging nettle (*Urtica dioica*)

A well-known troublesome weed originally from Eurasia but now widespread. The leaves are covered with stinging hairs when fresh but are quite safe to eat when dried or cooked. Nettles are rich in vitamins A and C, chlorophyll and mineral salts such as iron, calcium, potassium, silicon, manganese and sulphur; they may be sprinkled over salads or eaten as a cooked green vegetable. Sometimes used to treat anaemia, they are also useful for people on low salt diets and as a general tonic and blood purifier. Nettle tea is a diuretic useful for cystitis, and also helps to relieve high blood pressure. It stimulates the digestive system and helps to increase the milk flow in nursing mothers. Regular doses will control frequent nosebleeds and internal haemorrhaging. Nosebleeds can also be stopped by applying the fresh juice on a piece of cottonwool.

NEW JERSEY TEA, wild snowball, red root (*Ceanothus americanus*)

A small shrub from the USA with root bark which can be made into an infusion helpful for coughs and respiratory problems, and used as a gargle for tonsillitis and mouth sores. The American Indians made the whole plant into a tea used for all kinds of skin problems, including skin cancer.

NIGHT BLOOMING CEREUS (*Cereus grandiflorus*)

A small Jamaican cactus used in decoction to stimulate the heart and give relief from palpitations, as well as being used as a diuretic and for prostate disorders.

NIGHTSHADE, BLACK, common nightshade (*Solanum nigrum*)

A much smaller plant (about 30 cm or 1 ft high) than the deadly nightshade which grows up to 1.5 m (5 ft) tall. It too is poisonous and not recommended for domestic use, but it is used by homeopaths in a tincture for epilepsy. Externally the crushed leaves will relieve pain and inflammation in tumours and skin problems.

NIGHTSHADE, DEADLY — *see Belladonna*

NIPPLEWORT (*Lapsana communis*)

A common wild plant similar to the dandelion and eaten fresh in salads. Its dried leaves were traditionally made into a warm infusion for sore nipples.

NONI (*Morinda citrifolia*)

A Hawaiian plant, the ripe yellow fruit of which is mashed and placed directly onto sores and boils to bring them to a head. It can also be taken internally for asthma and high blood pressure, and gargled for a sore throat.

NUTMEG (*Myristica fragrans*)

The kernel of the fleshy fruit of the nutmeg tree which is native to the Moluccas and other islands of the East Indies. Used by the Persians 1000 years ago, it is now best known as a flavouring but is also a carminative helpful for vomiting, flatulence and to aid digestion. It can also be used for severe diarrhoea. In small doses nutmeg is a tonic, but large doses can have a narcotic effect due to the myristicin it contains. A liniment of nutmeg butter can be used as a counterirritant to treat arthritis.

O

OAK (*Quercus robur*)

A well-known large spreading tree, the powdered bark of which, taken in decoction, is a powerful astringent useful for

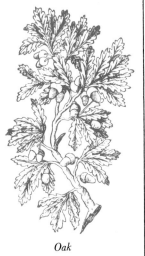

Oak

diarrhoea, vomiting and bleeding from the mouth. It is also antiseptic and can be used externally for bleeding piles, as a douche for leucorrhoea, a gargle for a sore throat, or a wash for infected sores. Used both internally and externally it is said to be good for varicose veins. Acorns are rich in protein and can be ground into a meal to make bread. Some people use them as a substitute for coffee.

OATS *(Avena sativa)*

A commonly cultivated cereal crop which can be made into an easily digested gruel suitable for patients with fever or gastro-intestinal inflammations. The seeds can be made into a decoction or a tincture and used as a nerve tonic which allays spasms and is good for the heart muscles. A homeopathic tincture from the flowering plant can be used for arthritis. Oat straw can be made into a tea for chest complaints or used in a bath for rheumatism, liver complaints, aching or cold feet, and for a variety of skin complaints. Oatmeal can also be made into a poultice for skin irritations or freckles, and is used in many commercial soaps and cosmetics.

OIL

The active ingredient of a herb extracted by combining it with vegetable oil. The pounded herb is heated with an oil such as olive oil in a covered pot for 2 hours, then strained and stored in a glass container, preferably with a small amount of vitamin E added to preserve the oil. Alternatively, the herb may be mixed with the oil (50 g of herb to 500 ml of oil) and left to stand for 2 weeks in a sealed container which is shaken daily. Oils are usually used externally.

OINTMENT

A solid, fatty substance prepared by mixing herbal oils with melted beeswax, lard, suet, paraffin or any other substance which will liquefy when rubbed onto the skin. An ointment may also be referred to as a salve or paste.

OLIVE *(Olea europaea)*

A Mediterranean tree grown mostly for its fruit, which is eaten or crushed for cooking oil. The oil is also a demulcent and laxative, increases bile secretion and peristalsis, and has been claimed to help break down cholesterol. It can be used as an enema or on burns, bruises and insect bites. It is very effective as a lotion to soften dry skin and dry cuticles, and is used as a base for many liniments and ointments. Mixed with alcohol it makes a good hair tonic, and combined with oil of rosemary it is an effective treatment for dandruff. The leaves are antiseptic and astringent, and can be made into an infusion which will calm general anxiety and lower fever.

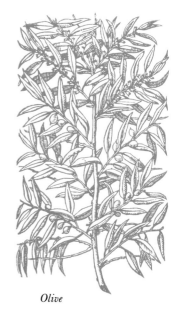

Olive

ONION *(Allium cepa)*

The numerous varieties of onion are cultivated mostly for cooking, but they also have significant medicinal value and many people believe they should be eaten daily to help prevent colds and coughs. Onions stimulate the appetite and digestion, though they may cause flatulence in some people. A remedy for gaseous indigestion pains is to eat half a raw onion with bread. The antiseptic and expectorant qualities of onions make the raw juice (mixed with honey) an excellent cough medicine, and homeopaths prescribe a tincture for hay fever. Onion juice is also said to lower the blood pressure and strengthen the heart. Applied externally it is helpful for skin infections and bee stings, to relieve the pain of rheumatism and arthritis, and even to strengthen brittle fingernails. Some people believe the high phosphorus content of onions stimulates creativity and improves concentration.

OXALIS, creeping oxalis, yellow wood-sorrel (*Oxalis corniculata*)

A creeping plant with shamrock-shaped leaves and yellow flowers. In Australia it is generally regarded as a troublesome weed, but in some countries of southern Asia the leaves are taken in infusion for fevers, dysentery and nausea, or used externally as an eyewash, as a soothing paste to relieve heat rash, and in a more concentrated form to remove warts and corns. In southern Africa it is used as a cough remedy and an antidote to poisons, particularly snakebite.

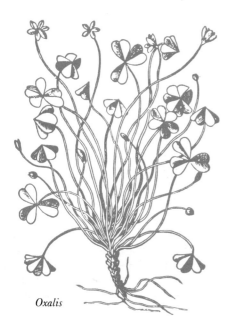
Oxalis

OXYTOCIN

A substance which facilitates childbirth by speeding up the contractions of the uterus. Examples include cotton, ergot, Peruvian bark and blue cohosh.

P

PAEONY, peony (*Paeonia officinalis*)

A large red garden flower which grows wild in southern Europe. Its powdered root was traditionally taken for liver and kidney problems, and can also be used as an antispasmodic to treat spasms, convulsions, epilepsy and whooping cough. The plant is poisonous, particularly the flowers. In Victorian England children sometimes wore necklaces made from the plant called piney beads; they were said to help with teething and prevent convulsions.

PANSY, wild pansy, heart's ease, heart of trinity, garden violet (*Viola tricolor*)

A well-known garden annual which has been cultivated for centuries for its pretty flowers and is also found wild in temperate areas of the northern hemisphere. It can be distinguished from other members of its family by its colours (purple, yellow and white), and the fact that the two upper petals are erect instead of leaning forward. The medicinal qualities of the pansy have been known since the Middle Ages, when it was used as a purifying tea believed to benefit the heart. The powdered leaves can be made into an infusion helpful for children's skin eruptions, asthma, catarrh and urinary problems. It has also been used for children suffering from bedwetting, hysteria and cramps.

The powder can be sprinkled directly onto a wound or mixed with honey to make a healing ointment. Some people have found relief from rheumatism by adding it to their bathwater.

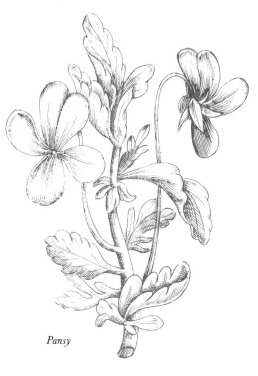

Pansy

PAPERBARK, broad-leafed paperbark (*Melaleuca quinquenervia*)

A well-known Australian tree with corky bark which peels off in sheets. It is found in swampy areas and is often grown in suburban areas along the eastern coast. The new leaves can be chewed to give relief from head colds, or made into a decoction for headaches, nasal congestion and the general feeling of nausea associated with colds. Other *Melaleuca* species can be used in a similar way — *see Tea-tree.*

PARASITICIDE

A substance which can be used to kill parasites. Examples include blackberry for ringworm, columbine for head lice, nasturtium for worms and pennyroyal for fleas.

PARSLEY (*Petroselinum crispum*)

A very popular herb, native to Europe but now cultivated worldwide and found in several different varieties. Although it has been used widely since the time of the Roman Empire, the ancient Greeks did not eat it but considered it a symbol of death, and in medieval England it was often used in black magic. Perhaps because of its long germination period, it was believed that the seed had to go to the devil and back seven times before the plant would grow. Parsley is a very nutritious food, rich in iron, calcium, iodine, manganese and copper, and in vitamins, particularly A and C, and is especially recommended for those suffering from anaemia or general poor health. The seeds contain the essential oil called apiol, which stimulates the appetite and increases the blood flow to the uterus and digestive system. A decoction of the root is a diuretic used to stimulate the kidneys and bladder, to dissolve gravel and stones, and help some lower back pain. In greater strengths it can be used for irregular menstruation and for liver and gall bladder problems. It should not be taken in large doses or for a long period of time as it may overstimulate the kidneys and can even cause abortion. Parsley tea, made from the leaves, is a digestive aid and a diuretic. Used externally it is said to fade freckles, help remove warts and make dark hair glossy. Used as a skin freshener it helps to close enlarged pores and reduce puffiness round the eyes.

PARSLEY PIERT (*Aphanes arvensis*)

A low-growing European herb with tiny green flowers; it is not related to common parsley. It is used in infusion for urinary complaints, especially cystitis, and to help dissolve kidney stones.

PASQUE FLOWER, Easter flower *(Anemone patens)*

A prairie plant from the USA which can be dried and used to help wounds heal. The fresh plant is an irritant.

PASSION FLOWER, maypop *(Passiflora incarnata)*

A climbing vine which grows wild in southern parts of the USA. The stem and leaves are used in professionally prepared medicines for insomnia, nervous headache and spasmodic complaints, and can be given in a tincture to restless children.

PATCHOULI *(Pogostemon cablin)*

A Malaysian plant used in bath herbs, soaps and cosmetics, and said to have a rejuvenating effect when inhaled. Its distinctive odour is used to mask other strong smells and it is also an insect repellent.

PAWALE, giant dock *(Rumex giganteus)*

A Hawaiian plant, the root bark of which is used to treat skin infections.

PAWPAW, papaya, melon, zapote *(Carica papaya)*

A well-known yellow tropical fruit with glossy black seeds. The milky juice of the unripe fruit contains the protein-digesting enzyme papain, which is similar to the enzyme pepsin produced by the gastric juices of the stomach, and so is helpful for dyspepsia and other digestive problems. It is used to make indigestion tablets and meat tenderisers. The juice can also be used to remove freckles and to kill intestinal worms. The leaves can be used on infected wounds. Pawpaw can be helpful in relieving allergies which are caused by inadequate protein breakdown.

PEACH *(Prunus persica)*

A well-known, widely cultivated fruit tree thought to come originally from China. The oil from the kernels can be used as a substitute for almond oil. The leaves can be used as a mild sedative, diuretic and expectorant for chronic bronchitis, and have been successfully used for whooping cough. They are also used for inflammatory bowel diseases and gastritis, and in small doses to relieve morning sickness in pregnancy. The powdered leaves can be used externally to help heal sores.

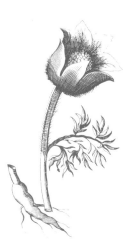

Pasque flower

PEANUT TREE *(Sterculia quadrifida)*

An Australian tree with unusual large seed pods which are bright red inside and contain glossy black seeds. The leaves can be crushed and applied to wounds, or an infusion can be made from the bark and used to soothe sore eyes.

PEAR *(Pyrus communis)*

This is the wild pear tree from which the commercial varieties have been cultivated. Pear juice is recommended for catarrh, colitis, hypertension, constipation and skin problems. It is particularly rich in vitamins A, B and C.

PECTORAL

A substance used to treat pulmonary and other chest disorders. Examples include lungwort, eucalyptus, plantain, Iceland moss and fenugreek.

PELLITORY OF SPAIN *(Anacyclus pyrethrum/Anthemis pyrethrum)*

A perennial plant rather similar to chamomile. The powdered root is made into lozenges which increase salivation and are excellent for a dry mouth and throat. As a tincture it is very effective for toothache.

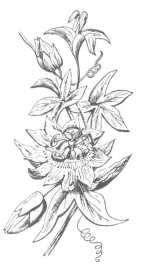

Passion flower

PELLITORY OF THE WALL *(Parietaria officinalis)*

A tall European weed with clinging black seeds. It is particularly effective in increasing urine production and as a remedy for urinary tract stones. It can be used as a tincture or an infusion.

PENNYROYAL, European pennyroyal *(Mentha pulegium)* American pennyroyal *(Hedeoma pulegioides)*

A member of the mint family characterised by its whorls of pale purple flowers. It is most often used in infusion to promote menstruation, and has also been traditionally used to cause abortion. It is very effective for flatulence and colic pains, and can be given to children with stomach upsets and feverish illnesses. Pennyroyal is a good insect repellent and will also soothe bites and itching skin.

American pennyroyal has similar qualities.

PEPPER *(Piper nigrum)*

Now one of the most widely used spices, it was also probably the earliest known to man. The bright red berries of this tropical vine, originally from India, were once a costly luxury and played a very important part in the spice trade. Black pepper is made from the dried unripe berries, while the stronger white pepper is made from the ripe berries with the skin removed. Both kinds are digestive stimulants and very helpful in relieving flatulence as well as helping nasal congestion and fevers. They are also antibacterial and repel insects. Pepper is also available in pills.

PEPPERMINT, brandy mint, white mint *(Mentha x piperita)*

A relatively modern herb which is now a very well known aromatic. It was first noted in England in 1696 and is a cross between spearmint and wild water mint. Its cool taste and fresh minty smell have made it widely used commercially in flavouring products such as toothpaste, sweets and cigarettes. Peppermint is useful for all sorts of digestive problems such as nausea, vomiting, dyspepsia, flatulent colic and diarrhoea. Although renowned for its cool taste, it generates internal heat and increases perspiration. Peppermint tea is often taken for colds, flu and headaches, and the oil can be inhaled for catarrh and bronchitis. The oil can be applied directly for toothaches or rubbed onto rheumatic joints. The leaves can be scattered around to keep away rats and mice.

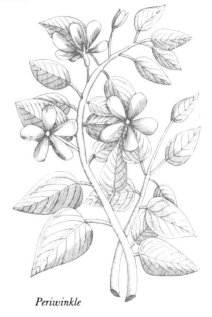

Periwinkle

PERIWINKLE, GREATER *(Vinca major)* lesser periwinkle *(Vinca minor)* Madagascar periwinkle *(Catharanthus roseus)*

A pretty blue-flowered creeping plant from Europe which is often grown in gardens. It has astringent and sedative qualities, and is used for excessive menstruation, haemorrhage, bleeding in the mouth and nose, or for bleeding piles and diarrhoea. Chewing on a leaf can cure toothache. Periwinkle has also been used to treat diabetes and leukaemia. The Madagascar periwinkle is the source of 2 anti-cancer drugs, vincristine and vinblastine.

PERU BALSAM (*Myroxylon pereirae*)

A bitter-tasting leguminous tree from El Salvador used as a stimulant and expectorant for catarrh and bronchitis, and as a disinfectant for skin diseases.

PERUVIAN BARK — *see Cinchona bark*

PICHI (*Fabiana imbricata*)

A small-leafed South American herb used in infusion as a stimulant and diuretic to treat liver and kidney complaints, and also thought to be good for catarrh.

PILEWORT — *see Celandine*

PIMPERNEL — *see Saxifrage*

PINEAPPLE (*Ananas comosus*)

A well-known tropical fruit, the juice of which is recommended for sore throats and which is said to increase the effectiveness of antibiotics when taken simultaneously.

PINE TREE — *see Fir*

PINKROOT, Carolina pink, starbloom (*Pigelia marylandica*)

A herbaceous North American plant used by the American Indians to expel intestinal worms. It is extremely poisonous in large doses.

PIPSISSEWA (*Chimaphila umbellata*)

A creeping woodland plant from temperate areas of the northern hemisphere, used in infusion as a diuretic helpful for dissolving bladder stones and other urinary problems. It can be used externally for sores, blisters and swellings.

PITCH

The resin from some coniferous trees such as the Norway Spruce, *Picea abies*. It is used as a base for plasters and also to treat chronic inflammation of the respiratory mucous membranes and chronic skin conditions like eczema and psoriasis.

PITCHER PLANT (*Sarracenia purpurea*)

A North American swamp plant famous for its ability to trap and consume insects. It was used by some American Indians for protection against smallpox, and also as a tonic to stimulate the appetite and digestion, but it is no longer widely used.

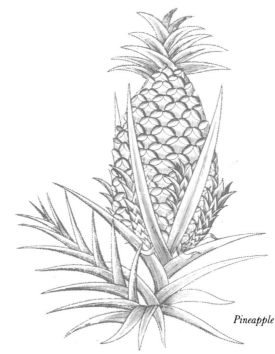

Pineapple

PLANTAIN, greater plantain
(Plantago major)

A very common lawn weed in temperate parts of the world and known since ancient times. There are several species of plantain, all of which have similar properties, though greater plantain is the one most commonly used by herbalists. It is a cooling, soothing diuretic which acts on the mucous membranes and can be used to treat diarrhoea, haemorrhoids, urinary disorders (especially cystitis), menstrual problems, coughs and bronchitis. The seeds, known as psyllium seeds, are a useful laxative. Plantain's astringent qualities make it excellent for all kinds of wounds and bleeding, both internal and external, and for skin infections, boils, burns and insect bites. The leaves can be used either fresh or in a poultice and have antibacterial qualities and stimulate healing. The root can be chewed for toothache and a decoction of the seeds can be given to children suffering from thrush.

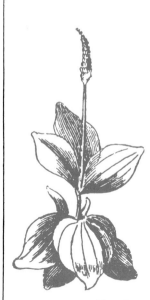

Plantain

PLASTER

Sometimes used as a synonym for poultice, though the herbal material is usually combined with a thickening agent such as flour to form a paste — *see Poultice.*

PLEURISY ROOT, swallow
wort *(Asclepias tuberosa)*

A North American plant found in dry sandy soils. Its dried root is taken in decoction or tincture for colds, flu, bronchitis and pleurisy, and to reduce pain and ease breathing.

PLOUGHMAN'S SPIKENARD *(Inula conyza)*

A tall yellow-flowered European roadside weed, the juice of which will soothe itching skin. An infusion can be taken to promote menstruation, to ease wheeziness and to help heal some internal injuries.

PLUM, wild plum *(Prunus domestica)*

The many varieties of plum are best known for their edible fruit. When dried (as prunes), they are a well-known laxative. Plum juice is also a laxative, as well as a digestive tonic, and is sometimes recommended for dyspepsia, obesity, piles and skin disorders. The dried leaves are laxative and diuretic, and are sometimes used to bring down fevers, as well as being used in a gargle or mouthwash.

POKEWEED *(Phytolacca americana)*

A tall North American plant which has been introduced to Europe. The young leaves are rich in minerals and the dried root is used as a laxative, to relieve pain and inflammation, and for skin diseases, rheumatism, and arthritis. The juice of the fruit has been used to treat cancer and haemorrhoids.

POLYBODY *(Polypodium vulgare)*

A perennial fern, the root of which is laxative and can be given in infusion as an appetite stimulant and digestive tonic, and also for coughs and chest infections.

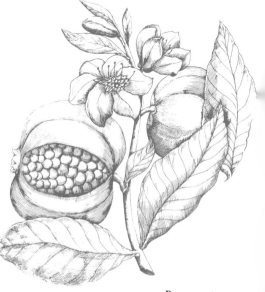

Pomegranate

POMEGRANATE *(Punica granatum)*

A small tropical tree originally from western Asia. The juice of its many-seeded fruit has been used since the time of the ancient Greeks to expel tapeworms, and is now sometimes used to treat high blood pressure and arthritis. The rind of the fruit is high in tannin and is an excellent astringent for skin problems; it can also be used in a gargle for sore throats and diarrhoea, and as a douche for leucorrhoea. Large doses can cause cramps and vomiting.

POPLAR, BLACK *(Populus nigra)*

A European deciduous tree with small yellowish-green flowers with red stamens. These are made into an ointment for haemorrhoids and skin disorders; this ointment can also be rubbed onto the chest for bronchitis and onto rheumatic and arthritic joints. The buds can also be taken internally for urinary problems. White poplar, *Populus alba*, can be used in a similar way, as can European aspen *(Populus tremula)*. *See also Quaking aspen.*

POPLAR, WHITE — *see* Poplar, black

POPPY, WHITE, opium poppy *(Papaver somniferum)*

A white-, mauve- or purple-flowered plant originally from central Asia and the eastern Mediterranean, but now cultivated elsewhere. The drug opium can be extracted from the ripening poppy capsule for up to 3 weeks after flowering. The sedative properties of this drug have been known since the time of the ancient Egyptians, and it was widely used for pain relief, to treat cholera and dysentery, and even to quieten restless children. The seeds, which contain no opium, have been used as a spice since the Middle Ages. They can also be made into a lotion for skin and mouth irritations, and toothache. Opium has become a widely abused drug and is now illegal in most countries. It is grown commercially as a source of the powerful painkilling drugs morphine and codeine which are used in orthodox medicine.

POPPY, WILD *(Papaver rhoeas)*

A red-flowered poppy which grows wild in Europe. Herbalists use an infusion of the petals to treat asthma, bronchitis, catarrh and angina, and also make the flowers into a soothing cough syrup which causes drowsiness.

POULTICE

A soft, wet, heated mass of herbs applied directly to the skin to ease pain or inflammation, or to act as an antiseptic or counterirritant. Fresh herbs are first bruised or crushed, while dried ones need to be softened in hot water. The poultice is usually placed between 2 pieces of fine cloth or in a bag, then held onto the skin while hot. A fresh poultice is usually applied several times a day.

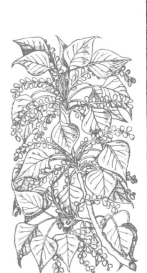

Poplar, black

PRICKLY ASH, toothache tree *(Zanthoxylum americanum)*

A native North American tree, the bark of which was widely used in infusion as a toothache remedy and sometimes as a wash for itching skin. It is also said to be good for rheumatism and indigestion.

PRICKLY PEAR *(Opuntia species)*

A fleshy cactus-like plant which is best known for the terrible destruction it caused when it spread out of control in some farming areas of Australia. The mucilaginous juice can be used to relieve coughs, and also as a base for ointments. A decoction of the pods will lower the blood sugar level and has been used in the treatment of diabetes.

PRIDE OF CHINA (*Melia azedarach*)

A deciduous tree originally from south-western China but now growing also in southern USA. A decoction of root bark is used in India as a general tonic. The seeds and oil of the fruit will get rid of worms.

PRIMROSE (*Primula vulgaris*)

A well-known European woodland plant with pale yellow flowers, traditionally used in infusion to relieve rheumatism and gout. Used either as a tincture of the whole plant or an infusion of flowers, it is a sedative which is very good to soothe tension headaches and for insomnia. It can be made into snuff to clear the nose and also into a facewash.

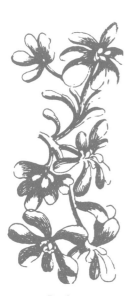

Purslane

PULSATILLA, wind flower, pasque flower (*Anemone pulsatilla*)

A large European weed with purple flowers. The leaves can be prepared as a sedative and antispasmodic infusion helpful for menstrual problems, insomnia, tension headaches and some skin problems. The plant stimulates secretions from the mucous membranes, the sweat glands and the bladder. It is poisonous in large quantities.

PUMPKIN (*Cucurbita pepo*)

A well-known vegetable which grows on a large creeping vine. The seeds can be used to expel tapeworms, for urinary complaints, and as a demulcent for the bowels. They are said to be effective against tumours and are used for treatment of an enlarged prostate. Many health-store patent remedies contain pumpkin seeds.

PURGATIVE

A substance which causes vigorous evacuation of the bowels. Examples include prune, aloe, hyssop, hellebore and castor oil.

PURSLANE, COMMON, green purslane (*Portulaca oleracea*) yellow purslane (*Portulaca sativa*)

A hardy, fleshy-leafed plant found in sandy soils, often near the sea. It is very rich in vitamins and minerals, and the young leaves are recommended by herbalists as a nutritious salad herb. The leaves can be made into a tonic tea which is good for blood disorders, and the juice can be used either internally or externally to treat skin diseases.

PYRETHRUM — *see Feverfew*

Q

QUAKING ASPEN, Canadian aspen (*Populus tremuloides*)

A deciduous North American tree with flowers growing in slender catkins. The sticky buds of these flowers are very similar to those of the poplar and can be used in the same way: as an ointment for rheumatism, arthritis, haemorrhoids, wounds and bronchitis, or taken internally as a tea for coughs, or a gargle for sore throats. The bark and leaves can be made into a diuretic infusion which is used to relax the intestinal tract, improve digestion, and relieve some headaches and fevers.

QUASSIA, bitter ash (*Picraena excelsa*)

A tall tree native to Central America and the West Indies which looks rather like an ash tree. The bitter-tasting wood chips are used to make bitters and to flavour tonic wines and aperitives; they will sharpen the appetite and help digestion. In infusion they can be used for fever, rheumatism, cramps, dyspepsia and to kill intestinal worms. The tea is also sometimes drunk to prevent a craving for alcohol. Externally it is good for dandruff and as a rinse for blond hair.

QUEEN OF THE MEADOW, gravel root, kidney root (*Eupatorium purpureum*)

A North American woodland plant used in infusion as a diuretic for kidney and urinary complaints, and rheumatism. The root can be used as an astringent.

QUEENSLAND SANDALWOOD, plumwood (*Santalum lanceolatum*)

A parasitic tree, the leaves and bark of which were made into a decoction and drunk as a purgative and to relieve respiratory complaints. An infusion of the leaves could be used externally for rheumatism or to soothe itching skin, and the leaves could be burned to repel mosquitoes.

QUINCE (*Cydonia oblonga*)

A fruit tree orginally from Iran. The seeds can be boiled in water to produce an astringent mucilage which is soothing for the intestinal tract. The down of the fruit was once used as a hair restorer and to prevent hair from falling out.

QUININE — *see Cinchona bark*

R

RADISH, COMMON, garden radish (*Raphanus sativus*)

A well-known salad vegetable originally from China. Its juice is rich in potassium, sodium, iron and magnesium, and can be used as a liver tonic and to stimulate bile production and treat gallstones. It should not be taken by people with inflammations of the stomach or kidney disease. Radish juice has also been used for coughs, bronchitis, headaches and flatulence. *See also Horseradish.*

RAGGED CUP (*Silphium perfoliatum*)

A North American plant with yellow flowers like sunflowers. Its gum is used as a stimulant and antispasmodic, and the rootstock is used for fevers, liver problems and general debility.

RAGWORT (*Senecio jacobaea*) American ragwort (*Senecio aureus*)

A common European weed with yellow flowers. Although not recommended for internal use as it may damage the liver, ragwort can be used externally as a lotion for ulcers and wounds, as a gargle for sore throats, and as an ointment for inflamed eyes. A homeopathic tincture is sometimes prescribed for cystitis.

American ragwort was used by the Indians for suppressed menstruation, to speed childbirth, and for urinary problems.

RASPBERRY, European raspberry (*Rubus idaeus*)

Best known for its delicious edible fruit, this plant is also useful because of its leaves, which have been used for centuries for a variety of women's dis-

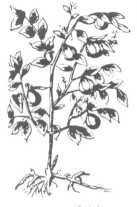

Quinine

orders. Raspberry tea, taken in early pregnancy, is a rich source of folic acid, iron, copper and vitamins A and C. Taken regularly it prevents morning sickness and is thought by some to reduce the likelihood of miscarriage. In later pregnancy it strengthens the pelvic muscles, regulates contractions and eases the pain of labour. It helps prevent haemorrhage, increases the milk supply, and can be used to bathe sore nipples. In nonpregnant women it strengthens the muscles supporting the uterus and is good for painful menstruation and vaginal discharge. Raspberry tea is a useful astringent to cure diarrhoea and can be gargled for sore throats or used to wash wounds, burns and skin infections. It is safe to give to children and is helpful for colds, flu and fever.

RED ASH *(Alphitonia excelsa)*

A common scrubland tree in eastern and northern Australia. Some Aborigines rubbed an infusion of the bark and leaves onto aching muscles and joints, or used it as a gargle for toothache. The leaves crushed in water were said to make a soothing bath to relieve headaches and soothe sore eyes, and a decoction of the bark could be taken as a tonic.

RED CEDAR *(Toona australis)*

A rainforest tree eagerly sought by the early Australian settlers for its beautiful timber. Its bark can be used to treat fevers and diarrhoea, and the flowers can be made into a tea to bring on menstruation.

RED CLOVER, wild clover *(Trifolium pratense)*

An important grazing crop grown for cattle in all temperate climates. It was not used medicinally by ancient herbalists, but its usefulness was discovered by the Americans after the plant had been introduced by the Europeans. They found it an excellent wash to heal sores and took it internally for skin diseases. Red clover contains high concentrations of lime, silica, iron, copper and other minerals, and has been found useful for treating chronic skin diseases such as eczema; applied externally, is said to heal ulcers, burns and skin cancers. It can be taken in infusion for anaemia and to stimulate the appetite and the liver. It is not recommended in large doses or for long periods, and is usually taken together with other herbs.

REFRIGERANT

A substance used in fevers to cool the body. Examples include chickweed, sorrel, purslane, currant and tamarind.

RESTHARROW, cammock, prickly restharrow *(Ononis spinosa)*

A thorny European shrub with reddish-pink flowers. It is used mainly as a diuretic, particularly by French herbalists who make a decoction of the roots and flowers for urinary-tract infections. A decoction of the root can be used for eczema and itching skin, and an infusion of the flowers makes a gargle for sore throats and gums.

RESTORATIVE

A substance which restores consciousness and normal physiological activity. Examples include borage, fenugreek, rosemary, hyssop and sarsaparilla.

RHATANY *(Krameria triandra)*

A red-flowered shrub from Peru, the root of which is a strong astringent used in infusion for diarrhoea and to stop internal and external bleeding.

RHUBARB, Chinese rhubarb
(Rheum palmatum)
culinary or tart rhubarb (Rheum rhaponticum)

Native to China and Tibet, this plant is also cultivated as an ornamental garden plant which resembles common rhubarb but has a huge flower stem over 2 m high. It is widely used in pharmaceutical preparations available at chemists and health food stores. Small doses of the powdered root are astringent and stop diarrhoea, while in large doses it is a purgative. It is not recommended for pregnant or nursing mothers, or those with chronic constipation. It is used in a tincture to stimulate the appetite.

Culinary rhubarb is the variety with red stems used for food. In large amounts it acts as a laxative. The powdered root can be given to stop diarrhoea, improve the appetite and regulate the bowels; because of its mildness, it can be given to children. The leaves are poisonous.

RICE (Oryza sativa)

A well-known staple cereal food. Brown rice is rich in vitamins B and E, and is generally considered nutritionally superior to refined white rice. Rice water is a common treatment for diarrhoea and is also sometimes taken for fevers and painful urination. It is made by boiling 15 g (½ oz) of rice in 600 ml (1 pint) of water, then straining and adding honey if required. Powdered rice can also be mixed into a poultice for skin inflammation.

RIVER MINT (Mentha australis)

A sprawling, bright green, peppermint-smelling plant which grows in swampy areas throughout Australia. It was used by the Aborigines and early settlers as a general tonic and as a tea to give relief from colds and coughs. Some Aborigines used it to bring on abortion.

ROCK-ROSE (Helianthemum canadense)

A yellow-flowered North American plant sometimes used as a tonic and astringent for skin inflammations, mouth sores and as an eyewash.

ROSE (Rosa species)

Members of the genus *Rosa* are prickly shrubs which grow wild in temperate parts of the northern hemisphere but are also widely cultivated. Several species, particularly red ones, have been traditionally used in European folk medicine. An infusion of dried rose petals can be taken for headache and dizziness, and a decoction mixed with wine is thought by some to be a stimulating tonic which also eases menstrual pain; the latter can also be used as a mouthwash and for toothache.

One of the most commonly used is *Rosa canina*, the wild dog rose, so named because its root was said to cure rabies contracted from mad dogs. Its egg-shaped hips or 'false fruit', left after the flower has died, are an extremely rich source of vitamin C, containing 10 times the amount contained in oranges. They also contain vitamins A, B, B2, E, K and P, as well as iron and copper compounds, and make a very valuable tonic and general vitamin supplement useful in convalescence and for those in a generally debilitated state. There is archaeological evidence that rosehips have been used in Britain for nearly 4000 years, but it was only during World War II that they became recognised as an important medicinal source of vitamin C. Rosehips also have astringent qualities and are useful for treating bleeding gums, diarrhoea and leucorrhoea. The seeds are diuretic and can be used for fluid retention and kidney complaints. The leaves are a mild laxative and can also be used in poultices to help external wounds to heal.

Rosa californica is a wild rose used by the American Indians to treat colds. Its seeds are helpful for alleviating muscular pains. *Rosa damascena*, damask or Moroccan

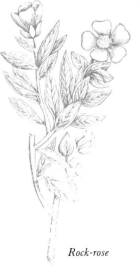

Rock-rose

rose, is mainly valued for its perfume, attar of rose, which is said to be rejuvenating and to regulate the menstrual cycle. Inhaling this perfume is said to cause drowsiness. This is the variety used to make oil of rose, which herbalists use in eye lotions. *Rosa centifolia*, cabbage rose, is found in eastern Caucasia and is the commercial source of rosewater, which can be made into a good ointment for roughened skin. It is also said to be useful for haemorrhage. *Rosa eglanteria*, sweetbriar, is a widely cultivated rose; it is used to relieve colic and diarrhoea.

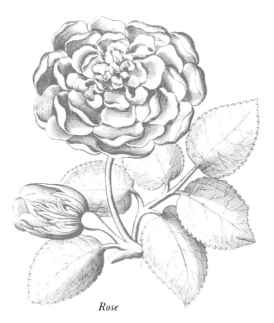

Rose

ROSEMARY (*Rosmarinus officinalis*)

A well-known aromatic herb native to the Mediterranean coast. It is regarded as a symbol of remembrance, fidelity and friendship, and was believed to strengthen the memory. In fact Greek students often wore garlands of it in their hair when taking exams. It is traditionally supposed to grow only in the garden of the righteous. Rosemary is best known for its culinary uses, but it also has considerable medicinal value and is used to treat a wide variety of ailments. Taken in infusion it is a good general tonic which stimulates the heart and blood circu-

lation, and is good for nervous depression, coughs and colds. It stimulates the digestive system, increasing the production of bile from the liver and reducing flatulence and indigestion pains. Some people use it instead of aspirin to relieve headaches, and it is sometimes said to strengthen the eyesight. Externally rosemary is used to treat rheumatism, neuralgia, sores, eczema, bruises and wounds. It is often used in shampoos and hair rinses to prevent dandruff, leave hair shiny, and prevent baldness by encouraging new hair growth. Rosemary leaves can be added to the bathwater and used as a skin freshener. If placed under the pillow they are said to keep away bad dreams. Rosemary is poisonous if taken in large doses and the essential oil should not be taken internally. The leaves are sometimes smoked in herbal cigarettes with coltsfoot to relieve asthma and bronchitis.

ROUGH TREE FERN (*Cyathea australis*)

A common tree fern in south-eastern Australia. The young fronds were roasted and eaten as a tonic by the Aborigines to aid recovery from an illness.

ROWAN, European mountain ash (*Sorbus aucuparia*)

A deciduous tree with white flowers which develop into clusters of berry-like false fruits; these are often made into an astringent jam said to be useful for diarrhoea. The fresh juice is slightly laxative, soothes inflamed mucous membranes, and makes a good gargle for a sore throat. It can also be used externally as a face mask to get rid of wrinkles.

RUBEFACIENT

A local irritant which stimulates and reddens the skin. Examples include nettle, hellebore, horseradish and thyme.

RUE, herb of grace (*Ruta graveolens*)

A shrubby plant, originally from southern Europe, used by the ancient Greeks and Romans as a bitter aromatic to season food, or to relieve indigestion and eye strain. It was once the custom for judges to carry a spray of herbs including rue into the courtroom to protect themselves from infection by the prisoners. The dried herb is taken in infusion as a tonic to prevent flatulence, to bring on menstruation, to relieve rheumatism, and for headache, dizziness and palpitations, especially in women going through menopause. Externally it can be used in an ointment for rheumatism and sciatica. In China it is used against malaria.

S

SACRED BASIL (*Ocimum sanctum*)

An aromatic plant with clusters of small purple flowers regarded as sacred by Hindus and often planted near temples in India. It is found in tropical areas from Asia to northern Australia. It was used by Aborigines as a blood tonic and the crushed leaves in water were used to reduce fevers. In India the leaves are used to treat catarrh and bronchitis, and the roots are made into a decoction for fever. The plant is sometimes used as an insect repellent.

SAFFLOWER, wild saffron (*Carthamus tinctorius*)

An annual plant with bright orange-yellow flowers, native to Mediterranean countries. The flowers are laxative and induce sweating. They can be used in infusion for colds, children's complaints such as measles, for eruptive skin diseases and to stimulate menstrual flow. The seeds are crushed to make safflower oil, which is used in cooking.

SAFFRON (*Crocus sativus*)

An extremely expensive spice made from the orange-red stigmas of the crocus flower, which came originally from Asia Minor (a region which today corresponds largely with Turkey). It is now mainly used for flavouring and colouring food, but it can also be taken to prevent flatulence, to increase perspiration, to stimulate menstruation, and to ease painful periods. It can be used in herb liquors to stimulate the appetite.

SAGE, garden sage (*Salvia officinalis*)

A well-known culinary herb originally from southern Europe. It has been used since ancient times for medicinal purposes and was so highly regarded that an Arab proverb asks, 'Why should a man die who grows sage in his garden?' Sage is an astringent and antispasmodic which slows down the secretion of fluids. It is especially useful for sinusitis, colds, excessive perspiration, diarrhoea and clear vaginal discharge, and to dry up the flow of milk in nursing mothers. Because it is so powerful it should not be used for more than a week at a time, and never by pregnant women. Sage can be made into a gargle which is very effective for sore throats, laryngitis and mouth sores, and helps to keep the teeth white. It will also help digestion, particularly of fatty foods, and can be combined with peppermint and rosemary to treat headaches. It is helpful for conditions like anxiety, depression and general fatigue, and is sometimes used to treat loss of memory associated with old age. Externally sage can be used in infusion to improve the condition of the skin and hair, and as a douche for vaginal discharge. The leaves will protect stored clothes from insects and can be rubbed onto insect bites to soothe the irritation.

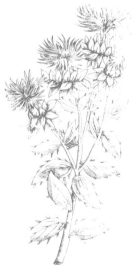

Safflower

ST JOHN'S WORT *(Hypericum perforatum)*

A wild plant, native to Europe and Western Asia, with yellow flowers which produce red oil when crushed. It has long been associated with magic; if hung on doors and windows, especially on St John's Day 24 June, it was believed to keep evil spirits away for a year. The flowers, steeped in olive oil for a fortnight, make the famous red oil used by the Crusaders in the Middle Ages to heal their battle wounds. It is still a highly prized healing oil which can be rubbed onto strained muscles, bruises, arthritic or rheumatic joints, ulcers, skin rashes, burns and haemorrhoids, as well as all kinds of cuts and wounds. Modern research has confirmed the antibacterial qualities of the oil. It can also be used to prevent brown age spots and soften the skin. Taken internally the oil can be used for colic, worms and lung congestion, but it should be used with caution as St John's Wort has been known to poison cattle and to make their skin very sensitive to light.

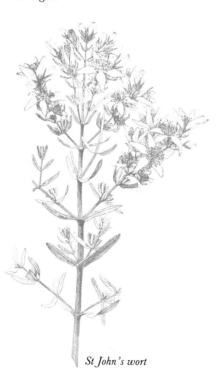

St John's wort

SALVE

A healing or soothing ointment.

SANDALWOOD, white sandalwood *(Santalum album)*

A small Indian tree, the wood of which contains an oil that is antiseptic and can be used for bronchitis and inflammations of the mucous membranes. It is widely used in soaps, perfumes and bath herbs because it is good for the skin. A decoction of the wood can be used for fever and indigestion.

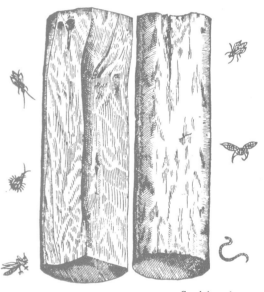

Sandalwood

SANICLE *(Sanicula europaea)* American sanicle *(Sanicula marilandica)*

A European woodland plant with umbels of pinkish flowers and seeds contained in sticky burrs. The whole herb is taken in infusion for diarrhoea, leucorrhoea, internal bleeding and mucous congestion in the chest. It is a good gargle for mouth sores and throat infections, and can also be used for wounds and skin eruptions.

American sanicle is also an astringent and can be used for similar purposes. Its powdered root is sometimes used for intermittent fevers.

SARSAPARILLA (*Smilax* species)

There are several species of this tropical climbing plant with red or black berries which has been used in European medicine since it was introduced from Mexico in the sixteenth century. The rootstock is prepared in infusion and used as a blood purifier and tonic especially helpful for rheumatism and chronic skin diseases like psoriasis. It is also used for colds, fevers, catarrh and flatulence, and has been used successfully against syphilis. An American species contains sarsapogenin which is used to make progesterone.

SASSAFRAS, ague tree, cinnamon wood (*Sassafras albidum*)

A North American deciduous tree; its bark is made into a hot tea recommended as a 'blood purifier' which will promote perspiration and urination, and is prescribed for rheumatism, arthritis and skin problems, and to ward off colds. It can also be used externally as an eyewash, for skin diseases and for poison ivy irritations. The bark of the roots has been used to relieve pain and bring down fever. Sassafras bark can be chewed or made into a tea to help break the smoking habit.

SAVIN (*Juniperus sabina*)

An evergreen shrub from the mountains of central Europe. It is poisonous and can easily cause abortions in pregnant women, but it is sometimes used to bring on menstruation, to expel worms and to treat warts and ulcers.

SAVORY, summer savory (*Satureia hortensis*) winter savory (*Satureia montana*)

A hardy Mediterranean plant widely cultivated as a kitchen herb. Its peppery taste makes it a useful seasoning and it has a strong volatile oil which aids digestion. Savory tea is often taken to relieve flatulence, indigestion, nausea, lack of appetite and most gastric complaints. It is also used as an expectorant and a gargle for sore throats, and is thought by some to be an aphrodisiac. Winter savory has similar properties.

SAW PALMETTO (*Serenoa serrulata*)

A shrubby plant from the eastern coast of North America. The purplish-black berries have expectorant properties and are used in infusion or tincture for colds, asthma, bronchitis and catarrh. The tea can be taken as a general tonic for convalescents, and is also thought by some to be an aphrodisiac.

SAXIFRAGE, great burnet, pimpernel (*Pimpinella major*) small burnet, burnet saxifrage (*Pimpinella saxifraga*)

A white-flowered European plant found in damp woodlands. Its root can be taken in decoction as a powerful diuretic, and also for colds, bronchitis, catarrh, heart palpitations and children's diseases such as measles. It makes a good gargle for mouth and throat infections.

Small burnet is a smaller plant with purple flowers. Its fresh peppery root can be used to ease toothache, stop diarrhoea, and dry up mucus, and acts as a diuretic. It also makes a good gargle and can be used to cleanse wounds and help them heal. It is more commonly used by modern herbalists.

SCABIOUS, lesser field scabious (*Scabiosa columbaria*)

A blue-flowered plant found in European meadows and cornfields; it is sometimes used to make a homeopathic remedy for chronic skin diseases such as eczema.

SCOTCH BROOM (*Cytisus scoparius*)

A leguminous shrub which grows wild in Europe and North America. The seeds and twigs can be used as a diuretic and also as a cardiac stimulant, but are poisonous in large doses. The flowering tops are sometimes smoked in cigarettes and can be hallucinogenic.

SEA HOLLY — *see Eryngo*

SEDATIVE

A soothing agent that calms nervous excitement, distress or irritation. Examples include opium, hops, peach, peony and saffron.

SELF-HEAL, woundwort, all-heal (*Prunella vulgaris*)

A small common weed, from the northern hemisphere, with hairy stems and purplish flowers. It is an excellent astringent useful for diarrhoea, internal bleeding, piles and leucorrhoea, and may be used as a gargle for sore throats. As its name suggests, it is a good remedy for external wounds. It can also be used for fits and convulsions.

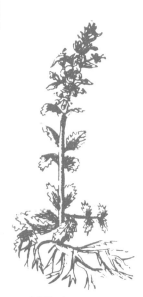

Self-heal

SENNA, TINNEVELLY (*Cassia angustifolia*)
American senna (*Cassia marilandica*)

The leaves and pods of Tinnevelly senna are used in pharmaceutically prepared laxatives. The dried leaves can be made into a paste with vinegar and used on pimples.

American senna is also used as a laxative, mostly in combination with other herbs. It is also used to get rid of intestinal worms and for rheumatism and biliousness.

SEVEN BARKS, wild hydrangea (*Hydrangea arborescens*)

A North American shrub with clusters of creamy-white flowers. The root can be used as a mild diuretic and is thought to be helpful in preventing bladder and kidney stones.

SHEPHERD'S PURSE (*Capsella bursa-pastoris*)

A common garden weed in temperate parts of the world. It has small white flowers and heart- or purse-shaped fruit pods. It is one of the best herbs for stopping bleeding, either internal or external, and can be used either fresh or dried. The large quantities of vitamin C it contains are thought to help blood clotting. It regulates blood pressure and disturbances of the circulation, and is helpful for varicose veins and hypertension. Shepherd's purse is especially useful for controlling excessive menstruation and reducing menstrual pain, and can also be used for diarrhoea and as a diuretic. For external wounds it can be made into an ointment, but the fresh juice on a piece of cotton wool is usually enough to stop nosebleeds. It can also be helpful for rheumatism.

SHINLEAF, wild lily-of-the-valley (*Pyrola elliptica*)

A North American plant with white flowers smelling like lily-of-the-valley. It is a mild astringent and can be used as a mouthwash, gargle or douche. The leaves make a good poultice for insect bites, bruises and other skin disorders.

SIALAGOGUE

An agent that stimulates the flow of saliva.

SIDA RETUSA, Paddy's lucerne
(Sida rhombifolia)

A widespread plant usually regarded as a weed. It is a well-known remedy for diarrhoea, said to be extremely effective if only the young tips are chewed, though it can also be taken in decoction. In some countries it is used to treat respiratory complaints such as asthma and even tuberculosis. The plant is widely used in Malaysia, where the leaves or roots are pulped and used as a poultice for sores and ulcers, and to relieve headache, toothache and fevers. It is also believed to have magical powers and to give protection to elephant hunters.

SILVERWEED, goose grass
(Potentilla anserina)

A European roadside plant with serrated leaves and yellow flowers like large buttercups. It is a useful astringent and can be taken for diarrhoea and skin disorders, as a lotion for haemorrhoids, and as a mouthwash. It is also antispasmodic and useful for stomach cramps, and has been used for fever and sciatica. Homeopathic practitioners prescribe silverweed for painful periods and stomach inflammation. *See also Cinquefoil.*

SKULLCAP, blue pimpernel,
helmet flower *(Scutellaria laterifolia)*

A perennial plant from North America used by the American Indians and then introduced to European herbalists. It is a sedative and an antispasmodic, and is regarded as a specific for epilepsy, spasms, twitching, and general excitability, and even hiccoughs. It has also been used for rheumatism and delirium tremens. The American Indians used it to bring on menstruation and to cure rabies.

SKUNK CABBAGE, collard,
meadow cabbage *(Symplocarpus foetidus)*

An unpleasant-smelling plant which looks like a cabbage and grows in swamps of North America. The root is an expectorant and antispasmodic, and can be used in a sweetened infusion for respiratory complaints, particularly coughs and asthma.

SLIPPERY ELM *(Ulmus fulva)*

The inner bark of this large North American tree can be used in infusion as a diuretic, for inflamed mucous membranes, and as a nutritive food for convalescents. Ground into a powder it makes a good poultice for ulcers, wounds and skin diseases.

SLOE, blackthorn, wild plum *(Prunus spinosa)*

A type of small plum, the flowers of which are a mild laxative and diuretic, and may be taken in infusion for urinary diseases such as cystitis and for rheumatism. The dried unripe fruits can be boiled in water and taken for diarrhoea.

SMALLAGE, smilage, wild celery
(Apium graveolens)

A similar plant to the well-known vegetable garden celery, except that it has an unpleasant odour. The seeds and stems are used as a tonic and to flavour other medicines. The juice can be used for rheumatism, arthritis, skin problems, flatulence, catarrh, lack of appetite, and to bring on menstruation. A decoction of the seeds can be used for bronchitis and, often combined with skullcap, as a sedative. The yellowish oil from the root is said to restore sexual potency after an illness.

SOAP BARK *(Quillaja saponaria)*

The bark of the soap tree, native to Chile and Peru, which forms a lather in water and is used for cleansing skin eruptions, as a hair tonic, to reduce fever, as an expectorant for bronchitis, and as a local anaesthetic.

SOAPWORT, soaproot, bruisewort *(Saponaria officinalis)*

A common pink-flowered weed which lathers in water like soap, and was used in Europe to wash tapestries and curtains. A decoction of the root can be used to wash itching skin conditions such as dermatitis. It is taken internally as an expectorant for respiratory congestion, but should be used cautiously as it is also a purgative and can cause side effects such as a dry mouth, tremors and tongue paralysis.

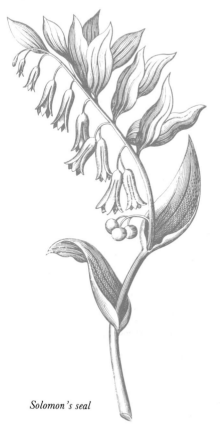

Solomon's seal

SOLIDAGO — *see Goldenrod*

SOLOMON'S SEAL, dropberry, sealroot *(Polygonatum multiflorum)* scented Solomon's seal *(Polygonatum odoratum)*

A white-flowered plant which looks like lily-of-the-valley. The astringent powdered root is used in a poultice for bruises, inflammations and wounds, and in a wash for other skin problems, painful piles and as an antidote to poison ivy. It can be taken internally for gastric inflammations, diarrhoea and neuralgia, American Indians used it as a tea for women's complaints.

Scented Solomon's seal has similar properties and also lowers the blood sugar level. It is used in the Orient for diabetes.

SORREL, COMMON, garden or wild sorrel *(Rumex acetosa)*

A type of dock often found wild along European roadsides and used as a seasoning or a salad herb rich in vitamin C. Since the time of the ancient Greeks the leaves have been used as a diuretic. They can also be used for feverish illnesses and to soothe mouth and throat ulcers. Externally they can be used as a wash for skin diseases. A decoction of the root (used externally) is recommended for boils, eczema and acne, and also for internal bleeding and excessive menstruation. The plant contains oxalic acid and is not recommended for people suffering from rheumatism; it should not be taken in large quantities as it can irritate the kidneys. Other types of sorrel have similar properties.

SOUTHERNWOOD, old man, old man's tree, lad's love *(Artemisia abrotanum)*

A woody-stemmed garden herb originally from southern Europe. It can be used as a tonic, astringent and stimulant, and is often used to bring on menstruation; it is sometimes used for intestinal worms. Combined with rosemary it is a good hair tonic to encourage hair growth. In Italy it is used to flavour cakes. The dried leaves can be used as a moth and insect repellent.

SOWBREAD, swinebread, cyclamen *(Cyclamen hederifolium)*

An attractive alpine flower often grown as a pot plant. It is not used by herbalists because it is a drastic purgative, but the fresh corm is made into a homeopathic tincture and used for rheumatism, migraine and diseases of the uterus.

SPEARMINT, common mint, garden mint *(Mentha spicata)*

A popular herb known since ancient times and used for both medicinal and culinary purposes. Mint tea is a traditional Arab social drink which is also thought to increase virility. The Romans introduced spearmint to Britain as an appetite stimulant and flavouring, and it is still one of the most widely grown kitchen herbs. The medicinal properties of spearmint are similar to those of peppermint, but less powerful. Because of its more pleasant taste it is often prescribed for children and babies. It aids digestion and is particularly helpful for relieving nausea, vomiting, colic, wind and hiccoughs. Unlike peppermint, spearmint is a diuretic and can be used to treat urinary disorders, particularly painful urination. Fresh leaves can be applied externally to relieve headaches and rheumatic pains, and an infusion makes a good skin lotion to improve the complexion and soothe roughened skin.

SPECIFIC

Any herb which has an effect on a specific organ or disease. For example, quinine is a specific for malaria.

SPEEDWELL, fluellen, Paul's betony *(Veronica officinalis)*

A common weed in Europe and North America with flowers rather like those of the snapdragon. The dried plant is used as an expectorant tea for bronchitis and catarrh, and as a tonic for stomach ailments and headaches. The fresh juice can be used externally for chronic skin problems.

SPIKENARD *(Aralia racemosa)*

An Indian plant also common in North America, Japan and New Zealand. Its dried root is used in infusion for rheumatism, asthma and coughs, and externally for skin diseases. It is sometimes taken before childbirth to ease labour. American Indians used it internally for backache and externally for chest pains, wounds, bruises and inflammations.

SPRUCE— *see Fir tree*

SQUILL, sea onion *(Urginea maritima)*

An onion-like bulb native to sandy soils near the Mediterranean. The fleshy inner scales of the bulb are a good soothing remedy for coughs and catarrh, and are included in many prepared mixtures. However, they are very dangerous and not recommended for home use. Squill also contains glycosides which stimulate the heart in much the same way as digitalis, and were used by the ancient Egyptians in 1500 BC for heart disease.

STAR ANISE *(Illicium verum)*

A small tree with a star-shaped fruit and seeds which are used in the same way as anise seed, to promote digestion and relieve flatulence and nausea, and as a stimulant and diuretic. In China, where the tree grows wild, the seeds are recommended for constipation, lumbago, hernia and bladder troubles.

STAR GRASS, ague grass, colic root *(Aletris farinosa)*

A North American grass, the dried root of which is used for flatulence and indigestion. It has also been used for menstrual problems.

STAVESACRE, housewort *(Delphinium staphisagria)*

A plant which is similar to the larkspur. The poisonous seeds are used to make lotions to kill head lice. Homeopathic practitioners sometimes prescribe pills made from the plant to cure impotency.

STERNUTATORY

A substance which causes sneezing — *see Errhine.*

STICKLEWORT — *see Agrimony*

STILLINGIA, queen's root *(Stillingia sylvatica)*

A perennial plant which grows in sandy soils in the southern states of the USA. Its dried root can be used in small doses for chronic skin and liver problems, and it was once used to help clear up syphilis. The oil from the root can be combined with sarsaparilla and used to treat bronchitis and sore throats.

STIMULANT

A substance which temporarily increases the activity of some organ or physiological process. Examples include tea, coffee, kola nuts, fennel and lavender.

STINGING NETTLE — *see Nettle*

STOMACHIC

Any herb which has a stimulating effect on the stomach. Examples include Iceland moss, chamomile, spearmint, sage and cumin.

STONE ROOT, horseweed *(Collinsonia canadensis)*

A North American woodland plant often combined with other plants as a diuretic. The fresh leaves can be used in a poultice to heal wounds and bruises.

STORAX TREE *(Styrax officinalis)*

Storax is a resinous balsam obtained by slitting the bark of these trees. It is a stimulating expectorant and one of the ingredients in friar's balsam, which is useful for treating asthma, bronchitis and catarrh. Storax is also used in ointments to treat ringworm and scabies.

STORKSBILL, pin clover, alfilaria *(Erodium cicutarium)*

An annual plant originally from the Mediterranean, now grown in parts of North America for hay. It can be used to control excessive menstrual bleeding, particularly when the uterus is inflamed. In small doses it is said to raise blood pressure, while in larger doses it will lower it.

STRAWBERRY *(Fragaria vesca)*

A plant best known for its fruit, which is rich in vitamin C and iron. The astringent leaves can also be used in infusion for diarrhoea, as a diuretic for urinary diseases, and in a tea which is said to heal spongy gums and loose teeth. It is also a good gargle for sore throats and a useful douche. When added to bathwater it is said to soothe aching hips and thighs. Strawberry juice is sometimes used in cosmetics and soaps to improve the complexion.

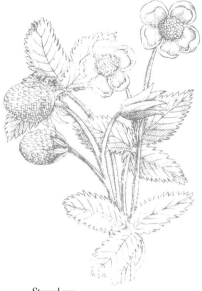

Strawberry

STROPHANTHUS KOMBE *(Strophanthus)*

A highly poisonous East African herb once used to make poisonous arrow heads. It can be used medicinally as a heart stimulant rather like digitalis.

STYPTIC

Any herb which contracts body tissue, particularly one that slows bleeding by contracting the blood vessels. Examples are woundwort, spotted cranebill and shepherd's purse. *See also Astringent.*

SUCCORY, chicory *(Chicorium intybus)*

A blue-flowered plant belonging to the dandelion family. Its dried root can be ground and added to coffee, and the fresh green leaves used in salads. The juice ·from the fresh root is a tonic, diuretic and laxative, and is often recommended for jaundice and for rheumatism. It stimulates the flow of bile and helps digestion.

The boiled leaves and flowers can be made into a poultice for painful inflammations.

SUDORIFIC

An agent which increases perspiration — *see Diaphoretic*.

SUMACH, sumac, smooth sumac *(Rhus glabra)* sweet sumach *(Rhus aromatica)*

A North American tree with leaves that turn red in autumn. The astringent and antiseptic bark can be used for chronic diarrhoea, for leucorrhoea, and as a gargle for sore throats. A tea made from the leaves and berries is a diuretic helpful for bladder inflammation, and a tea made from the berries alone is used for fever, sores and inflamed mucous membranes.

Sweet sumach is an ornamental shrub with astringent root bark which is sometimes used for diabetes and also for incontinence in the aged or bedwetting in children.

SUMBUL — *see Musk root*

SUNDEW, common, round-leafed sundew, dewplan *(Drosera rotundifolia)*

An unusual plant with reddish hairy leaves which exude a liquid capable of trapping insects. It contains a natural antibiotic regarded as a specific for whooping cough and also an effective remedy for other respiratory ailments such as coughs, asthma, bronchitis and laryngitis, and which also helps counteract nausea. It can be used as a herbal tincture or in homeopathic pills.

SUNFLOWER *(Helianthus annuus)*

A tall yellow flower originally from North and Central America and brought to Europe by the Spanish. It is widely used for its oil, which contains poly-

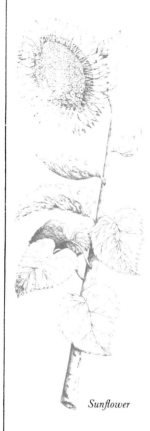

Sunflower

unsaturated fats and so is particularly recommended for people with high cholesterol levels. The seeds are very rich in vitamin B and are believed in parts of Russia to preserve male potency if eaten daily; they also have diuretic and expectorant properties. About 16 drops of oil can be taken 3 times a day to treat coughs and bronchitis. American Indians used the oil and roots in a poultice for rheumatism, arthritis and bruises.

SWALLOW-WORT *(Asclepias syriaca)*

A common North American roadside weed, the powdered root of which is an analgesic used in infusion to reduce pain and give relief from coughing in asthma and bronchitis. The juice can be used on warts. *See also Pleurisy root.*

SWEET FERN, meadow fern *(Comptonia peregrina)*

A North American deciduous shrub used as a tonic and astringent, particularly for diarrhoea and skin problems.

SWEET-FLAG — *see Calamus*

SWEET GUM, liquidambar *(Liquidambar styraciflua)*

A tall deciduous tree originally from North America. The resinous gum from the branches can be made into an antiseptic ointment for wounds and skin problems, or taken in decoction as an expectorant for coughs and mucous congestion. The bark has been used to relieve diarrhoea.

SYNERGIST

A substance which increases the effectiveness of another substance when the 2 are combined.

T

TAMARIND *(Tamarindus indica)*

A tropical tree with yellow-veined flowers and soft brownish fruit enclosed in a light-brown oblong pod. The mildly laxative pulp of the fruit is used as a food and made into a refreshing drink particularly useful for those suffering from feverish illnesses, and is also used to mask the taste of unpleasant pharmaceutical preparations. The leaves can be used externally in a poultice for sores or skin infections.

TANSY *(Tanacetum vulgare)*

An attractive plant with feathery leaves and clusters of bright yellow flowers. The ancient Greeks considered it a symbol of immortality and its pungent scent of lemon and camphor made it popular as one of the 'stewing herbs' in Tudor England. The leaves and flowers can be made into a tea to induce menstruation and to expel worms in children, but it is poisonous in large quantities. It can be used externally for pimples, sunburn, freckles, bruises and rheumatism, and for toothache and sore eyes. If the leaves are rubbed over fresh meat it is said to keep longer without refrigeration.

TARRAGON, estragon *(Artemisia dracunculus)*

An important culinary herb, particularly in France. It stimulates the appetite and digestion, and can be taken in a weak tea to relieve flatulence, cure insomnia and sweeten the breath. It is also a diuretic and can help to bring on menstruation.

TEA

An infusion prepared by pouring boiling water over a herb and letting it stand in a covered container. It is then strained and used medicinally or as a refreshing drink.

TEA *(Camellia thea)*

A Chinese evergreen shrub about 2.4 m (8 ft) high, also grown in Japan, Sri Lanka and India. The leaves are dried and roasted, then packaged and used as the familiar household drink. Green tea is dried for less time than black tea. Because it is so widely used the medicinal value of tea is not always recognised. It contains tannin, which is an astringent and helps to control loose bowels, and caffeine, a stimulant which is well known for its reviving and invigorating effect. In large doses tea can cause sleeplessness and digestive disturbances.

TEASEL *(Dipsacus fullonum)*

A rigid, prickly roadside plant, the dried flower heads of which are often used in flower arrangements. Homeopathic practitioners make a tincture from the fresh plant for skin diseases and inflammations.

TEA-TREE *(Melaleuca alternifolia)*

A small Australian tree with papery bark and creamy, bottlebrush-like flowers. The oil distilled from its leaves contains a variety of organic compounds, among them viridiflorene, terpenes, cymones, pinenes, terpineols, cineol, sesquiterpines and sesquiterpene alcohols. Strongly antiseptic, the oil is ideal for treating septic wounds, carbuncles and pus-filled infections, and can also be used for throat and mouth disorders (especially pyorrhoea and gingivitis). It is also effective against a broad range of skin fungi and can be used as a household antiseptic for cuts and insect bites. It should be diluted in water (1:40). Tea-tree oil is also a very effective inhalant to clear the head and to relieve bronchial congestion. It will also kill fleas on the family dog if added to its bathwater.

THEOBROMA, chocolate tree *(Theobroma cacao)*

A Central American tree, the seeds of which are made into chocolate and cocoa butter. Cocoa butter is used in cosmetics, especially lip salves, to protect and soothe dry skin. Theobromine can be used against angina and as a mild nervine.

THORN APPLE — *see Jimson weed*

THUJA, white cedar, arborvitae, tree of life *(Thuja occidentalis)*

A type of pine tree often grown in parks; its leaves and tips are used as a counterirritant for muscular aches and rheumatism, and to kill warts. It is poisonous taken internally, but it is sometimes used in small doses for rheumatism and to bring on menstruation.

THYME *(Thymus* species*)*

There are many different species of thyme, all descended from wild thyme, *Thymus serpyllum*, which has similar properties to the common garden thyme, *Thymus vulgaris*, but is not as effective. For thousands of years thyme has been used as a flavouring which aids the digestion of fatty foods, but it has also had other uses. The ancient Egyptians used it in embalming, the Greeks burnt it as incense on their altars, and the Romans used it as a skin freshener. Thyme is a powerful antiseptic, rich in thymol. In the past this quality meant it was sometimes carried by the nobility to protect them from the diseases and odours of the people. Today it is widely used in commercially manufactured soaps, toothpastes and mouthwashes. A herbal tincture will destroy head lice and cure fungal skin infections such as athlete's foot. A strong infusion of thyme added to the bathwater is good for skin diseases, rheumatism and bronchitis. Thyme can also be taken internally for sore throats, coughs and respiratory complaints, and for diarrhoea and gastric disturbances. It will stimulate the appetite and relieve flatulence and colic, but should not be taken in very large doses as it may cause poisoning and overstimulation of the thyroid gland. Some people believe that an infusion of thyme poured over the head daily will prevent baldness.

TI *(Cordyline terminalis)*

A common Hawaiian plant used to wrap food for cooking and to make skirts. A leaf soaked in water and tied around the head is believed to cure headaches.

TINCTURE

A concentrated solution of a medicinal herb in alcohol. It is a suitable way of taking any herb which will not yield its special properties to water alone, or which has qualities that are destroyed by heat. Because the alcohol acts as a preservative, the mixture can be kept for a long time — usually several years — and is usually taken in very small quantities. A good method of preparing a tincture is to place 100 g of the herb in a sealed bottle with 500 ml of any spirit such as gin, brandy or rum. Set the bottle aside for 2 weeks, shaking it each day, then filter the contents through a fine cloth and bottle the liquid in a dark glass container. A tincture may also be made in vinegar.

TISANE

An infusion of herbs.

TOBACCO *(Nicotiana tabacum)*

The dried leaves of a widely cultivated plant originally from South America. Tobacco is not used in modern herbal practice because it is an addictive drug which has been associated with many diseases, particularly cancer and heart disease. However, it was used medicinally by the American Indians as a sedative and as an ointment for ulcers and tumours.

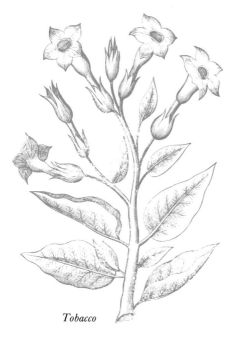

Tobacco

TOLU BALSAM *(Myroxylon balsamum)*

A Central American evergreen tree which yields a pleasant-tasting brown resin used in cough syrups as an expectorant and stimulant.

TONIC

A substance which stimulates and restores the whole organism and is particularly useful during convalescence. Examples include blackberry, dandelion, celery, sarsaparilla, ginseng, nettle and alfalfa.

TOOTHACHE TREE (*Euodia vitiflora*)

A rainforest tree, the leaves of which were crushed and placed directly onto a decaying tooth to ease the pain. This remedy was popular among some Queensland Aborigines.

TOOTHED RAGWEED (*Pterocaulon serulatum*)

An aromatic plant of the daisy family, the leaves of which have been used by Aborigines in different ways to treat head colds. They can be chewed, made into a decoction, or simply crushed and inhaled. They were also sometimes used to treat spear wounds.

TORMENTIL, shepherd's knot (*Potentilla erecta/Potentilla tormentilla*)

A yellow-flowered European plant, the root of which contains tannin and is an excellent astringent useful for diarrhoea, leucorrhea and haemorrhages, as a skin lotion, and as a gargle for sore throats. The root can be chewed to harden gums and keep them healthy.

TRAGACANTH (*Astragalus gummifer*)

A small thorny shrub from Turkey, Iran, Afghanistan and Russia, which forms a mucilage used pharmaceutically in lozenges and face creams, and also used to suspend heavy insoluble powders.

TREFOIL, clover (*Trifolium repens*)

A common grassland plant with white flowers which can be made into a sedative tea for bronchitis and coughs. The plant can also be made into a poultice for skin tumours. Modern herbalists usually use red clover — *see Red clover*.

TURKEY CORN (*Corydalis formosa*)

A North American plant with purplish-red flowers, the root of which can be made into a bitter tonic infusion used for digestive disturbances, as a diuretic and for skin diseases. It is poisonous in large doses.

TURMERIC (*Curcuma longa*)

A tropical plant, the dried rhizome of which is ground into a vivid yellow spice used as a flavouring, particularly in curries. It is used medicinally in India and some Asian countries as a remedy for flatulence and liver complaints and, when boiled with milk and sugar, to treat a head cold. In China it is used to stop haemorrhages.

TURNIP (*Brassica rapa*)

A cultivated plant with a globular, soft-fleshed tuber which is eaten as a vegetable. It can also be made into an ointment for chilblains.

TURTLEBLOOM, balmony (*Chelone glabra*)

A herbaceous white-flowered plant, the leaves of which are used in infusion for indigestion, to stimulate the appetite, and as a general tonic for convalescence. It can also be used externally for sores, eczema and piles.

TWIN LEAF (*Jeffersonia diphylla*)

A North American plant with a root which contains antispasmodic and expectorant qualities, and is used for chronic rheumatism and cramps, as a tonic, and as a gargle for sore throats. It can also be used as a poultice.

U

UVA-URSI — *see Bearberry*

V

VALERIAN, all-heal, wild or fragrant valerian *(Valeriana officinalis)*

A well-known herbal sedative made from the root of a pink-flowered plant native to Europe and western Asia. It has a characteristic strong smell which most people find unpleasant, though cats and other animals are attracted to it. The medicinal qualities of valerian are destroyed by heat, so the root is dried, then prepared in a cold infusion which is often sweetened with honey. It is used for all sorts of nervous conditions: hysteria, migraine, palpitations, high blood pressure and insomnia. Its antispasmodic qualities make it helpful for stomach cramps, menstrual pain, convulsions, epilepsy, rheumatism and neuralgia. Valerian should not be used in large doses or for a long period of time. Externally it can be applied as a lotion for sores, rashes and swollen joints.

VERBASCUM — *see Mullein*

VERBENA — *see Vervain*

VERMIFUGE

A substance which causes the expulsion of intestinal worms. Examples include nas-turtium, cyclamen, pawpaw and woundwort. A vermicide is an agent which destroys intestinal worms. Both are also known as anthelmintics.

VERVAIN, verbena, European vervain *(Verbena officinalis)*

A native European herb considered sacred by the ancient Greeks and Romans, and regarded as almost a panacea. During the Middle Ages it was thought to give protection against the plague, and was also used in love potions. It is now used as a sedative tea for anxiety, depression and other nervous conditions. It is also a general digestive tonic, especially helpful for liver and gall bladder problems, and is used to induce sweating in colds and flu, and to soothe asthmatic coughs. Vervain tea is sometimes used for menstrual difficulties and to increase the milk flow of nursing mothers. Externally it can be used on wounds and ulcers, as a mouthwash for sore throats and bad breath, and to bathe inflamed eyes. It can be applied hot to ease neuralgia or painful sprains, and can be dabbed on the forehead to soothe headaches.

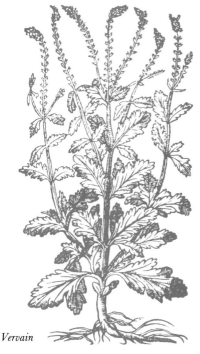

Vervain

VINE TREE — *see Grape*

VIOLET, sweet violet *(Viola odorata)*

A small wild plant, originally from Europe, now cultivated in many countries. Admired for its sweetly perfumed violet flowers, it has also been used medicinally since the time of the ancient Greeks. The leaves are antiseptic and can be crushed and applied directly to the skin or made into an infusion. If this is drunk daily and also used as a poultice, it has been claimed to cure some cancers. The flowers are expectorant and can be made into a good cough syrup. Their perfume is said to ease headaches and insomnia.

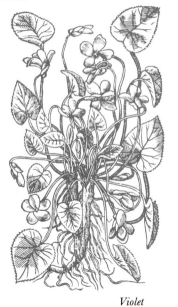

Violet

VIPER'S BUGLOSS *(Echium vulgare)*

A European coastal plant related to borage. The leaves can be made into an infusion which stimulates the kidneys, produces sweating in fevers, and reduces inflammations, headaches and general anxiety. The seeds are sometimes given in decoction to nursing mothers.

VIRGINIA SNAKEROOT *(Aristolochia serpentaria)*

A North American plant once considered an excellent remedy for snakebite. The chewed root was applied directly to the bite after it had been cut and the poison sucked out.

VIRGIN'S BOWER *(Clematis virginiana)*

A woody climbing plant, the leaves and flowers of which can be taken in infusion for severe headaches. Sometimes the same effect can be achieved by inhaling the scent from the bruised root or leaves.

VULNERARY

A substance which is used to help heal wounds. Examples include burdock, melilot, yarrow, aloe and woundwort.

W

WAFER ASH *(Ptelea trifoliata)*

A North American shrub, the root bark of which can be made into a general tonic particularly beneficial for stimulating the appetite.

WAHOO, arrow-wood, bitter ash, spindle tree *(Euonymus europaeus/ Euonymus atropurpureus)*

A small deciduous tree, the bark of which is used as an astringent, a tonic and a mild purgative. It was popular in the nineteenth century as an expectorant for chest congestion and a treatment for indigestion. In the early twentieth century it was discovered to have a similar effect to digitalis and became popular as a cardiac drug. The leaves can cause poisoning.

WALNUT, English walnut (*Juglans regia*)

A large tree grown mainly for its edible nuts. The dried leaves are astringent and can be used in infusion for acne, ulcers, chronic skin conditions like eczema, rheumatism and bleeding gums, and to dry up excessive milk flow. They can also be taken internally as a tonic and to stimulate the appetite. The nuts are a good source of manganese and the powdered bark can be taken in infusion as a laxative. Black walnut, *Juglans nigra*, which is common in the USA, also has astringent properties.

WATER AVENS (*Geum rivale*)

A hairy perennial plant found in moist places. Its rootstock can be taken in infusion to stimulate the appetite and improve digestion, and as a remedy for diarrhoea. An infusion from the whole plant can be used for respiratory congestion and nausea.

WATERCRESS, scurvy grass (*Nasturtium officinale*)

A European plant found wild in cold slow streams. It is exceptionally rich in vitamins C and E, and in the minerals iron, manganese and iodine. Used fresh it can help to prevent illnesses and is good to clear the skin, stimulate the digestive system, dissolve kidney stones and stimulate the glands, particularly the pituitary gland. It is a useful expectorant to help clear catarrh, and is also sometimes used for eczema. The juice should not be taken in large doses or too frequently as it can cause kidney and stomach inflammations.

WATER ERYNGO, button snakeroot, rattlesnake weed (*Eryngium aquaticum*)

A swamp plant from North America, the root of which can be chewed to aid digestion by increasing the flow of saliva. It is also an expectorant useful for chronic laryngitis, and a diuretic helpful for kidney stones and urinary inflammations.

WATERMELON (*Citrullus vulgaris*)

A well-known fruit which has been cultivated for about 4000 years. The fruit and seeds can be eaten as a diuretic for kidney and bladder disorders, and the seeds alone can be used to expel intestinal worms.

WAX MYRTLE, bayberry (*Myrica cerifera*)

An American shrub, the bark, leaves and fruit of which can be made into an astringent tea for sore throats, haemorrhages and diarrhoea, or used externally for wounds and bruises.

WHEAT (*Triticum* species)

A very well-known cereal originally grown in the Middle East, and now widely cultivated elsewhere. Wheatgerm is a popular health food which is particularly rich in vitamins and is often taken as a dietary supplement. Capsules of wheatgerm oil have a high content of vitamin E and are sometimes taken to improve circulation.

WHEATGRASS MANNA

The freshly prepared juice of wheatgrass (*Agropyron* species) is sometimes recommended as a method of treating cancer, leukemia and other ailments. It can be used in conjunction with other treatments.

WHITE PINE, soft pine *(Pinus strobus)*

A large North American evergreen tree; the bark and tips, steeped in boiling water, are a widely used remedy for coughs, chest congestion, tonsillitis, laryngitis and catarrh. The tea can also be used for rheumatism and kidney troubles. The heated resinous sap can be used externally to treat wounds, sores and insect bites, and to draw out embedded splinters. It can also be applied as a poultice for pneumonia, sciatica and sore muscles.

WHITE POND LILY, sweet-scented water lily *(Nymphaea odorata)*

A dark-green aquatic plant with white, many-petalled flowers which bloom above water. The astringent, antiseptic root can be used in infusion as a mouth gargle, an eyewash or a douche, and as a lotion to heal sores and soften the skin.

WILLOWHERB, rosebay *(Epilobium angustifolium)*

A tall pink-flowered European plant, the dried root of which is soothing and astringent, and is used in decoction for digestive upsets. The dried herb is sometimes used for whooping cough and asthma.

WILLOW TREE, white willow *(Salix alba)*

A well-known large deciduous tree, the bark of which has been used in decoction for thousands of years to relieve pain and reduce fever. It contains salicin, a substance which is closely related to the synthetic drug aspirin. Willow bark reduces inflammation and can be used to treat rheumatism. The bark and leaves make an astringent tonic useful for internal bleeding and also to prevent the recurrence of diseases such as malaria. It is also good for throat and mouth inflammations, as an external wash for sores and wounds, and even as a footbath for sweaty feet. An infusion of the leaves can be used as a digestive tonic and to soothe heartburn. Other types of willow such as *Salix nigra* and *Salix caprea* can be used in the same way.

WINTERGREEN, deerberry, teaberry, mountain tea *(Gaultheria procumbens)*

A North American evergreen shrub with leaves that exude an oil containing methyl salicylate, which was once used commercially to prepare aspirin. The sharply astringent leaves can be used in infusion to relieve headache, aches and pains, and to reduce fever. Externally they can be used as a mouthwash for sore throats and gums, as a compress for skin problems, and in a poultice to relieve rheumatism and aching joints. The oil is widely used as a flavouring.

WITCH GRASS, couch grass, dog grass *(Agropyron repens)*

A perennial grass, native to Europe but introduced elsewhere and often found as a weed. It can be used in infusion as a general tonic and is sometimes recommended for liver, gall bladder and urinary problems.

WITCH HAZEL *(Hamamelis virginiana)*

A deciduous shrub native to North America and used by the American Indians. It is now cultivated in gardens and grown for use in commercial preparations such as soaps and cosmetics, or as distilled witch hazel (hamamelis water). The leaves and bark are made into an astringent lotion which is also soothing and helps stop bleeding. It is used mostly externally for skin irritations, bruises, sprains, sunburn, insect bites, varicose veins, haemorrhoids, and tired feet, as a mouthwash for sore throats and gums, and as a douche for vaginitis. Well diluted, it is also sometimes taken intern-

Wintergreen

ally to help stop internal bleeding, and for diarrhoea.

WOLF'S BANE — *see Aconite*

WOODRUFF, sweet woodruff, master of the wood *(Asperula odorata)*

A European woodland herb with a distinctive smell rather like vanilla. In Germany it was traditionally used in infusion to make a type of punch said to be a refreshing drink as well as a digestive tonic. Woodruff tea can be used as a diuretic, to relieve stomach pains, and for restlessness and insomnia; it is also sometimes recommended for migraine. The fresh leaves are anticoagulant and can be used to help heal cuts and wounds; they also keep insects away from clothes.

WORMSEED, feather geranium, chenopodium, goosefoot *(Chenopodium ambrosioides)*

A yellow-flowered plant from Central America, the seeds of which can be used in infusion to treat worms in children. They should be used with caution as an overdose can be fatal.

WORMSEED, treacle *(Erysimum cheiranthoides)*

An annual plant with small yellow flowers and a hot taste similar to mustard. The seeds are laxative and can be used to kill intestinal worms. They are also sometimes used for rheumatism.

WORMWOOD, old woman, absinthe *(Artemisia absinthium)*

A bitter aromatic herb native to Europe. It has been used as a digestive tonic for centuries, and wormwood tea is still often recommended for indigestion, flatulence, dyspepsia and liver and gall bladder complaints. It is taken to promote menstruation and improve blood circulation, and

a tea from the flowers will expel worms. Externally wormwood can be used on sprains or bruises, and the oil relieves the pain of headaches, rheumatism and arthritis. Wormwood is now used to flavour vermouth. Two other varieties, Roman wormwood *(Artemisia pontica)* and sea wormwood *(Artemisia maritima)* have similar properties, but are not as strong.

WOUNDWORT — *see Self-heal*

Y

YARROW, milfoil, sneezewort, achillea *(Achillea millefolium)*

An aromatic feathery-leafed perennial native to Europe. Highly regarded as an all-healing plant, it was traditionally believed to give protection — both from disease and evil spirits — to homes and churches. It was said to be the herb which Achilles used to stop the bleeding of his soldiers' wounds. Yarrow was used by witches and was sometimes carried to weddings in the belief that it would bring 7 years of love. It has other much more orthodox uses: as a general tonic which will stimulate the appetite, improve digestion and liver function, and soothe intestinal disturbances. It is good for the heart and blood circulation, being particularly beneficial for high blood pressure, varicose veins, haemorrhoids and internal bleeding. Yarrow helps to regulate menstrual periods and reduce cramp and excessive bleeding, as well as helping to relieve the disturbances of menopause. A hot infusion promotes perspiration and can be used to treat colds and flu, and children's diseases like measles and chickenpox. The fresh juice is sometimes used to treat diabetes. Used externally yarrow is an excellent astringent and antiseptic which can be applied to wounds to stop bleeding, and makes a very good cleanser for greasy skin and pimples. It can also be used for chapped hands or sore nipples. The leaves can be chewed to alleviate toothache or added to the water to make a relaxing bath.

YELLOW DOCK (*Rumex crispus*)

A large-leafed weed native to Eurasia and well known in much of the world. It is particularly useful for chronic itching skin complaints such as eczema and psoriasis, especially when these are associated with constipation or liver disorders. It can be applied as an ointment made from the powdered root or taken in a decoction. Yellow dock is also helpful for improving the digestive functions, particularly by stimulating the liver and improving the flow of bile, and as a tonic rich in iron and useful for anaemia. It can also be used for rheumatism, gout and jaundice, or gargled for sore throats. Externally it can be applied to boils, wounds, haemorrhoids and parasitic infections such as ringworm.

YELLOW SPIDER FLOWER, tick weed (*Cleome viscosa*)

A strong-smelling, sticky-leafed plant found in hot, wet parts of Australia and often regarded as a weed. It has similar qualities to other types of capers and was used by the Aborigines to cure headaches. The leaves can be used on wounds and ulcers, or made into an ointment for earache; they have also been used to treat intestinal worms.

YERBA BUENA (*Micromeria chamissonis*)

A herb which grows on the sand dunes of the west coast of the USA, and was used by the Indians to relieve colic and purify the blood. It can be made into a tea for arthritis, or mixed with spearmint and taken for insomnia.

YERBA MANSA, yerba del pasmo (*Corynanthe johymbe*)

A North American plant, the leaves of which can be made into a tea to reduce swellings, cure colds and asthma, and purify the blood. It can be used as a bath herb for aching muscles or made into a poultice for cuts and bruises.

YERBA MATE, Paraguay tea (*Ilex paraguensis*)

An evergreen tea drunk by the Indians of Paraguay as a mild stimulant with a diuretic action.

YERBA SANTA, holy herb, mountain balm (*Eriodictyon californicum*)

An aromatic evergreen shrub from western USA; its leaves exude a gummy substance which can be smoked or chewed as a type of herbal tobacco recommended for coughs and catarrh. It can be taken as a tea for bronchitis, asthma and other respiratory complaints, and has also been recommended for headaches, sore throats, arthritis and rheumatism. Externally it can be used as a poultice for bruises, sprains and insect bites.

YEW, chinwood (*Taxus baccata*)

A large northern hemisphere tree with tiny yellow flowers and red or yellow berries. The tree is very poisonous, especially the berries, but the leaves are made into a homeopathic tincture which can be used for rheumatism and arthritis.

YUCCA, jucca (*Yucca gloriosa*)

An evergreen plant from the deserts of Central America which is also grown in gardens for its large white flowers. The juice is used in hair and scalp tonics.

TREATMENTS USING HEALING PLANTS

A

ABSCESSES — *see Boils*

ACNE

There are a number of factors which can contribute to acne, so the practitioner must decide which is the main cause before choosing the appropriate remedy. Acne which is due to glandular disturbances is often treated with burdock root taken in infusion or applied externally as an ointment or a wash. It can also be treated with a decoction taken 3 times a day and made from equal parts of burdock, dandelion root, red clover, and echinacea. For acne which is aggravated by nervous tension an infusion of chamomile flowers, lavender or limeblossom can be used either internally or externally. A steam bath of 2 parts elder flowers and 1 part each of marigold and eucalyptus flowers can be beneficial. Place the hot infusion in an open bowl, cover the head with a towel and lean over the bowl for 5 to 10 minutes. A lotion made from marigold flowers will reduce oiliness, while a cold infusion of comfrey leaves will soothe and help heal already inflamed skin.

ANAEMIA

Anaemia is a deficiency of haemoglobin which is often caused by lack of iron. Sometimes anaemia may be cured simply by adding to the diet herbs which are rich in iron such as chives, parsley, alfalfa, nettles, dandelion, chickweed or watercress. A tea made from hops and taken after each meal will help the body to assimilate the iron already in the diet. Some herbalists recommend a tea made from 2 parts of stinging nettle combined with 1 part each of dandelion root and alfalfa.

ANXIETY — *see Stress*

APPETITE, LACK OF

There are a number of herbs which can be taken to stimulate the appetite and to promote digestion. They are generally taken in infusion, ½–1 cup an hour before each meal. Peppermint tea is frequently recommended. An alternative is an infusion of equal parts of alfalfa, angelica, dandelion and fennel. Herbs such as mint, parsley, marjoram and watercress may be eaten fresh as part of the 'appetiser' at the beginning of a meal.

ARTERIOSCLEROSIS

Research has shown that raw garlic helps to control blood cholesterol and break down fatty deposits inside blood vessels. Garlic may also be taken in capsule form. Regular doses, taken 2 or 3 times a day, of limeblossom, hawthorn and nettle tea (either alone or in combination) are often recommended to reduce blood pressure and strengthen the arteries.

ARTHRITIS

Similar treatments can be used for arthritis, rheumatism and gout. Celery seeds, nettle and meadowsweet are often recommended, as are elder flowers, burdock, dandelion, cleavers, liquorice, corn silk, sarsaparilla, ginger and cayenne pepper.

Because these complaints are usually chronic, treatments must be taken for several weeks followed by a break of 2 or 3 weeks, and subsequently resumed. This pattern may need to be followed for several months. One recommended cure is to take 3 cups a day of an infusion of 1 part each of ginger root and celery seed, 3 parts burdock root and 5 parts dandelion root. An external treatment can be made from equal parts of dried mullein leaves and St John's wort heated in vinegar and applied as a compress. Ginger, cayenne pepper, angelica, fennel and chamomile can all be used externally as oils or in poultices.

It is often necessary, too, to make some changes to the diet.

ASTHMA

Herbal remedies for asthma usually include two types of herbs: expectorants such as coltsfoot, mullein, hyssop and comfrey to clear the lungs, and antispasmodic and sedative plants such as skullcap, chamomile and hops to calm the patient and help to restore normal breathing rhythm. These herbs are usually combined in a tea which should be taken in a dose of ½–1 cupful 3 times a day. An example of 1 of these teas is:

    angelica root (3 parts)
    coltsfoot leaves (3 parts)
    skullcap (2 parts)
    crampbark (2 parts)
    thyme (1 part)
    peppermint (1 part)

Sometimes herbal cigarettes made from dried herbs such as coltsfoot and mullein are recommended. Before going to sleep at night some asthmatic patients find it helpful to take a hot bath to which catmint or pine has been added.

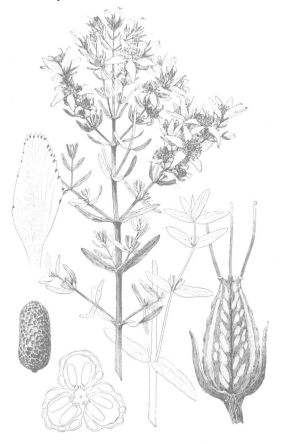

St John's wort — a remedy for bedwetting

ATHLETE'S FOOT

This is often a very troublesome infection. It is very important to wash and dry the feet thoroughly and keep them in the sun as much as possible. Some people find it helpful to soak their feet for half an hour in a footbath made from red clover and hot water (about 100 g to 1 litre). A foot powder can be made from gum benzoin and arrowroot and dusted on regularly.

B

BAD BREATH

This is usually due to some internal problem, but the symptoms can be alleviated by chewing a few leaves of mint, parsley, basil, rosemary or thyme. These herbs can also be taken in infusion and gargled frequently, as can lemon verbena, lavender, cloves or fennel seeds.

BEDWETTING

This is often due to some underlying emotional cause, but it may be helped by small doses of a tea made from horsetail herb, St John's wort or corn silk. Another remedy is to take 3 doses a day of ½ cup of a tea made from 1 part each of stinging nettle, St John's wort and lemon balm, and 2 parts of cramp bark.

BLOOD PRESSURE

Professional advice should be taken to determine the cause of high blood pressure, but there are several herbs which, if taken regularly, will tend to stabilise blood pressure. Among these are garlic, cayenne, hawthorn berries, limeblossom and nettle.

BOILS

To encourage boils to come to a head they should be bathed regularly in hot water. There are also a number of herbal poultices which can be applied; these should be changed 2 to 4 times a day. Boiled nettle leaves are suitable, as is a paste of powdered slippery elm with a pinch of capsicum, or a poultice or ointment made from mullein, burdock, chickweed, comfrey, marshmallow or plantain. For recurrent boils, herbal teas made from burdock root, yellow dock or fumitory should be taken regularly. An infusion of echinacea is said to be a good blood purifier.

BREASTFEEDING

Plants which help to increase the milk supply include milkwort, fenugreek, borage, anise, vervain, fennel and dill. Anise and fennel are also thought to pass into the milk and prevent the baby from developing colic. Garlic seems to upset some babies. Sore nipples can be soothed by an ointment of 2 parts marigold flowers and 1 part marshmallow root applied regularly. Some people recommend witch hazel to stop milk leaking from the nipples. To dry up the milk flow an infusion of sage or mint can be taken 3 times a day.

BRONCHITIS — *see Asthma*

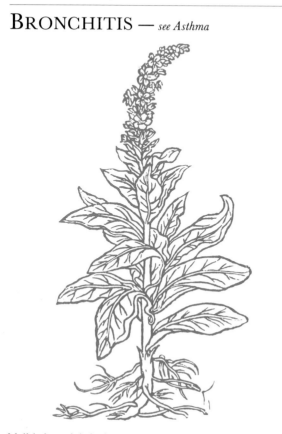

Mullein leaves help bruises

BRUISES

One of the simplest remedies is to break off a leaf of aloe vera and rub it on the bruise 3 or 4 times a day. A hot poultice is most effective, as is a compress or ointment made from either marigold flowers, hyssop, comfrey, mullein leaves or St John's wort. Witch hazel and a diluted tincture of arnica are both effective remedies which are easy to keep on hand. If there is a tendency to bruise easily it may be necessary to take some measures to improve the blood circulation.

BURNS

The affected area should be immediately immersed in cool water and left there for several minutes. Severe burns and those which cover a large area of the body should have medical attention as soon as possible, and the patient should be treated for shock. However minor burns can be treated with fresh aloe vera gel or with a poultice or ointment made from marigold flowers, comfrey, plantain, St John's wort, chamomile, marshmallow, burdock, chickweed, elder or even cabbage leaves.

C

CATARRH

A highly recommended remedy for catarrh is to take 3 cups a day of an infusion of mallow leaves. Other useful herbs which can be taken in the same way include anise seed, fennel, fenugreek, hyssop, agrimony and white horehound. Raw garlic or garlic capsules are often very helpful. For nasal catarrh and sinusitis, an infusion of equal parts of elder flowers and eyebright is often effective, while for chronic bronchial catarrh a tea of 2 parts each of coltsfoot and horehound leaves combined with 1 part of angelica root is preferable. Eucalyptus oil or a similar inhalant is often very helpful, especially at night.

COLIC

In babies — Probably the best known herbal remedy is dill water, but caraway, fennel and anise seed are also suitable. Catnip, lemon balm, chamomile or vervain can also be taken in infusion, a teaspoonful at a time.

In adults — Acute abdominal pain from gases in the bowel can be relieved by a hot infusion of peppermint or catmint. Some practitioners recommend wild yam.

CONJUNCTIVITIS — *see Eye problems*

CONSTIPATION

In many cases the cause of constipation is lack of dietary fibre, in which case the best cure is to eat foods containing more roughage. However sometimes constipation is aggravated by stress, and herbal remedies which have nervine and antispasmodic properties are often helpful. One such remedy is an infusion of 1 part each of liquorice root, anise seed and valerian root combined with 2 parts of chickweed herb. This should be taken 3 times a day. Stewed figs, senna pods, cascara and linseed all have laxative properties.

CORNS

Corns can be softened by regular application (at least twice a day) of any of the following: crushed marigold leaves, freshly crushed garlic, lemon juice, a leaf from the houseleek plant, or the milky sap from the fig tree *(Ficus carica)*.

COUGHS

Coughs are among the most common ailments and there are a large number of herbal remedies available. A good general cough medicine can be made from 2 parts each of coltsfoot, mullein, horehound, anise seed and marshmallow combined with 1 part each of thyme and liquorice root. A hard, dry cough can be loosened by a mixture of liquorice and marshmallow with a pinch of thyme and caraway, and also by an infusion of elecampane root. To soothe a tickling cough try a mixture of 3 parts each of coltsfoot, horehound and mullein combined with 1 part thyme, taken in small doses when necessary.

CRAMP

Suggested remedies to relieve muscle spasms include an infusion of 4 parts cramp bark combined with 1 part ginger, taken 3 times a day. An alternative is an infusion of equal parts of hop flowers and valerian root combined with 3 parts of skullcap flowers.

CROUP

This annoying barking cough which troubles so many young children can often be helped by small doses of a tea made from vervain and coltsfoot, strained and then drunk warm, mixed with honey. A teaspoon is sufficient for a small child, while a 5 year-old could take a dose of 1 tablespoon. Garlic and honey can also be helpful.

CUTS — *see Wounds*

CYSTITIS

There are several herbal remedies for this painful inflammation of the bladder, all of them having diuretic, antiseptic and demulcent properties. They include couch grass, cranesbill, meadowsweet and burdock root taken in infusion 3 times a day. Other suitable teas can be made from 2 parts burdock to 1 part blackberry or 1 part cleavers to 4 parts marshmallow.

D

DANDRUFF

This is often caused by poor general health and can be improved by regular doses 3 times a day of an infusion of nettle or cleavers. The scalp should also be massaged daily with a lotion made from nettle seeds, or from equal parts of nettle and burdock, or from rosemary, sage or thyme.

DEPRESSION

An infusion of lemon balm leaves can be taken 3 times a day for several weeks to help in the treatment of long-term depression. This may also be combined with equal parts of skullcap and vervain. Other useful herbs are lavender, borage, chervil and ginseng.

DIARRHOEA

There are a great many herbs which can be used for diarrhoea. One of the most commonly recommended is blackberry, taken in infusion 3 times a day. Others include: agrimony, raspberry, comfrey, geranium, plantain, meadowsweet, mullein and marshmallow. A pinch of cinnamon, ginger or caraway seeds can be added to an infusion of any of these to improve their effectiveness.

DIZZINESS

If this is due to anxiety rather than some physiological problem such as ear infection, anaemia or abnormal blood pressure, then an infusion of balm, taken 3 times a day, is a good remedy.

Other herbs used for dizziness include rosemary, sage and peppermint combined in equal quantities and taken in infusion, or cayenne, cinnamon and clove, prepared in the same way.

E

EARACHE

A few drops of any of several herbal oils can be placed in the ear or on a small wad of cottonwool inserted in the ear to alleviate the pain of earache. Marigold, garlic or almond oil are suitable, and in Europe mullein oil is highly regarded. Hyssop or yarrow herb can also be applied as a hot compress on cottonwool outside the ear. Some herbalists recommend an infusion of melilot taken 3 times a day.

ECZEMA

When this is due to a food allergy then the best remedy is to change the diet. However, there are several herbal remedies which are helpful in relieving itching. A soothing lotion can be made from an infusion of plantain leaves, or the leaves can be applied as a poultice to particularly bad patches. An alternative is an ointment or a lotion made from 2 parts chickweed combined with 1 part each of stinging nettle, marigold flowers and burdock root. For internal use, an infusion can be made from 2 parts each of stinging nettle, marigold flowers, vervain, dandelion root and burdock root combined with 1 part each of yellow dock root and red clover flowers. A cupful should be taken 3 times a day. For small children a lotion of Weleda Sambucus compound is often recommended, or small doses of a tea of 3 parts stinging nettle combined with 1 part each of burdock root, marigold flowers and lemon balm leaves. For dry eczema some practitioners recommend doses of sunflower seed oil and plenty of watercress.

EYE PROBLEMS

Conjunctivitis, styes or sore, tired or red eyes can be soothed by regular bathing with a lotion of 3 parts eyebright and 1 part marigold flowers. Similar lotions can be made from elder flowers, fennel seeds, raspberry leaves, chamomile flowers, plantain or chickweed.

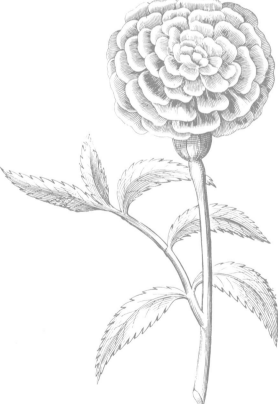

Marigold flowers — a lotion is helpful for conjunctivitis

F

FEVER

There are several herbal teas which can be taken to increase perspiration and help bring down a high temperature. They include yarrow, peppermint, elder flower, sage, meadowsweet, cleavers, catnip and lemon balm. These should be taken hot, a glassful every hour, and the patient should rest in bed till the fever has gone. Some herbalists prefer to combine the herbs. One example of this is a tea of 2 parts each of elder flowers and peppermint combined with 1 part of yarrow herb. For children only mild herbs such as chamomile, lemon balm and raspberry should be used.

Many herbalists recommend that no food should be eaten while the fever lasts.

FLATULENCE

There are many causes of flatulence and attempts should be made to find out and treat the background cause. However the pain and discomfort can be relieved by regular doses of herbal teas made from fennel, anise, caraway, catmint, ginger and other carminative herbs. One example is a combination of 4 parts fennel to 1 part ginger. Another is made from equal parts of anise seed, chamomile, lemon balm and peppermint.

FRACTURES

While it is necessary to seek medical attention when a broken limb is suspected, the healing process can be hastened by applications of comfrey, as a poultice if possible, or otherwise taken as a tea.

H

HAEMORRHOIDS

These very painful varicose veins of the rectum are often aggravated by lack of fibre in the diet. Herbal remedies which can be taken to alleviate piles include an infusion of 3 parts each of shepherd's purse, plan-tain leaves and marigold flowers combined with 1 part fennel seed, or alternatively a decoction of black-berry root bark can be taken. Soothing and astringent herbs such as witch hazel, pilewort, comfrey and mullein oil can be applied externally. A very effective ointment can be made from equal parts of witch hazel, plantain, marigold flowers, St John's wort and comfrey root. This can be applied several times a day.

HAIR LOSS OR POOR HAIR CONDITION

This may occur for a number of reasons — stress, poor diet, pregnancy, drugs, hormonal changes, old age or an inherited tendency to baldness. Attention should first be given to the diet, to make sure it contains sufficient vitamins and minerals, particularly vitamin B. Silica is especially important and can be obtained from an infusion of cleavers herb taken three times a day. Nettle tea is helpful and can also be rubbed into the scalp daily. Rosemary and sage are both used as a good tonic and conditioner for dark hair, while chamomile and yarrow are recommended for blondes. They should be rubbed into the scalp daily. Dry hair can be improved by an infusion of comfrey leaves, elder flowers and burdock, while oiliness can be reduced by lavender.

HAY FEVER

Acute attacks of hay fever can be helped by an infusion of 2 parts of sage combined with 1 part each of elder flowers and eyebright taken every few hours. For chronic hay fever, take regular doses of an infusion of elder flowers and eyebright. Other useful infusions can be made from yarrow, wood betony and eyebright or a mixture of eyebright, lungwort and golden seal.

HEADACHE

This is a very common ailment which may be caused by any of a number of different factors. If the head-aches are frequent then the patient should try to find out the underlying cause and treat that. However there are a number of different herbal teas which can be tried to alleviate the symptoms. These include a combination of equal parts of peppermint, sage and rosemary or yarrow, skullcap and vervain.

For migraine headaches an infusion of feverfew,

taken every hour or two, is often very helpful. A few drops of the essential oil of any herb such as rosemary, lavender, peppermint, wintergreen or ginger can be applied externally to the temples and will often bring soothing relief.

I

INDIGESTION — *see Flatulence and Colic*

INSECT BITES AND STINGS

A number of plants can simply be crushed and rubbed on the skin to relieve pain and itchiness. These include aloe vera, marigold flowers and the leaves of St John's wort, plantain, pennyroyal, rosemary and hyssop. If the discomfort is great an infusion of balm, borage, broom or fennel could be used. Many herbs will also repel insects. Fresh basil, horehound, stinging nettle and elder leaves will all keep away flying insects, as will a few drops of the esssential oils of citronella, lavender or pennyroyal rubbed onto the skin.

INSOMNIA

There are a number of herbs which can be used, either alone or in combinations, to brew a relaxing tea that will cause drowsiness. These include valerian, skullcap, chamomile, lavender, lemon balm, vervain, hop flowers and catnip. Some people recommend a herbal pillow containing lavender, chamomile, rosemary, limeblossom or hops. For small children a very mild tea of chamomile, lemon balm or vervain may be used.

ITCHINESS AND RASHES

The exact herbal treatment prescribed will depend on the cause of the itchiness, but there are a number of suitable herbs. These include chickweed, aloe vera, burdock and yellow dock root as well as meadowsweet, fumitory, cleavers, St John's wort and sarsaparilla. A lotion of either marigolds or elder flowers is very effective in relieving itching. For an inflamed, eruptive rash a tea of equal parts of burdock root, marigold flowers and stinging nettle can be taken three times a day.

L

LARYNGITIS

Frequent drinks of hot lemon juice and honey, or garlic and honey in hot water, are helpful, as is a teaspoon of liquorice root and honey taken 3 times a day. Soothing herbal teas can be made from marshmallow root, coltsfoot or mullein leaves. To ease the dry cough, every few hours take a tablespoon of an infusion made from a teaspoon each of sage, thyme and marjoram boiled in 300 ml (½ pint) of hot water with a stick of liquorice added. Some people recommend eating large quantities of boiled onions. An infusion of lavender flowers can be taken 3 times a day and also inhaled regularly.

M

MENSTRUAL PROBLEMS

Excessive menstrual discharge is often treated with a decoction of shepherd's purse, 1 cupful being taken every 2 hours. Other suitable herbs are yarrow, plantain and ladies' mantle. For period pain an infusion of 4 parts cramp bark to 1 part ginger can be taken. Other helpful herbs include chamomile or marigold flowers, vervain, melilot, lemon balm and raspberry. Delayed menstruation can be brought on by an infusion of 3 parts cramp bark combined with 1 part each of motherwort herb and marigold flowers. Premenstrual tension is often helped by evening primrose tablets or by regular doses of an infusion of equal parts of motherwort and lemon balm.

MIGRAINE — *see Headaches*

MORNING SICKNESS

The nausea of early pregnancy can often be relieved by a simple herbal remedy such as lemon balm or cinnamon tea, or a combination of spearmint, raspberry, meadowsweet and chamomile. Even these remedies should be used with care, and not more than 3 cups should be taken in a day.

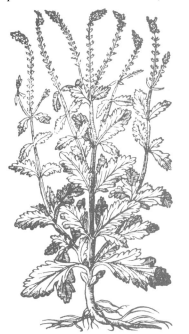

Vervain — a mild vervain tea helps induce drowsiness

N

NAUSEA

When nausea is accompanied by vomiting, it is generally considered best not to eat any food. However a tisane of chamomile, peppermint, mint or limeblossom taken several times a day may be helpful. Also recommended are an infusion of tarragon herb or small doses of Weleda's Melissa, a compound which includes coriander, clove, nutmeg and cinnamon. Some people find it helpful to chew crystallised ginger.

NERVOUS TENSION — *see Stress*

NIGHTMARES

Some people recommend a soothing herbal tea such as chamomile or wood betony taken at bedtime.

Other suitable herbs are rosemary, lavender, primrose and thyme.

NOSEBLEED

The head should be held back and the juice from fresh nettles, marigolds or shepherd's purse inserted into the nostril. Other plants which can be used in the same way are yarrow, herb Robert, cranesbill and golden rod. Distilled witch hazel is also effective.

P

PAIN

There are many herbs which can reduce pain — the remedy chosen will be determined by the cause of the pain. St John's wort is very effective for neuralgic pains and is applied externally. Comfrey leaves can be used in the same way and are often recommended for sprains. Rosemary, peppermint, cayenne, linseed, ginger, thyme and meadowsweet can all be used externally to relieve muscular pain.

PILES — *see Haemorrhoids*

POST-NATAL DEPRESSION

An infusion of vervain and lemon balm leaves taken 3 times a day is said to be an effective cure for post-natal depression.

PREGNANCY

Two excellent herbs, both widely recommended for pregnant women, are raspberry and chamomile. Raspberry leaf tea, taken regularly after the third month, is regarded as an excellent tonic to strengthen the pelvic and uterine muscles, prevent miscarriage and make delivery easier. Chamomile flowers make a very good tea which is especially helpful for cramps, indigestion and morning sickness. It is also very useful for babies' colic, teething and sleeplessness. Some herbalists recommend limeblossom tea for high blood pressure. *See also Morning sickness.*

PSORIASIS

This chronic skin disease with its characteristic scaly patches often responds well to herbal treatments if taken regularly. One recommended tea is made from equal parts of burdock root, dandelion root, yellow dock root, red clover flowers and cleavers. This can be supplemented by echinacea tablets. Balm, nettle and raspberry leaf teas are also used both internally and externally, and some people recommend a bath containing yarrow. Another alternative is an ointment or lotion made from 2 parts burdock root combined with 1 part each of chickweed, marigold flowers and marshmallow root.

S

SHOCK

When shock is accompanied by injuries which may need an anaesthetic, then nothing at all should be given to the patient. For other cases, sweetened peppermint tea is often recommended. So too is an infusion of 2 parts each of chamomile, hop flowers and vervain leaves. An alternative is a tea made from 4 parts skullcap to 1 part valerian root.

SINUSITIS — *see Catarrh*

SORE THROAT

The first symptoms of sore throats are often soothed by hot drinks of lemon juice, honey and water, and many practitioners recommend rest and little food. A teaspoon of fresh crushed garlic mixed with honey can be taken every few hours, and an infusion of equal parts of sage and thyme gargled frequently. An alternative remedy is a herbal tea of agrimony and raspberry, or an infusion of marshmallow flowers and leaves may be taken, a wineglassful 4 times a day. Some practitioners recommend painting the tonsils with a soft brush dipped in an antiseptic such as eucalyptus oil. An infusion of dried blackberry leaves makes a useful astringent gargle, and if fresh blackberries are available they can be eaten to prevent recurrent sore throats.

SPLINTERS

Deeply embedded splinters can often be drawn towards the surface of the skin by applying an ointment or poultice of marshmallow, agrimony, hawthorn or comfrey, covered with a dressing. One highly recommended ointment is made from 10 parts of plantain leaves combined with 1 part of cayenne pepper.

SPRAINS

The first treatment is to apply a compress of ice or cold water. This can be followed with a poultice of bruised comfrey leaves which should be changed three or four times a day and should quickly reduce the pain and inflammation. Distilled witch hazel or tincture of arnica are also often used on sprains.

STRESS

There are a great many herbal remedies which are recommended to ease nervous tension and general anxiety. Some of these are valerian, vervain, chamomile, rosemary, lavender and woodruff. Many herbal teas are a combination of several of these. A good general nerve tonic is a combination of equal parts of valerian root, gentian root, vervain, chamomile, catmint and skullcap. A teaspoonful is infused in a cupful of water for 10 minutes and then taken before meals.

STYES

A compress of elder flowers, marigolds or crushed nasturtium seeds will relieve the discomfort. *See also Eye problems.*

SUNBURN

The first remedy is to take a cool bath or shower as soon as possible. The sunburnt areas can be sponged with a cool infusion of nettles, elder flowers or chamomile flowers, or with olive oil and cider vinegar, aloe vera gel, vitamin E oil, or the oils from comfrey, elder leaf or St John's wort. Some natural health practitioners recommend applying a lotion of olive oil and cider vinegar before sunbaking, and claim that if sesame oil is added it will absorb the sun's ultraviolet rays.

T

TONSILLITIS — *see Sore throat*

TOOTHACHE

There are several home remedies which will alleviate the pain of toothache, at least until professional dental care can be obtained. A small piece of cottonwool soaked in oil of cloves or grated raw onion can be placed directly onto the cavity, or the mouth can be rinsed with a strong infusion of St John's wort and chamomile flowers or mallow leaves and flowers. A very simple remedy is to chew either fresh plantain leaves or yarrow.

TRAVEL SICKNESS

Many people recommend ginger root, either fresh or preserved (crystallised). An alternative is a paste made from powdered ginger, cinnamon and honey, eaten in small doses as required. Peppermint, spearmint or aniseed flavoured sweets are often helpful. So too is chamomile tea taken before the journey.

U

ULCERS

Mouth ulcers can be cleared by applying a tincture of myrrh several times a day or diluting it as a mouthwash. Alternatives are a mouthwash of bistort root, marshmallow root or blackberry leaves, or a combination of sage leaves and marigold flowers.

Leg ulcers and bed sores can be helped by aloe vera leaves, or by a poultice of comfrey, chickweed, marigold flowers or slippery elm, supplemented by a blood purifier such as echinacea tablets.

Gastric and duodenal ulcers can be helped by golden seal or papaya (pawpaw) tablets, or by regular doses of an infusion of 3 parts marshmallow root to 1 part marigold, or 10 parts marshmallow combined with 2 parts each of marigold and meadowsweet and 1 part lemon balm.

V

VARICOSE VEINS

A decoction of shepherd's purse, taken regularly for periods of up to 3 weeks, is sometimes recommended. So too is yarrow tea. External remedies include marigold flowers and distilled witch hazel which can be made into a lotion and applied when necessary.

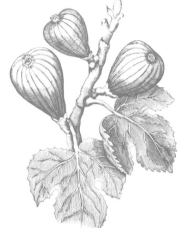

Fig sap is one of several treatments for warts

W

WARTS

Warts should disappear after a few weeks if painted twice a day with the milky juice of dandelion stems or freshly crushed marigold leaves. Other remedies are lemon juice, garlic, castor oil, and the milky sap of the fig tree *(Ficus carica)*.

WOUNDS

All wounds, cuts and grazes should first be washed with clean, tepid water. If bleeding is severe, pressure should be applied to the artery and medical attention sought. There are a number of herbs which are useful for treating injuries. Witch hazel, yarrow, stinging nettle and shepherd's purse are all good to stop bleeding. Other herbs with antiseptic and analgesic qualities are also helpful. A good all-purpose remedy can be made from equal parts of marigold flowers, plantain leaves, St John's wort and comfrey root. It can be applied several times a day, either as a poultice or an ointment.

PART 2

ALTERNATIVE HEALTH THERAPIES

ABDOMINAL SEGMENT

One of 7 body segments in Reichian therapy. The abdominal segment includes the large abdominal muscles: the rectus, transversis abdominus, latissimus dorsi and sacrospinalis. Sexual repression expressed in this segment may inhibit the normal wave-like motion of the abdomen during orgasm. Massage and deep breathing exercises are used in treatment. *See Reichian therapy.*

ABREACTION

In psychotherapy, the removal of emotions associated with forgotten or repressed ideas or events. Abreaction is a central goal of several alternative mind and body therapies including rebirthing and psychoperistalsis — *see separate listings for these subjects.*

ABSENT HEALING

A form of faith-healing that takes place without the healer being present. Absent healing usually involves the power of prayer or the 'projection' of positive and healing thoughts to the sick person.

ACCOMMODATION

In the Bates Method, a natural treatment for vision improvement. Accommodation is the act of adjusting eye focus from near to far in order to strengthen the eye muscles — *see Bates Method.*

ACU-POINT

A specific point on a meridian to which pressure is applied in order to rectify an imbalance of *chi* energy. Acu-points are also known as *tsubo. See Acupuncture, Shiatsu.*

ACUPRESSURE — *see Shiatsu*

ACUPUNCTURE

An ancient system of Chinese medicine based on the principle that health is achieved by balancing *yin* and *yang* energies in the body. *Yin* and *yang* are opposite polarities, *yin* being regarded traditionally as passive, negative and feminine, and *yang* as active, positive and masculine. The body is enlivened by the flow of *chi* (life-force) through energy conduits or meridians in the body, and the techniques of acupuncture are intended to ensure that any imbalances in the flow of *chi* are rectified. When imbalances are removed, disease — by definition — is eliminated.

Early accounts of acupuncture are provided in Szuma Chien's *Shi Ji*, dating from the Han Dynasty (about 200 BC), in the *Nei Ching Su Wen*, and in the biographies of Pien Chueh and Tsang Kung which date back about 2000 years.

In acupuncture, needles are used to stimulate specific points along the meridians. The original needles were made of stone; later, they were fashioned from iron and silver, and contemporary acupuncturists now make use of stainless steel needles.

In Chinese medicine, the body is divided into 5 elements and these are associated with the 5 so-called Ts'ang organs:

liver (wood); heart (fire); spleen (earth); lungs (metal), and kidneys (water). There are also two 'metaphysical' organs referred to in acupuncture as the 'triple warmer' and the 'gate of life'.

Twelve major meridians are identified in acupuncture, although practising acupuncturists make use of 59 major and minor meridians and up to 1000 acupuncture points along these channels of life-energy. The principal meridians are as follows:

MERIDIAN	ORGAN
Arm Sunlight Yang	Large intestine
Leg Sunlight Yang	Stomach
Arm Greater Yin	Lungs
Leg Greater Yin	Spleen
Arm Lesser Yang	Triple warmer
Leg Lesser Yang	Gall bladder
Arm Absolute Yin	Gate of life
Leg Absolute Yin	Liver
Arm Greater Yang	Small intestine
Leg Greater Yang	Bladder
Arm Lesser Yin	Heart
Leg Lesser Yin	Kidneys

The meridians in acupuncture provide a different framework from that understood in modern western medicine, but it is evident that acupuncture is effective in reducing pain: it sometimes allows complicated surgery to be performed on patients while they are still conscious.

The British acupuncturist Dr Julian Kenyon believes that acupuncture activates 'electrical pathways' which weave through the neuroglia, or connective tissue of the nervous system. Similarly, Canadian researcher Professor Ronald Melzack has noted that there is a 71 per cent correlation between visceral, cutaneous and nervous reflexes — which he calls 'trigger' points — and the traditional acupuncture points used to relieve pain. It is also noteworthy that the heart meridian runs along the internal cutaneous nerve and ulnar nerve, the bladder meridian corresponds in part to the sciatic nerve, and the gate of life meridian lies along the median nerve.

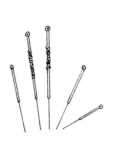

Originally, acupuncture needles were made from stone; these are modern stainless steel

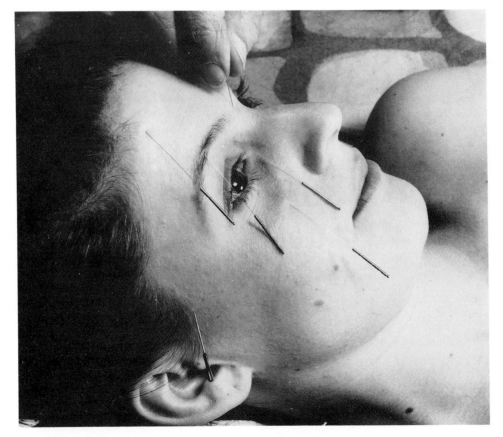

Acupuncture needles are inserted at precise locations on the meridians

Following systematic research in Sweden, Scotland, the United States and Canada, it is now thought that acupuncture stimulates production of endorphins, or natural opiates, in the brain and that these endorphins produce a strong analgesic effect. However, practitioners of acupuncture believe that their techniques are effective in treating a wide range of health complaints — including arthritis, lumbago, asthma, gout, obesity and even paralysis — and that the scope of acupuncture extends well beyond pain control. Accordingly, it will take many years of further scientific research before acupuncture is fully understood within the frameworks established by Western medicine.

A traditional Chinese drawing showing an acupuncture meridian, or chi *channel*

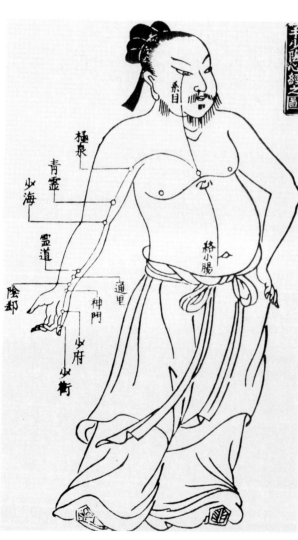

ADJUSTMENT

A term used in chiropractic to refer to the thrust delivered by the therapist in order to move a misaligned vertebra to its proper position. The term was coined by the founder of chiropractic, D. D. Palmer.

AFFIRMATION

A positive thought, statement or image used to reinforce a desired health condition. Affirmations are used in many visualisation and self-hypnosis therapies, and are a form of positive reinforcement. They derive originally from the work of the French psychotherapist Emile Coué who believed strongly in using hypnotic instructions to the subconscious mind to eliminate disease and imbalance. *See also Auto-suggestion, Hypnosis.*

AIKIDO

A Japanese martial art which advocates non-aggressive self-defence and holistic well-being. The term itself means 'The Way of Harmony' and includes a variety of practical exercises featuring both attack and defence. In aikido emphasis is placed as much on the activation of *ki* (life-force) and correct breathing, as on physical strength itself, and the key is to learn how to channel power both to avert an attacker and to maximise inner balance and vitality.

ALEXANDER TECHNIQUE

A bodywork approach formulated by Australian-born actor and recitalist F. Matthias Alexander (1869–1955). Alexander joined a dramatic arts company in Melbourne, but was annoyed by bouts of hoarseness which interfered with his performances. He decided to observe the patterns of recurrence and noticed that when using his voice in recitals he produced a series of muscular contractions around his neck and head. Alexander became increasingly interested in posture and over the next 10 years evolved a technique of adjusting 'body use' patterns. In particular he emphasised a basic movement called 'the Primary Control' from which proper body movement flowed. His formula was to 'let the neck be free to let the head be forward and up, and the back widen and lengthen'.

After leaving Australia for England in 1904 Alexander became well known in London and in due course was able to demonstrate his technique to such distinguished figures as Lillie Langtry, George Bernard Shaw and Aldous Huxley — among many others.

The Alexander Technique, as it is now presented internationally, teaches self-awareness of the body and places special importance on the relationship of the head to the neck and the two of these to the torso. Subjects learn to sit, stand and walk in a way that maximises efficient body use, and the technique is particularly effective in helping those who have lordosis (hollow back), kyphosis (round back) or scoliosis (spinal curvature).

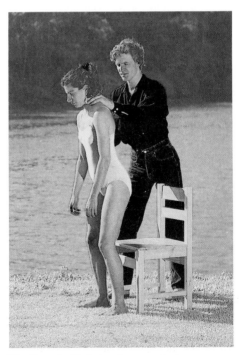

The Alexander Technique focuses on posture

ALLOPATHIC MEDICINE

A form of medicine based on the notion of allopathy, a general term used by naturopaths to describe orthodox western medicine, and specifically the viewpoint that disease is external to the body and requires treatment of an external nature (medicines, pills, ointments) to combat a presumed disease entity in the organism. *See Allopathy; compare with Naturopathy.*

ALLOPATHY

A term introduced by Samuel Hahnemann, the founder of homeopathy, to describe the curing of disease by introducing treatments which are unrelated in nature to the disease itself. According to Hahnemann, allopathic treatments increase the burden on the diseased organism — *see Allopathic medicine.*

ALTERED STATE OF CONSCIOUSNESS

A state of consciousness different from normal, everyday consciousness, the latter sometimes being referred to as the 'consensus reality' on which normal patterns of communication are based. Altered states exclude or minimise the external world, allowing subconscious imagery to rise into consciousness. Altered states include dreams, trance and hypnotic states, and are utilised by practitioners of clinical hypnotherapy, guided imagery and psychosynthesis to allow new perceptions to arise in the subject undergoing therapy.

ALTERNATIVE MEDICINE

Health modalities and therapies which are regarded as a viable alternative to mainstream, orthodox medicine. Alternative medicine encompasses a wide range of approaches to body, mind and spirit, some of which have more scientific credence than others. Among the best known forms of alternative medicine are chiropractic, osteopathy, naturopathy, acupuncture and herbalism. *See also separate listings for these subjects.*

AMBIENT MUSIC

Non-intrusive music conceived for relaxation or meditation. Ambient music is generally muted and abstract in form, featuring subtle textures and tonal colours rather than pronounced melodies. The music may be used for visualisation purposes to enhance meditations on specific symbolic elements (for example, earth, water, fire, air, spirit), to arouse *kundalini* energy, or to relax different parts of the body. Leading contemporary musicians in this genre include Brian Eno, Steven Halpern, Aeoliah, Kitaro and Geoffrey Chandler. *See also Music therapy.*

ANMA

An early form of Japanese and Chinese massage, the main function of which was to stimulate blood circulation. Anma was traditionally used to treat stiff shoulders and back tension, and has now been largely replaced with shiatsu — a more all-encompassing form of body therapy — *see Shiatsu.*

ANTHROPOSOPHICAL MEDICINE

A medical approach developed by German mystic Rudolf Steiner (1861–1925). Steiner was the founder of anthroposophy, a breakaway esoteric movement derived from theosophy.

Much of Steiner's thinking hinges on what he considered to be the three-fold pattern in man and nature. He believed that the dynamics of health operated through three interrelated systems:

- the nerves and senses (linked to the faculty of thinking);
- the metabolism and limbs (linked to the will);
- the circulation and respiration (linked to feeling).

Steiner also drew on the occult notion of 'etheric' and 'astral' energies, in turn associating the etheric with the metabolism, and the astral with the nerves and senses. According to Steiner, the astral was associated with what he called the 'upper pole' in man, and the etheric with the 'lower pole'. These two poles needed to be in balance for a state of true health to prevail. People with excess upper-pole energy tended to suffer from health complaints involving sclerosis and crystallisation, whereas those with excess lower-pole energy were more likely to suffer from inflammatory conditions and fever.

Steiner believed that the plant kingdom supplied the basic etheric energies which nourished man and restored vitality to diseased organs. However, different parts of any given plant were associated with different functions in the body. The flowers of the plant were linked to the metabolism, the roots to the nerves and senses, and the leaves to the circulatory system. This explained how some of the etheric energy from plants could be made available to the upper pole in man, nourishing his thought processes and allowing for the evolution of consciousness.

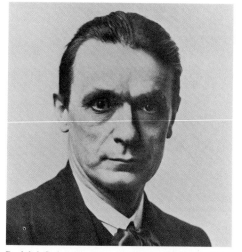

Rudolph Steiner, founder of anthroposophical medicine

APPLIED KINESIOLOGY

During the 1960s the chiropractor Dr George Goodheart advocated the principle that disease had 3 potential components: biochemical (nutritional), mental (psychological and spiritual) and structural (physical), and that all three aspects had to be heeded to regain health or balance. Goodheart's research led to the finding that muscle spasm was not a primary but a secondary factor in disease, and that correct muscular treatment involved balancing contracting (hypertonic) muscles as well as slackening (hypotonic) muscles. Weakened muscles could result from stress factors impinging upon the autonomic nervous system, and dietary and chemical imbalances. *See also Touch for health*.

ARICA SYSTEM

A training programme in self-development formulated by Bolivian-born mystic Oscar Ichazo. The arica system combines aspects of the Eastern esoteric traditions with western humanistic psychology and is sometimes known as 'scientific mysticism'. Arica includes breathing and movement exercises, encompassing what is called 'psycho-calisthenics', and a framework of the psyche based on 9 levels of consciousness. Each level is regarded as a way of unifying the physical, emotional and mental aspects of existence, and each has its own exercises and meditations.

The overriding aim of the Arica Institute, now based in New York, is to help transform society so that all mankind has a scientific understanding of the psyche.

AROMATHERAPY

A term coined by the French chemist René Maurice Gattefossé to describe essential oils and resins which can be used to treat the skin, cause stimulation or relaxation, prevent bodily infection, or maintain bodily resistance to disease. The oils and resins applied in aromatherapy derive from flowers, plants and trees, and superficially this type of treatment resembles herbalism. However, practitioners of aromatherapy maintain that they are dealing with the *essence* of a plant rather than its specific curative components, and that quite different healing properties may be involved.

Gattefossé discovered the beneficial effects of plant essences by accident, while working in his laboratory. He burned his hand severely and found that by using some lavender oil which happened to be nearby, he was able to soothe his hand effectively — and the burn healed much more swiftly than he would have expected. He later continued his research with essential oils, concluding that many of them had antibacterial qualities which could be useful against infections. They were also appropriate for treating skin conditions like acne, boils and dermatitis.

Aromatherapy makes use of a wide range of essential oils, including chamomile, lemon, eucalyptus, garlic, geranium, hyssop, mint, sage, lavender, fennel, rosemary and thyme. *See also herbal listings, Bach flower remedies*.

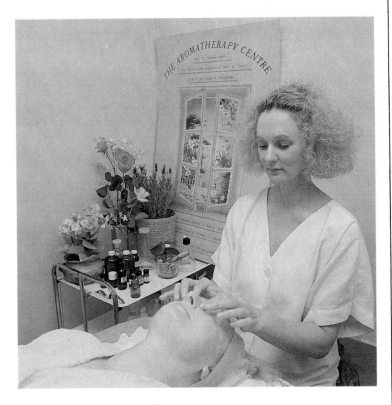

Aromatherapy utilises healing oils

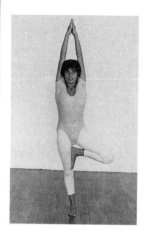

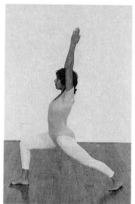

Yoga asanas

ASANAS

Yogic postures associated with the practice of meditation. There are many different asanas, the most famous being the 'lotus', in which the meditator sits upright with the legs crossed and the hands resting palm upwards on the knees. Asanas are said to assist the process of meditation by allowing currents of psychic energy to flow more readily, for example the arousal of *kundalini* through the channel *sushumna*, which corresponds to the spinal cord. Other asanas include the 'lion', 'serpent' and 'bow' postures. *See also Kundalini, Yoga.*

ASTROLOGICAL DIAGNOSIS

An ancient and medieval system — now purely of curiosity value — of correlating diseases with different signs of the zodiac. Astrology was practised by the Babylonians, Assyrians, Egyptians, Greeks and Romans, and in the Middle Ages tended to merge with other traditions like herbalism and alchemy. According to astrology, one's sun sign (or birth sign in the zodiac) highlights potential disease conditions.

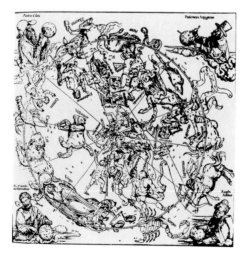

Astrological signs are said to correlate with different diseases

SIGN	DISEASES
Aries	Those of the head and face, smallpox, epilepsy, apoplexy, paralysis, measles, convulsions
Taurus	Tumours and afflictions of the neck and throat (for example tonsillitis)
Gemini	Those of the arm and shoulders, aneurisms, frenzy and insanity
Cancer	Those of the breast and stomach, cancers, consumption and asthma
Leo	Those of the heart, the back and the vertebrae of the neck, as well as fevers, jaundice and pleurisy
Virgo	Those of the viscera or internal organs (for example, the intestines)
Libra	Kidney complaints
Scorpio	Afflictions affecting the sexual organs
Sagittarius	Those of the hips and muscles, including rheumatism
Capricorn	All cutaneous diseases, those affecting the knees and 'melancholy' ailments like hysteria
Aquarius	Those of the legs and ankles, including lameness, swelling and cramps
Pisces	Those of the feet

AURA

In certain meditative and faith-healing practices, the psychic energy field that surrounds both animate and inanimate bodies. The aura can be dull or brightly coloured, and psychics — those who claim to perceive the auric colours directly — interpret the quality of the person or object according to the energy vibrations. Bright red, for example, is said to indicate anger; yellow, strong intellectual powers, and purple, spirituality. Faith-healers and psychics generally believe that the halos depicted around the head of Jesus Christ and the saints are examples of mystically pure auras. *See also Faith-healing, Kirlian photography.*

AUTOGENIC TRAINING

A method of medical self-regulation developed by Berlin-based psychiatrist Johannes H. Schultz in the late 1920s. Schultz drew on research by brain physiologist Oskar Vogt as well as Eastern mystical practices like yoga and Zen, with which he was familiar.

Dr Schultz evolved a series of 6 standard expressions designed to induce a state of deep relaxation. The subject was required to concentrate on each of the following expressions passively, while lying with the eyes closed in a quiet room. Each of the basic expressions was combined with a visualisation as follows:

1 'My right arm is heavy' (concentrate on the limb in question and repeat for the left arm, right and left legs, neck and shoulders).
2 'My right arm is warm' (repeat as above, including visualisations of each limb in turn).
3 'My heartbeat is calm and regular' (tune-in to the rhythm of the heartbeat or pulse).
4 'My breathing is calm and regular' (tune-in to the breath pattern; usually the expression induces slow, deep breathing).
5 'My solar plexus is warm' (visualise the abdomen as the centre of the body). *Note:* this visualisation should be omitted if the subject is suffering from any abdominal abnormalities and some practitioners recommend medical guidance for this exercise.
6 'My forehead is cool' (focus on the forehead and experience the sense of relaxation this exercise induces).

The series of visualisations ends with a 'return phrase':

'I am refreshed and alert'.

Autogenic training is recommended as an adjunct to other meditative visualisation approaches.

AUTO-SUGGESTION

A therapeutic technique, often used as an adjunct to hypnosis, in which the subject uses suggestion to bring about psychological or physical changes in himself. The suggestion may be an affirmation or a positive thought, and is often intended to boost self-esteem or eliminate fears or phobias. Some types of auto-suggestion can be used in hypnotherapy to overcome psychosomatic illnesses or unwanted habits like smoking or bedwetting. Auto-suggestion was developed by the Frenchman Emile Coué (1857–1926), who is famous for advising his patients to repeat the affirmation: 'Each day, and in every way, I am getting better and better'. (They were to do this silently before going to sleep each night and on awakening every day, some 15–20 times on each occasion.)

AWARENESS THROUGH MOVEMENT — *see Feldenkrais System*

AYURVEDIC MEDICINE

From the Sanskrit words *ayur* ('life') and *veda* ('knowledge'), an ancient Indian system of medicine. The *Ayurveda* is also the name of one of the four *Vedas*, Hindu sacred texts.

The ayurvedic physician divides the universe and all living things into 5 elements: *akasha* (spirit), *vayu* (air), *tejas* (fire), *apas* (water) and *prithivi* (earth). The human body is said to be made up of 7 basic constituents, or *dhatus*: *rasa* (food), *rakta* (blood), *mamsa* (bone), *meda* (fat and perspiration), *asthi* (bone marrow), *majya* (viscidity) and *shukra* (satisfying movements). As long as these elements are in balance the person remains healthy.

Ayurvedic practitioners treat the patient as a whole, advising on personal lifestyle habits, diet and choice of sexual partner, as well as taking into consideration astrological factors and evaluating the quality of urine, sweat and the voice.

Treatments include a wide range of traditional Indian remedies coupled with yogic breathing techniques, mantras, fasting, cleansing diets, bathing and enemas.

B

BACH FLOWER REMEDIES

English wildflower remedies discovered by Dr Edward Bach (1880–1936). Bach graduated from Birmingham University and University College Hospital, London, and became a Harley Street physician. However, he became increasingly convinced that medicine should not be preoccupied with disease symptoms so much as with the mental conditions underlying them.

After working for a time at the Royal London Homeopathic Hospital, he abandoned his practice altogether and in 1930 went to live in the countryside. He believed that he would be able to identify medicinal healing agents in the wildflowers growing in the fields and meadows for, as he wrote in his book *Heal Thyself*, 'Among the types of remedies that will be used will be those obtained from the most beautiful plants and herbs to be found in the pharmacy of Nature'.

Over a 7-year period Dr Bach identified 38 flowers which appeared to have healing qualities and which he believed could be used to treat emotional afflictions. Bach would take the heads of the wildflowers and place them upon the surface of water contained in a glass bowl. They were then left for 3 hours to absorb sunlight and transfer their essence to the water. Later the flowers would be removed and the water retained. With flowers growing on trees, Dr Bach adopted a different method, removing the blossoms, covering them with water and boiling them gently in a sterile saucepan for 30 minutes. The flowers were then removed and the water retained as before.

Dr Bach classified his 38 remedies under 7 headings, as follows:

For fear: rock rose, mimulus, cherry plum, aspen, red chestnut
For uncertainty: cerato, scleranthus, gentian, gorse, hornbeam, wild oat
For insufficient interest in present circumstances: clematis, honeysuckle, wild rose, olive, white chestnut, mustard, chestnut bud
For loneliness: water violet, impatiens, heather
For despondency or despair: larch, pine, elm, sweet chestnut, Star of Bethlehem, willow, oak, crab apple
For over-care of the welfare of others: chicory, vervain, vine, beech, rock water

Dr Bach believed his remedies should be taken singly, rather than in combination, but some practitioners in more recent times prefer the latter approach. Whereas the original Bach flower remedies were water-based, these days the essences are made up and preserved in alcohol.

BAREFOOT SHIATSU

A form of shiatsu originating from anma, or Chinese massage, and extended in modern practice to the whole body. While the practitioner may indeed use the naked feet to apply massage-pressure, the therapy may also involve the thumbs, elbows, knees and hands. In applying back massage the practitioner may stand on the sacrum and use the foot to work along the side of the spine and shoulder blades. Another variant, used to relieve shoulder tension, involves standing on the subject's outstretched hand and working gently on the shoulder and down the arm, again by applying pressure with the foot.

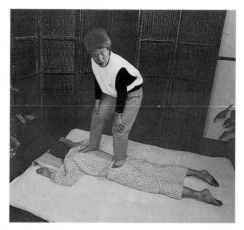

Barefoot shiatsu

BATES METHOD

A treatment developed by American eye physician and ophthalmologist Dr William H. Bates (1860–1931) who taught in the New York Postgraduate Medical School. After many years of practice, during which he examined 30 000 pairs of eyes, Bates came to believe that effective vision was substantially mental as well as physical. Defective vision could be caused as much by stress and anxiety as by deterioration of the lens. He therefore instructed his patients in relaxing the muscles around their eyes.

Dr Bates developed several specific therapeutic techniques, including *palming* and *sunning*, and was praised by English novelist Aldous Huxley — who was himself almost blind and who used the Bates Method to great personal advantage.

BIER'S HYPERAEMIC TREATMENT

A treatment developed by German physician August Bier (1861–1949) in which additional blood flow is enforced in a specific part of the body. The area to be treated is placed in a special box and hot air (62–110°C or 144°–230°F) introduced through a tube. This treatment does not extend for more than an hour on any single day.

Bier's hyperaemic treatment is recommended for sciatica, arthritis and varicose veins, and some practitioners have found it useful for cases of gangrene.

BILLINGS METHOD

Named after its discoverers, Drs John and Evelyn Billings, a technique of natural birth control based on the fact that body symptoms change at different stages of the menstrual cycle. One of the most significant changes occurs in the vaginal mucus.

During the normal menstrual cycle the mucus secreted by the cervix follows this pattern:

1 Menstrual period.
2 A few days with no mucus discharge. The interior of the vagina is moist but there is no exterior wetness.
3 A few days of 'infertile' mucus discharge, which is thick and white-yellow. This mucus is 'tacky' and sticky to touch.
4 For 4–5 days a 'fertile' mucus is discharged, and this is now thin and watery. This period indicates the approach of ovulation and sexual intercourse at this time could lead to conception since sperms can swim through the mucus.
5 Peak fertility time. The mucus is more profuse and has a texture similar to raw eggwhite. It can be stretched between the finger and the thumb.
6 After ovulation the mucus becomes cloudy, white-yellow and 'tacky', and then ceases altogether.

By observing these patterns, a woman can systematically monitor the likelihood of conception or contraception. The method is also known as the Cervical-mucus Method. *See also Natural birth control.*

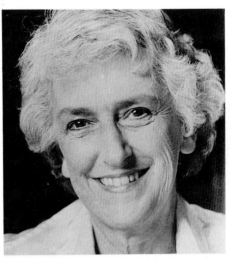

Dr Evelyn Billings

BIOENERGETICS

A term used to describe the specific form of psychotherapy developed by Alexander Lowen in the United States as an offshoot of Reichian therapy. Bioenergetics differs in emphasis by specialising in the following 3 areas:

Grounding This has to do with the subject's emotional security and provides a means of discovering one's personal sense of identity. A specific stance is employed so that the subject has positive contact with the ground.

Breathing Normal breathing patterns may be inhibited by muscular tension as a result of early emotional trauma. Breathing skills are developed by placing the body in a stressful position or by intense kicking while in a prostrate position etc.

Character Structure Bioenergetics recognises 5 character structures — the *Schizoid* (characterised by muscular patterns related to the fear of falling apart); the *Oral* (muscular patterns related to the fear of isolation or abandonment); the *Psychopathic* (muscular patterns related to the fear of failure); the *Masochistic* (muscular patterns related to inadequately asserting rights and needs) and the *Rigid* (muscular patterns related to the fear of emotional heartbreak).

In all cases the therapist guides the subject towards confronting the particular problems associated with muscular hold-ing patterns, and developing increased self-awareness. *See also Reichian therapy, Body armour.*

BIOENERGY

A term used in Reichian therapy to describe the flow of energy or life-force in the body. In Reich's view, disease or imbalance resulted from the blockage of bioenergy in different muscular segments — *see Reichian therapy.*

BIOFEEDBACK

A technique of using electronic equipment to provide visual or auditory feedback relating to physical symptoms or processes. Biofeedback machines can monitor changes in the electrical activity at the surface of the skin, which in turn reflects increases in muscle tension. These changes are interpreted electronically as light flashes, clicking noises or some similar sensory signal.

Biofeedback equipment can be used by subjects who wish to gain some degree of control over involuntary or 'autonomic' processes in the body — such as heart

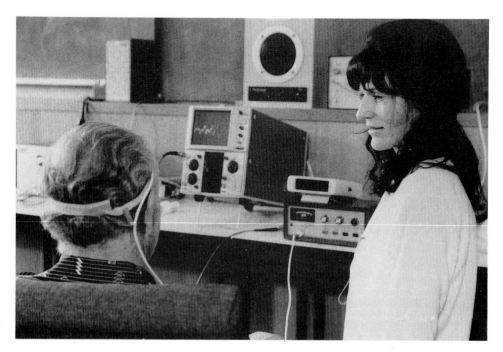

Monitoring pain and tension with biofeedback

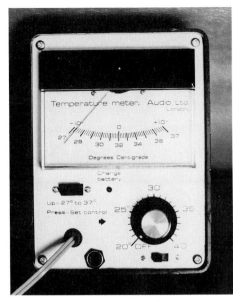

A temperature meter used in biofeedback

rate and blood pressure. The equipment is also useful as a meditative device, providing feedback when a certain brainwave frequency (for example, alpha or theta) comes to the fore in one's spectrum of consciousness.

Biofeedback equipment was pioneered in San Francisco by Dr Joe Kamiya and has been used widely in relaxation therapy. Sophisticated biofeedback machines have been developed in Britain by C. Maxwell Cade and Geoffrey Blundell and these are able to monitor a number of physiological functions, including cortisone levels in the body. Dr Elmer Green of the Menninger Institute in Kansas also believes biofeedback is useful in treating migraines, gastrointestinal disorders, asthma, epilepsy and cerebral palsy.

BIORHYTHMS

A concept of energy cycles which influence personal effectiveness, creativity and general health patterns from day to day. Biorhythms were discovered independently by two scientists, Dr Hermann Swoboda, Professor of Psychology at the University of Vienna, and Dr Wilhelm Fliess, who later became President of the German Academy of Sciences. Dr Swoboda kept records of his patients' health patterns and distinguished 2 specific cycles — the first *physical*, extending over 23 days, and the second *emotional*, extending over 28 days. Dr Fliess, working in Berlin, also found substantial evidence to support the concept of these cycles.

A third biorhythm, the *intellectual*, was discovered by Alfred Teltscher, an Austrian engineer who tested patterns of academic performance at a college and high school in Innsbruck. This biorhythm was based on a 33-day cycle.

According to the principle of biorhythms, life is a series of progressive 'ups' and 'downs'. The physical cycle includes resistance to disease, strength, and coordination. The emotional includes sensitivity, mood, perceptions and mental balance, and the intellectual affects memory, alertness and logic. Because the cycles are of varying length, they rarely overlap. For example, while the intellectual cycle may be peaking, the emotional cycle may be in decline, and the physical cycle a variant somewhere in between. The 'highs' of the cycles are times of maximum effectiveness, and tend to produce positive thoughts and moods, while the 'lows' are times of negativity and possible risk — because one is prone at these times to make errors of judgement.

The concept of biorhythms allows each person to highlight periods which feature combined positive aspects (or their negative counterpart) on any given day. Each individual cycle begins from zero on the day of birth, and tables are available which show specific rhythm-patterns on a day-by-day basis. The cycle does not return to a baseline or zero position for 58 years and 67 (or 68) days.

The concept of biorhythms has been succinctly explained by American public relations analyst Bernard Gittelson in his book *Biorhythm* (New York, 1977).

BODY ARMOUR

Concept in Reichian Therapy that different muscles in the body record the memory of past traumatic events. Repression of negative emotions blocks the flow of life-energy through the body and, in addition, the muscles 'armour' themselves as a protection against the recall of these repressed feelings to consciousness. According to Reich, 'the body is frozen history'. *See also Reichian therapy.*

Bodywork — encompassing physical movement and massage

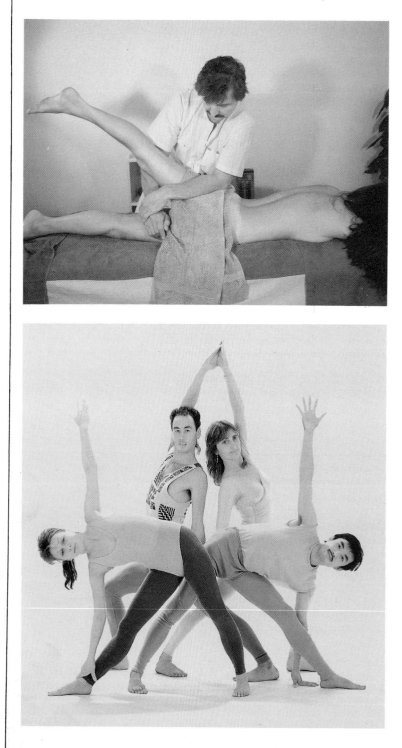

BODYWORK

A general term used to describe a wide range of physical therapies effective for freeing muscle spasms, correcting poor posture and maximising efficient body use. It also includes cathartic techniques which release emotional trauma expressed in the musculature of the body. Bodywork techniques include the many different forms of massage and therapeutic yoga, as well as the Alexander Technique, chiropractic, osteopathy, shiatsu, Reichian therapy, Rolfing, Trager therapy, deep tissue muscle therapy, rebirthing and shintaido — *see separate listings.*

BO-SHIN

A traditional Chinese system of analysing health conditions through facial analysis. By this method, indicators in different parts of the face provide clues to the health of the internal organs and body systems.

The face is divided into 3 horizontal zones: the nervous system corresponds to the area above the eyes, the circulatory system to the area from the eyes to the top of the lips, and the digestive system to the area of the mouth and chin. In other correlations the eyes are linked to the liver and spleen, the ears to the kidneys, and the nose to the lungs and heart. The ear, meanwhile, is considered in Chinese medicine to be the major diagnostic organ, epitomising the body as a whole. Here the inner ear or concha relates to the digestive tract, the middle section or anti-helix provides keys to the health of the nervous system, and the outer ear, or helix, relates to the circulatory system.

BRAZILIAN TOE MASSAGE

A form of massage which utilises acupuncture meridians ending in the toes. In acupuncture theory the meridians connected to the organs all end in the toes: the spleen and liver connect with the big toe, the stomach with the second biggest toe, the bladder with the central toe, the gall bladder with the second smallest toe and the kidney with the small toe. By holding the toes, a *chi* energy connection is made between practitioner and patient, the masseur being able to channel energy and in turn influence the organs of the other person.

The masseur holds both central toes lightly at their tips with his central fingers and thumbs, and retains this position for 3 minutes. He then proceeds to treat the other toes for the same length of time, using specific fingers in combination with the thumb. In the case of massage applied to the big toe, the first 2 fingers and the thumb are used conjointly because there are 2 meridians in this toe.

Brazilian toe massage is deeply relaxing and has also proven to be effective in treating insomnia and headaches.

BREAST SELF-EXAMINATION

A precautionary 3-step method for women to detect early signs of breast cancer. The method involves monitoring the breasts for changes and should be carried out once a month, during the week following menstruation.

BUDO

A general term for Japanese martial arts, also used in describing aspects of bodywork therapies which have derived from them; for example aikido, shintaido.

C

CALCIUM RING — *see*
Sodium ring, Iridology

CALISTHENICS

A form of light gymnastic exercise including sit-ups, stretching movements, jumps and push-ups, intended to build the muscles and promote physical health and well-being.

CANCER PERSONALITY

A concept developed by Dr Lawrence LeShan, Dr Carl Simonton and others, proposing a relationship between psychological factors, stress, and the outbreak of cancer.

Dr LeShan compared 250 cancer patients with 150 non-cancer subjects and found the following patterns:

- 77% of cancer subjects but only 14% of healthy subjects showed extreme tension over the loss of a close relative or friend.
- 64% of cancer subjects, as opposed to 32% non-cancer, showed signs of not being able to adequately express anger, resentment or aggression towards other people, but instead bottled up their feelings.
- 69% of cancer patients had low personal esteem, while only 34% of the control group showed this characteristic.
- Typically, cancer subjects experienced a major emotional trauma 6 to 18 months prior to the development of the disease.

Dr Simonton believes that the most pronounced characteristics of cancer subjects are:

- a tendency to hold resentment and a marked inability to forgive;
- an inclination towards self-pity;

- a poor ability to develop and maintain meaningful, long-term relationships;
- a poor self-image.

CELLULAR MEMORY

A concept in Reichian therapy and deep tissue muscle therapy that fears and negative emotions are carried in the body at a deep muscular level. The body in turn forms a bond of protective muscle 'armour' which shields the body from the outside world. Therapeutic deep tissue massage is designed to work through these layers of body armour and release the fear trapped at the cellular level. *See also Reichian therapy, Deep tissue muscle therapy, Body armour.*

CERVICAL-MUCUS METHOD — *see Billings Method*

CERVICAL SEGMENT

One of 7 body segments in Reichian therapy. The cervical segment includes the deep muscles of the neck, the platysma, the sternocleido and the tongue. Common emotions associated with armouring in this segment are sadness and fear. These may derive from childhood memories of parental rage (threatening to 'cut the child's throat') or the stoic attempt to 'keep one's head above water' — an emotion which often results in a stiff neck! Reichian therapy in this segment includes forceful yelling and a variety of tongue exercises. *See Reichian therapy.*

CHAKRAS

A term used in kundalini yoga to denote the spiritual nerve-centres that align with the central nervous column, *sushumna*. The yogi learns to arouse kundalini energy through the chakras from the base of the spine to the crown of the forehead. The chakras, from the lowest to highest in sequence, are *muladhara* (located near the genitals), *svadisthana* (solar plexus),

manipura (spleen), *anahata* (chest), *visuddha* (neck) *ajna* (between the eyebrows) and *sahasrara* (crown of the head). The meaning of the Hindu word *chakra* is 'wheel', but the symbolism implies a spiritual centre. The chakras do not correspond literally to any organ and are mystical rather than physiological in nature. *See also Yoga, Kundalini.*

CHELATION THERAPY

Chelation, from a scientific viewpoint, is the incorporation of a metallic or mineral ion into a heterocyclic ring structure. In chelation therapy small amounts of the amino acid disodium ethylenediamine tetra-acetic acid (3.0 g infused as a 0.5% solution) are injected into the bloodstream, usually to treat vascular disorders and conditions relating to calcium tissue deposits. According to Drs Morton Walker and Gary Gordon, in *The Chelation Answer* (1982), this form of therapy has an average 82 per cent success rate for improving blood circulation. It also appears to temporarily lower blood calcium levels, stimulating the body to draw on calcium sources elsewhere in the organism, especially pathological deposits. Chelation therapy seems also to assist in restoring metabolic health by removing toxic heavy metals like lead and mercury and restoring normal enzyme functioning. This therapy may also be suitable for treating arterial spasm, blood clots, plaque formation and arthritis. Many practitioners believe it to be the main alternative to coronary bypass surgery (there are now around 200 000 bypass operations in the United States each year).

CHI (or CH'I)

In traditional Chinese medicine, the flow of energy in the body. It is also known as 'the breath of life'. Practitioners of acupuncture believe that *chi* flows through channels of the body known as 'meridians', and that an imbalance of *chi* leads to disease. Stimulation of acupuncture points along these meridians helps to rectify this imbalance. In Japan, *chi* is designated *ki. See also Acupuncture, Meridian.*

CHI KUNG

A technique of 'Standing Zen' in which the mind directs the breath, thereby activating the *chi* energy which vitalises the entire body. Chi Kung utilises a vertical stance and a variety of arm and hand gestures accompanied by strict breath control. During the in-breath, through the nose, the stomach expands but the upper chest and shoulders do not move. The lungs are filled with air, held for a slow count of 3 and the air is expelled through the nose.

CHINA

A homeopathic remedy derived from the yellow bark of the Peruvian cinchona tree, *Cinchona officinalis*, which is also used to produce quinine. The substance is of special historical significance because the founder of homeopathy, Samuel Hahnemann, used cinchona in an experiment on himself. In this experiment he compared the similarity in symptoms between an unhealthy person suffering from malaria and a healthy person taking cinchona. This led him to formulate the homeopathic Law of Similars.

China is now used in homeopathic potencies to treat weakness caused by loss of blood, exhaustion following pneumonia or influenza, fevers accompanied by chills, and states of dizziness and nervous irritability. It may also help those suffering from tinnitus, or ringing in the ears. China is indicated for chronic rather than acute disease conditions. *See also Cinchona bark* (Part 1).

CHIROPRACTIC

A modern technique of physical therapy developed by Daniel David Palmer (1845-1913). The word 'chiropractic' derives from the Greek *cheiro* and

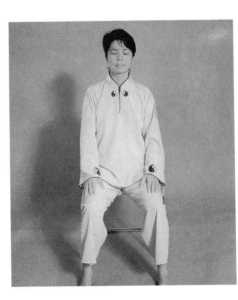

Chi Kung — meditative breathing

practikos, meaning 'done with the hands'. As a therapy, chiropractic focuses primarily on complaints related to irregularities of the spinal column — as well as other bones and joints — and on manipulative techniques that can rectify these problems.

Chiropractic is used to treat a wide range of disorders. These include complaints like sciatica — caused by a 'pinched nerve' resulting from displaced vertebrae exerting pressure on sensitive nerve-endings — as well as occipital and facial neuralgia, circulatory problems, postural disorders like kyphosis, scoliosis and lordosis, lumbago, and various types of spasm.

Some practitioners maintain that they can also treat conditions like bronchial asthma, colitis, constipation and appendicitis through chiropractic — especially where such disorders are related to postural problems or spinal misalignments.

Chiropractic bears some resemblance to osteopathy, and it is not uncommon for practitioners to hold qualifications in both therapies. Chiropractic tends to place more emphasis on the role of the nervous system, whereas osteopathy emphasises the relationship of blood circulation to healthy tissue. Both chiropractic and osteopathy remain 'alternative' health-care therapies, but within this range of treatments they are among the least controversial. Many orthodox doctors now accept the role of chiropractic and osteopathy as an adjunct to physiotherapy and therapeutic massage.

CHROMOTHERAPY — *see Colour therapy*

CLINICAL ECOLOGY

A study of the links between environmental factors and illness, which also encompasses the apparent connection between nutritional deficiencies and some forms of mental illness. It also includes the study of diseases caused by food allergies which may in turn be linked to chemicals, environmental pollutants or other similar factors. Illnesses which may sometimes be associated with food allergies or environmental factors include asthma, depression, eczema, migraine, obesity, hypertension and schizophrenia.

COLONIC IRRIGATION

A naturopathic technique of cleansing the colon with water, usually to treat chronic constipation, biliousness, diarrhoea or indigestion. The patient lies relaxed on a table and the practitioner introduces water into the colon with a syringe, cleansing it. The water is allowed to flow back out again. Mineral oils may also be used as lubricants. *See also Enema.*

COLOUR BREATHING

A technique of visualisation combining aspects of colour therapy and meditation. The subject relaxes using a slow and even breathing rhythm, and visualises him/herself feeling happy and positive. He/she then imagines a beam of coloured light entering the solar plexus with the inward breath, and spreading through the body beneath the skin. The outward breath is used to visualise the release of toxic substances from the organism.

The colour selected for visualisation depends on the healing function required: different colours have different therapeutic applications *(see table)*.

COLOUR THERAPY

A therapeutic technique of applying coloured light to the body for a healing purpose. Some aspects of colour therapy are quite orthodox. A study at the New England State Hospital in the United States showed that during a half-hour period, staff members bathed in blue light universally recorded a drop in blood pressure, whereas red light caused the blood pressure to rise.

Other variant therapies are more controversial, and more mystical. Dr Dinshah Ghadiali believed that his patients would benefit from drinking water irradiated by different coloured light. Swiss-born therapist Theo Gimbel, who now resides in England, believes blue is the most healing colour, but that orange can serve as an antidepressant and turquoise can be used to rest the nervous system and reduce inflammatory conditions. Gimbel has extended his research to include techniques of colour visualisation and diet control using foods of a specific colour. *See also Colour breathing.*

COMPLEMENTARY MEDICINE

An expression preferred by some to the term 'alternative medicine'. The emphasis here is that the alternative health modalities like herbalism, osteopathy, chiropractic, acupuncture, iridology and naturopathy, should complement orthodox medicine, rather than compete with it as a direct alternative. Some practitioners of holistic health, for example, emphasise that the role of orthodox medicine is primarily curative, and that many of the 'alternative' therapies emphasise preventive health care, sound diet and nutrition, and the psychosomatic aspects of disease — areas of medicine that have not been considered important until comparatively recently.

COLOUR SELECTION CHART

RED

Properties: Warm, the ray of strength and vitality, a stimulant.
Opposite colour: Blue.
Therapeutic action: Increases the temperature, heart beat, circulation and stimulates the liver and spleen.
Use for: Lumbago, rheumatoid arthritis, sciatica, anaemia, colds, paralysis. Raises blood pressure, releases adrenalin. Stimulates hearing, seeing, smelling, tasting, touching. Exhaustion. Cleans blood.
Negative action: Should not be used by alcoholics or ruddy, overweight types, people with high blood pressure or on inflamed conditions.
Red foods: Beetroot, tomatoes, red cabbage, spinach, silverbeet, cherries, currants, watermelon, grapes, whole wheat, liver, radishes.
Variants: Scarlet — courage, sex stimulant, helps potency and frigidity, raises blood pressure, renal, heart, kidney and adrenal stimulant.
Pink — raises emotional vibrations, the colour of universal healing. Useful in rejuvenating the skin, removing wrinkles, acne, puffiness and sagginess. Removes scars caused by surgery or childbearing. Reduces weight.
Magenta — boosts vitality rate, cardiac and adrenal tonic, stimulates genitals, revitalises spine.

ORANGE

Properties: Warm, the ray of energy, a stimulant.
Opposite colour: Indigo.
Therapeutic action: Energises the thyroid gland, increases vital energy, depresses para-thyroid action, expands lung action, activates respiratory system. Has emetic effect. Can be used when red cannot.
Use for: Coughs, colds, bronchitis, cramps or muscle spasms. Toning up digestive system, stimulating milk-production after childbirth, relieving asthma and ulcer conditions. Increases enthusiasm, stimulates pancreas.
Negative action: Should not be used in acute inflammatory states.
Orange foods: Carrots, pumpkins, oranges, peaches, apricots, canteloupe, mangoes, eggs and dairy products.
Variants: Orchid — for spiritual attunement.
Gold — for healing in general, helps put a gloss and shine to the hair. Colour breathing of orange ray will transmute brown and grey moods.

YELLOW

Properties: Warm, the ray of intellect. It activates the motor nerves and generates energy for muscles. A stimulant.
Opposite colour: Violet.
Therapeutic action: Stimulates the mind, relieves lethargy, activates digestive system, liver and kidneys. Increases skin secretion. Acts as a tonic and blood cleanser. Activates colon and sluggish lymphatics.
Use for: All sluggish conditions, revitalising the whole system, fluid retention, constipation, increasing mental capabilities, strengthening the nervous system, paralysis of all kinds.
Negative action: Should not be used in hyperactive states, overexcitement, nausea, diarrhoea, irritability or by those who suffer from insomnia.
Yellow foods: Corn, bananas, pineapples, lemons, grapefruit, parsnips, butter, eggs, cheese.
Variant: Lemon — relieves colds, stimulates thymus gland, increases brain activity, blood cleanser, tonic, stimulates motor nerves. Removes toxic waste. Bone and tissue builder. Useful where congestion is present.

GREEN

Properties: Cool, the ray of harmony and the master healer, a relaxant.
Opposite colour: Magenta.
Therapeutic action: A tonic, it strengthens without stimulating or sedating. Helps combat infection, builds cell tissue. Excellent for insomnia and irritability. Soothes stomach and liver inflammation. Improves vision. Calms nerves.
Use for: Relieving exhaustion and inflamed conditions. Insomnia, hypertension, headaches, sore eyes, emotional upsets.
Negative action: Should not be used in anaemic conditions.
Green foods: All green vegetables, celery, asparagus, peas, beans, cabbage.
Variant: Turquoise — cools fevers, reduces weight, prime skin builder, hastens formation of new skin, relieves pain, has quietening effect on overactive mental states. For treating sunburn, relieving itching and a general tonic to the skin.

BLUE

Properties: Cool, the ray of inspiration and a relaxant.
Opposite colour: Red.
Therapeutic action: Relieves inflammation and fever, heals burns and pain of all kinds. It has a calming, soothing effect and is an astringent, and antiseptic.
Use for: Burns, itching, eczema, laryngitis. Activating the pituitary gland and the etheric body. For pain of any kind. Lowers the blood pressure.
Negative action: Should not be used when fatigue, depression, paralysis or constipation is present.
Blue foods: Berries, grapes, prunes and plums.
Variant: Dark blue — mends bones.

INDIGO

Properties: Cool, the ray of intuition and a relaxant.
Opposite colour: Orange.
Therapeutic action: Has sedative and pain-relieving qualities. Stimulates the para-thyroid gland. Depresses the thyroid gland and respiratory system. Helps reduce bleeding and excessive menstrual flow. Stimulates formation of white blood cells in the spleen.
Use for: Diseases of the eye, ear and nose. Cornea, styes, deafness and cataracts. Pneumonia, pain and inflammation. Swelling, convulsions, tonsillitis, whooping cough, haemorrhages. Toning muscles, nerves and skin. Relieving the pain of colitis.
Negative action: Should not be used when chills are present.
Indigo foods: Blueberries, blue plums, blue grapes.
Variant: Purple — depresses the sex drive, activates without irritating the liver, lungs and kidneys. An inspirational colour.

VIOLET

Properties: Cool, the ray of spirituality and a relaxant.
Opposite colour: Yellow.
Therapeutic action: Stimulates the pineal gland, sedates the mind and nervous system. A powerful bactericide and parasiticide. Encourages bone growth, activates white blood-cell production. Depresses lymph and motor nerves, maintains potassium-sodium balance in body.
Use for: Bladder trouble, cramps, concussion, epilepsy, neuralgia, nervous and mental disorders, sciatica, dandruff, dermatitis. Lowering heart rate, inducing sleep. Soothing tired nerves and overactive adrenals.
Negative action: Should not be used when energy is required, when chills are present or when depressed.
Violet foods: Eggplant, red cabbage, blackberries.
Variant: Lavender — eases tired nerves, relaxes the muscles. Induces sleep.

From Fai Chivell Hast, 'Colour Healing and Colour Breathing' in N. Drury (ed.), *Inner Health*, Harper & Row, Sydney, 1985.

COMPRESS

A pack of compressed wet linen or towelling used to reduce inflammation. Packs of this type can be applied to areas of the body which are sprained, bruised or swollen. Cold compresses relieve pain and congestion in swollen areas by repelling excess blood which has been drawn to the region. Hot compresses are useful for areas where there is pain but no swelling. Sometimes herbs like witch hazel or homeopathic treatments like arnica are also used with compresses.

CONNECTED BREATH CYCLE

In rebirthing, a type of breathing pattern in which there is no pause between the in-breath and the out-breath. This form of breathing causes hyperventilation and tetany, and is used in rebirthing to allow a patient to overcome subconscious traumas and emotional blockages — *see Rebirthing*.

Connected breathing in rebirthing

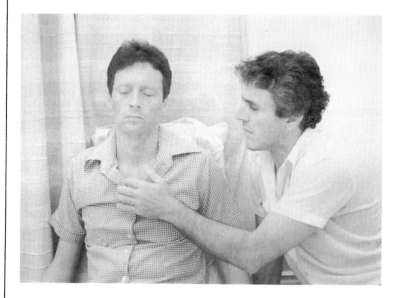

CONTRAINDICATION

A symptom or condition which indicates that a given treatment could be inadvisable.

COPPER

A metal with apparent healing qualities. Copper bracelets and bangles are often worn to alleviate bodily aches and pains — especially rheumatism. Professor W. R. Walker of the University of Newcastle, Australia, believes that traces of copper possibly dissolve in the perspiration, merge with a natural amino acid, and enter the veins — thereby reaching the source of inflammation. Copper bracelets seem to be especially effective for people living in damp or humid conditions.

COUEISM

A therapeutic approach developed by Emile Coué, the French hypnotherapist. *See Auto-suggestion*.

CRANIAL OSTEOPATHY

A branch of osteopathy specialising in the study of the bones of the skull (cranium) and their relationship to ill-health. Pioneered by Dr William G. Sutherland, cranial osteopathy recognises that the skull is not solid but consists of several interlocking bones. Surrounding each of these bones is a layer of membrane which allows a slight amount of movement in the sutures, or joints. Distortions, or lesions, in these sutures can interfere with fluid motion in the craniospinal compartment and have an adverse affect, in turn, on the spinal cord. Dr Sutherland's 'cranial concept' includes recognition of the inherent motility of the brain and spinal cord; fluctuations in cerebro-spinal fluid; mobility of the dura mater (reciprocal tension membrane) within the skull and spine; articular mobility of the cranial bones, and involuntary mobility of the sacrum between the ilia.

Cranial osteopathy has proved effective in treating a variety of disease symptoms including deafness, sinusitis, facial pain and lower back pain. Practitioners believe that some forms of apparent retardation may also be associated with a rigid cranium, perhaps compressed during birth, and that cranial manipulation may facilitate normal patterns of development.

CUPPING

In massage, a technique of tapotement in which the thumb is fully stretched and the fingers and the palm of the hand are slightly domed. The tip of the thumb should also touch the index finger. In cupping, the wrists are held rigid and the main movement is from the elbow, down. The hands alternate in their contact with the patient's body. *See also Tapotement.*

CUPPING

An ancient technique used to cause blood to rise to the surface of inflamed areas of the skin. Thick glass or metal cups are taken and herbs or cottonwool burnt inside them. After the burning process is complete the warm cups are placed on the skin, creating a partial vacuum as the cup cools. Blood now flows more readily through the small blood vessels as the cups are left in position for up to 10 minutes. The process may be repeated several times on different parts of the body.

D

DEEP TISSUE MUSCLE THERAPY

A form of therapeutic massage designed to adjust the skeletal system and return the body to its natural postural alignment. Poor diet and stress factors can cause the muscles to shrink, restricting elasticity and body movement. Deep tissue muscle therapy (DTMT) seeks to restore full rotational movement to the joints and improve the blood circulation to all parts of the body. Because muscular shrinkage often derives from emotional factors and psychological holding patterns, it is not uncommon for DTMT sessions to produce a strong emotional and cathartic response in the patient. To this extent DTMT resembles some aspects of Rolfing and Reichian therapy, and employs related terminology. As American DTMT therapist John Cottone has expressed it, 'The DTMT process works through the armament and liberates the body, allowing the blocked emotional and psychological energy and cellular memory fears, to be brought to the surface and dissipated.'

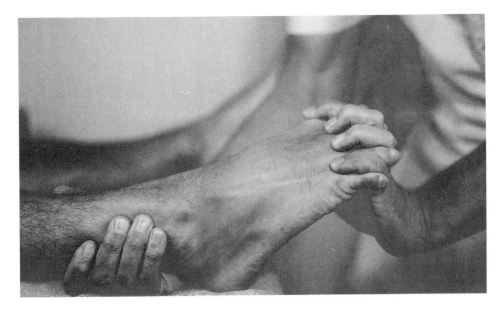

Applying pressure in deep tissue muscle therapy

DIAGNOSTIC WITNESS

A selection of tissues, organs and disease entities in homeopathic potency, which can be used in dowsing practices, counterposed against a blood sample from the patient. A diagnostic witness is used by practitioners of psionic medicine, who utilise a W. O. Wood chart. The witness is placed in the left-hand corner of the chart, directly opposite the blood sample on the right. *See W. O. Wood chart, Psionic medicine, Dowsing, Radiesthesia, medical.*

DIAPHRAGMATIC SEGMENT

One of 7 body segments in Reichian therapy. The diaphragmatic segment includes the diaphragm, stomach, pancreas, solar plexus, gall bladder, liver, duodenum, kidneys and the muscles of the lower thoracic vertebrae. Fear held in this segment may manifest as lordosis, and body armour here may lead to the sensation of 'knots in the stomach'. Peptic ulcers, liver conditions and diabetes may also have their origin in this segment, in some instances. *See also Reichian therapy, Lordosis* (Part 3).

Dowsing more than 400 years ago, from George Agricola's De Re Metallica

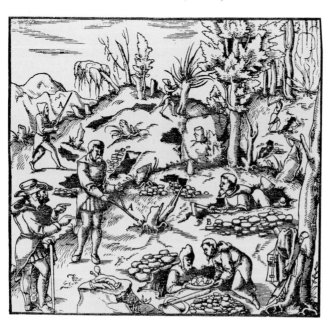

DILUTIONS, HOMEOPATHIC

When a homeopathic medicine is added to a solution of distilled water and alcohol in the ratio of 1 part medicine to 9 parts water, it is known as a 1x dilution. In a 1:99 ratio, such a medicine is referred to as an 1c dilution. Many homeopathic remedies are of a 6c strength and are taken at 4-hourly intervals until an improvement in health occurs. Examples include *Nux vomica* 6c for stomach upsets, *Arsenicum album* 6c for diarrhoea, and *Gelsemium* 6c for influenza.

DO-IN

A form of shiatsu that can be performed on oneself (the term means 'self-stimulation'). Like acupuncture and shiatsu, do-in stimulates acupuncture points on the meridians and is intended to provide relief from specific symptoms associated with an imbalance of *chi* energy. *See also Shiatsu, Acupuncture, Meridian.*

DOUCHE

A strong spray or jet of water directed onto the body — either generally or to a specific location — for the purpose of cleansing. The bathroom shower is a common form of douche, while the Scotch douche consists of a stream of hot water applied for 1 to 5 minutes, followed by a cold stream of 5 to 30 seconds. The douche is a useful way of cleansing a body cavity such as the vagina.

DOWSING

A traditional practice of locating underground water by means of a divining rod. The rod is Y-shaped and is usually made of hazel, metal, or substitute woods like rowan or ash. As the dowser walks above the location of the underground water, the rod jerks in an involuntary and spontaneous manner, indicating the depth and location of the water.

The dowsing principle has also been applied in a medical context to the practice of radiesthesia, which utilises a pendulum that is allowed to sway above the patient's body. The different movements of the pendulum are believed to indicate the presence or absence of life-force and vitality, and disease is regarded in this situation as a form of energy imbalance. *See Radiesthesia, medical.*

E

EFFLEURAGE

In massage, a technique of rubbing or stroking the body with gliding movements, usually at the beginning or end of a session. Effleurage has a calming-down effect, and is applied with soft to medium pressure in a slow and rhythmic manner.

ELECTRO-ACUPUNCTURE

A form of acupuncture stimulation using electronic equipment. One form involves the use of a TENS machine (transcutaneous electrical nerve stimulation), in which specific acu-points are stimulated to trigger an endorphin response in the brain. Electro-acupuncture is especially beneficial for treating both chronic and acute pain conditions, and for reducing the need for analgesic drugs after surgical operations. The preferred frequencies are 10–200 Hz for acute levels of pain, and 2–3 Hz for chronic pain. *See also Acupuncture.*

ENCOUNTER THERAPY

A therapeutic approach which developed from humanistic psychology during the 1960s. Associated with such figures as Carl Rogers, Fritz Perls and Will Schutz, encounter therapy emphasises the 'self-actualised' person and seeks to uncover processes which enable participants to rediscover pleasure, joy and self-fulfilment.

In encounter groups, between 10 and 15 people may sit in a circle, without a specified leader, and seek to 'reach' and perceive each other in a real and genuine way. Such therapy depends on developing honest relationships with the other participants and expressing one's feelings — verbally or physically.

Gestalt therapy, as practised by the late Fritz Perls, was an especially direct and confronting form of encounter therapy.

ENEMA

A single, direct stream of water propelled into the colon with a fountain syringe, for cleansing purposes. The method resembles, but is less gentle than, colonic irrigation — *see Colonic irrigation.*

Encounter therapy — baring the soul

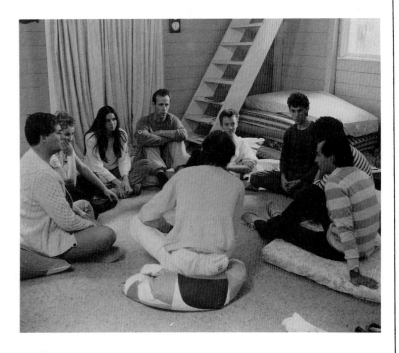

F

FACE MASK

In natural cosmetic health care, a hydrating treatment in which a face-cloth or piece of foam is wrung in hot water and applied over the face after it has been massaged with a vitamin-enriched cream oil. Holes may be cut in the mask for the eyes and nose, and a typical treatment takes 10 minutes. Face masks make the face soft and smooth.

FACIAL STEAM BATH

A remedial steam bath used to cleanse the face and rejuvenate the skin. Just over 1 litre of boiling water is used, together with ½ cup of dried herbs (alternatively, 1–2 cups of fresh herbs). The hair is tied back and the face held about 30 cm above the bowl containing the hot water. The lowered head and bowl are then covered with a draped towel and the person allows the steam-vapour to rise up onto the face for 4–10 minutes. The face can later be sponged with cottonwool which has been dipped in lavender water. Herbs recommended for the facial steam bath include marigold, chamomile and lime flowers, sage or peppermint.

FAITH-HEALING

A form of healing in which both healer and patient appeal to some form of spiritual authority — a god, ancestor spirit, the Holy Ghost, etc. — to intercede in a person's illness and restore health. *See Spiritual healing, Psychic surgery.*

FASTING

A health practice in which food intake is eliminated for purposes of internal bodily cleansing, weight reduction and the elimination of toxins.

The body consists of five-eighths water; when the person fasting stops eating there is a sodium reduction — sodium helps retain water in the body — and for this reason alone, fasting causes a dramatic drop in body weight. However, the body also begins to draw on its reserves, which are contained in food stocks in the body cells, glycogen in the liver, protein in the blood, and fat deposits which have been stored. This, too, causes weight reduction.

Fasts should be carefully controlled, preferably with the aid of a specialist nutritionist. Usually transitional stages are involved in a fast. For example, solid foods may be restricted to fruit, then replaced by diluted fruit juice, and then — for 1 or 2 days — water alone. Fasts should be adapted to individual requirements and usually last for 7–10 days.

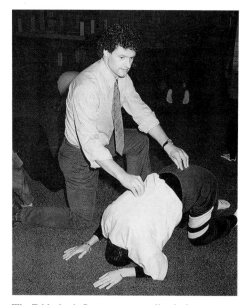

The Feldenkrais System — expanding body awareness

FELDENKRAIS SYSTEM

A system of 'Awareness Through Movement' and 'functional integration' developed by Russian-born Israeli educator Moshe Feldenkrais. Feldenkrais based his method on the importance of awareness in human functioning. According to his approach we live in 4 possible states: asleep, awake, conscious and aware. Consciousness is a higher level of being aware, but awareness has to be developed.

Awareness cannot be taught verbally, but has to be experienced, and Feldenkrais' method involved creating appropriate situations for non-coercive, non-cerebral learning. In particular, Feldenkrais advocated the idea that movement was both the essence of life and the embodiment of intention — a direct expression of the brain. His lesson involved both habitual and non-habitual body movements, and he would encourage participants to accomplish movements and postures which they had previously thought were unattainable. People in his classes felt exhilarated, more alive, when they were able to move and express themselves in new ways. Always, however, participants learned through experience, rather than by being taught specific details. 'You only learn what you already know', said Feldenkrais, '. . . learning is the crystallisation of experience.'

Feldenkrais' work with functional integration involved treating the nervous system primarily through the skeletal structure, by using gentle physical manipulation. Here physical support would be given to sections of the body to offset gravity, returning the body to an early childhood state. Feldenkrais' aim was to undo the emotional and cultural programming inflicted on people from childhood, and to teach new ways of expressing natural impulses. For him, physical distortions were as much in the brain as in the body, and it was not until outmoded perceptions and inhibitions in the cortex could be broken down that new types of physical behaviour could be developed. 'People are not a bunch of properties', he once said, 'They are a process. All life is a process. Improve the quality of the process and the rest will take care of itself.'

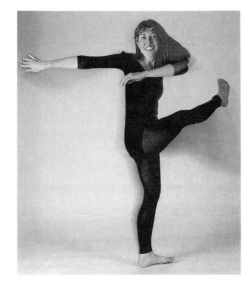

Fitness and exercise aid well-being

FITNESS

Current scientific research shows that while physical fitness does not guarantee cardiovascular health, it certainly tones the muscles, can help develop resistance to debilitating diseases, generally improves efficiency and stamina, and can even enhance emotional well-being.

Fitness is generally attained through regular aerobic exercises, which in turn are designed to promote the use of oxygen to burn fuel in active muscles. In principle, aerobic exercises are designed to leave the practitioner refreshed rather than exhausted, and they include jogging, lap swimming, fast cycling, aerobic dancing, rope jumping and brisk walking. These activities, performed continuously for around 20 minutes, significantly increase the heart and breathing rate. The heart becomes more efficient in its action, pumping more oxygen-rich blood into the working muscles with less effort. In addition, conditioned lungs hold more air and those who are fit need fewer breaths to sustain a given type of physical activity.

The main benefits of exercise are as follows:

• It increases the quality of high-density lipoproteins (HDLs) which remove cholesterol from the blood vessels and help to excrete it. To this extent, therefore, exercise lowers blood cholesterol levels.

- It reduces the quantity of triglycerides, an artery-damaging type of blood-fat.
- It helps reduce the incidence of clots that might clog the blood vessels and thus lead to a heart attack or stroke.
- It enables practitioners to work off excess body fat.
- It helps reduce muscular tension and anxiety, and therefore promotes a sense of well-being.

See also Aerobics, Jogging.

FLICKING

In massage, a technique of tapotement in which the fingers are slightly bent and kept loose and flexible. Body contact is made with the edge of the little finger, followed by the top of the ring finger and the tip of the middle finger — in that order. In this form of tapotement the wrists are kept flexible. *See also Tapotement.*

FLOAT TO RELAX

A practice of floating naked inside a sensory isolation tank. The original tanks — which utilised seawater — were pioneered by Dr John Lilly in the 1950s while he was working for the National Institute of Mental Health in the USA. Dr Lilly believed that because the experience gave an impression akin to floating gravity-free in space, that it would lead to 'inner security and a new integration . . . on a deep and basic level'.

Lilly's design was modified by Glenn Perry to replace the seawater with Epsom salts, which had no effect on the skin or hair. The new tanks developed into the samadhi tanks that are now available for commercial purchase or hire.

In Float to Relax tanks the participant floats for around 45 minutes in salinated water heated to 'ambient skin temperature' (35.2°C). During the float, the idea is to surrender one's stress and tensions, and retreat for a time from the pressures of the outside world. To this extent the Float to Relax system resembles medi-

tation. However, it also has other health benefits. Freeing the musculo-skeletal system from gravity eases pressure on the back and joints, and allows energy to be released to other parts of the body. Floating also stimulates right-hemisphere brain function, enhancing one's capacity for creativity and intuition. *See also Samadhi tank.*

'FULL LOTUS' POSTURE — *see 'Lotus' posture*

FUNCTIONAL INTEGRATION — *see Feldenkrais system*

G

GEM THERAPY

The use of gems for a healing purpose. Gems are often used by spiritual healers to focus energies in their patients, and can also be worn touching the skin, to allow their subtle vibrations to penetrate the body. Gems also equate with the signs of the zodiac and in this capacity are referred to as 'birthstones'. Examples of healing gems are as follows:

Ruby (Aries) *Virtues:* strength and vitality. May be used for its assertive qualities or to reinforce physical health and well-being.

Emerald (Taurus) *Virtues:* purity and stability. May be used to cool inflammation (especially in the eyes) and to develop the power of love.

Citrine (Gemini) *Virtues:* clarity and insight. May be used to develop the intellectual faculties of the mind and also to reduce pain.

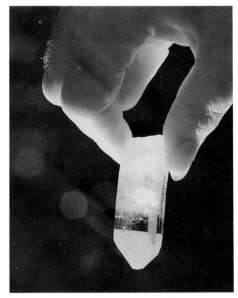

Gems have specific healing qualities

Pearl (Cancer) *Virtues:* patience and inner strength. Usually associated with feminine principles, it may be used to enhance the maternal instincts and the capacity for enduring love.

Golden topaz (Leo) *Virtues:* virility and safety. May be used to arrest flagging inspiration, strengthen the mind, and impart general good health. Traditionally it was worn by pilgrims to ward off evil.

Peridot (Virgo) *Virtues:* purity and balance. May be used to aid digestion, dispel feelings of negativity, and induce tranquillity.

Diamond (Libra) *Virtues:* longevity and strength. A symbol of endurance, the diamond may be used to develop strength of mind and constancy in love (hence its popularity as a wedding stone), but it can also ensure good health and long life.

Garnet (Scorpio) *Virtues:* as a cleanser and stimulant. May be used to cleanse the blood and to treat prostate problems and rheumatoid arthritis. Garnet is used generally against wounds, infections and inflammations.

Amethyst (Sagittarius) *Virtues:* calmness and serenity. Traditionally the amethyst is used to dispel nightmares, prevent drunkenness and relieve insomnia. It is also used by meditators to help develop psychic powers.

Blue sapphire (Capricorn) *Virtues:* wisdom and enlightenment. It may be used in spiritual healing to develop wisdom and moral insight.

White zircon/rock crystal (Aquarius) *Virtues:* independence and protection. May be used to ward off hostility from others and to bring wisdom to its wearer. It also helps induce sleep.

Aquamarine (Pisces) *Virtues:* stability and purity. May be used to overcome negative emotions, develop insight and psychic awareness.

GELSEMIUM

A homeopathic remedy used as a treatment for influenza characterised by fever, sore throat, fatigue, lethargy and dizziness. Increased potencies may be required (up to 200c potency) to treat severe cases of influenza, but lower potencies (6–30c) are preferred.

GESTALT THERAPY

An approach to gaining self-awareness practised by psychotherapist Frederick ('Fritz') Perls, most notably at Esalen Institute, California, during the 1960s. Perls developed several techniques which would allow people to recognise their projections and disguises as real feelings, and subsequently be able to fulfil themselves. The underlying principle of Gestalt psychology is that an analysis of parts does not lead to an understanding of the whole, for parts by themselves have no meaning. Perls urged his clients to be aware of *how* they were experiencing existence *now* — and he believed in cutting through the niceties of social interaction to the person behind the image. This often involved exercises in role-play and strict self-observation.

Although he trained as a psychiatrist, Perls came to believe there was no need to delve into analysis per se. People revealed themselves through their being and through their behaviour. 'All relevant gestalten,' wrote Perls, 'are emerging, they are on the surface, they are obvious like the emperor's nakedness.'

GRAPHO-THERAPY

A technique for treating personality and character problems through handwriting analysis. Grapho-therapists believe that handwriting is influenced by the brain, and vice versa, so the act of monitoring and making adjustments to the handwriting style can be used for a positive, therapeutic purpose. Characteristic features include:

T-bars T-bar crossing indicates the degree of determination, self-confidence and willpower; the position where the stem is crossed is considered significant.
Angle Forward-leaning or backward-leaning writing may provide insights into the expression of feelings and emotions.
Loops These indicate through their size and abundance the extent to which the personality is expressed through the emotions.
Size Larger writing is usually characteristic of self-confidence, whereas smaller writing may indicate attention to detail and higher levels of concentration.

Grapho-therapy is often used in police survey work and is a popular adjunct to psychotherapy, especially in Europe.

GUIDED IMAGERY

A visualisation method in which the therapist guides the patient into an altered state of consciousness through progressive relaxation, and then through sequences of healing imagery. This technique is excellent for overcoming phobias, stress-related conditions, and diseases of psychosomatic origin. It is commonly used in clinical hypnosis. *See also Hypnosis, Progressive relaxation.*

H

HACKING

In massage, a technique of tapotement in which all the fingers are stretched and kept rigid, and body contact is made with the edge of the hand and the little finger. The wrists are held rigid and the main movement is from the elbow, down. The hands alternate in their contact with the patient's body.

'HALF LOTUS' POSTURE

In yoga, a variant on the well-known 'full lotus' asana. In the 'half lotus', the legs are crossed but the feet are not pulled up to rest on the thighs. Western devotees of yoga sometimes find the posture easier to maintain without discomfort. *See also 'Lotus' posture, Yoga.*

HANDWRITING ANALYSIS — *see Grapho-therapy*

HARA

A Japanese concept of the vital centre in man. Traditionally the *hara* is located just below the navel, and the word itself translates both as 'belly' and also as 'vital culture'. The *hara* is the symbolic focus of one's being — both from a physical and a spiritual viewpoint — and is a central concept in many bodywork and meditative practices of Japanese origin.

HEALING CHANNEL

A term used in spiritual healing to describe a person who has become a channel for healing energies which can then be transmitted to another person.

Sometimes this is done mentally, sometimes physically through laying-on-of-hands. Practitioners of psychometry and some forms of massage also refer to themselves as 'intuitive channels' and feel guided by a higher, divine source in their work. *See also Psychometry, Spiritual healing.*

HEALING CRISIS

Term used by some homeopaths to refer to the initial aggravation of symptoms during treatment, prior to improvement. This situation may arise where a homeopathic remedy is given in too great a strength, or in a general situation where the body is especially sensitive to a particular substance or effect used in therapy. *See Homeopathy.*

HELIOTHERAPY

Any form of therapeutic treatment utilising the direct rays of the sun. The main health value of sunlight comes from the ultraviolet rays it contains — the oils on the skin are converted into vitamin D during their exposure to these rays. However in most cases, bathing in direct sunlight is not recommended for lengthy periods — 2 hours is usually the maximum. Sore skin, blistering and skin cancers can result from excessive exposure to the sun.

HIGH COLONIC IRRIGATION

The complete flushing of the colon with water. *See Colonic irrigation.*

HIPPOCRATIC OATH

An oath attributed to Hippocrates (c.460–c.375 BC), often referred to as 'the Father of Western Medicine'. The Hippocratic Oath is regarded by many naturopaths and doctors as the central dictum of holistic health. This is the complete text:

I swear by Apollo the Healer and by Aesculapius, by Hygeia and Panacea, and by all gods and goddesses, making them my witness, that I will fulfil according to my power and judgement this oath and this covenant. I will look on him who taught me this art as I do my own parents, and will share with him my livelihood. If he be in need, I will give him money. I will hold his offspring as my own brethren, and will teach them this art, if they wish to learn it, without fee or written bond. I will give them instruction by precept and by lecture and by every other mode to my sons, to the sons of him who taught me, and to those pupils who have taken the covenant and sworn the physician's oath, and to none other besides. According to my power and judgement, I will prescribe regimen in order to benefit the sick, and do them no injury or wrong. I will neither give on demand any deadly drug, nor prompt any such course, nor, similarly, will I give a destructive pessary to woman. In holiness and righteousness I will pass my life and practise my art. Into whatever houses I enter, my entrance shall be for the benefit of the sick, and shall be void of all intentional injustice or wrongdoing, especially of carnal knowledge of woman or man, bond or free. And whatsoever, either in my practice or apart from it in daily life, I see or hear which should not be spoken of outside, thereon will I keep silence, judging such silence sacred. If then I fulfil this oath and do not violate it, may I enjoy my life and art and be held in honour among all men forever; but if I transgress and prove false to my oath, then may the contrary befall me.

HOLISTIC HEALTH

From the Greek *holos*, meaning 'whole', a branch of medicine which holds that true health stems from the balance of body, mind and spirit, and that emotional and stress-related factors account for a large proportion of disease. A holistic doctor therefore evaluates the whole person, not merely the physical symptoms of disease, in guiding that patient back to health. Holistic health care encompasses a wide variety of modalities which attend the different aspects of the human condition. These include dietary therapy, exercise regimes, oriental medicine, hypnotherapy, spiritual counselling and meditation, as appropriate.

HOME BIRTH — *see Natural childbirth*

HOMEOPATHY

A school of medicine conceived by German doctor and scholar, Samuel Christian Hahnemann (1755–1843). Hahnemann was interested in translating medical texts from English, French and Italian, and it was a work titled *Treatise on Materia Medica* by Scottish physician William Cullen that led him towards the principles of what would become known as homeopathy. According to Cullen, the symptoms produced by quinine in a healthy body were similar to the symptoms it helped remove in illness. From this, Hahnemann conceived the idea that 'like could be used to treat like' in medicine. Hahnemann adopted the word 'homeopathy' — which derives from the Greek *homoion pathos*, meaning 'to treat disease with the same substance' — and he also coined the term 'allopathy' to describe the use of *unlike* substances to remedy a complaint. This distinction is still made by naturopathic practitioners.

Hahnemann tested the homeopathic principle on himself by taking small doses of potent poisons like aconite, belladonna and strychnine, and also an extract from the bark of the Peruvian cinchona tree — a substance used at that time to treat malaria. In this way he produced artificial disease conditions in his body which he then treated with dilutions of the same substances.

Homeopathy is based on the idea that the body contains innate defence and healing mechanisms which can be activated to dispel illness. Hahnemann believed that diseases were imbalances of the whole mechanism and that these diseases expressed themselves through symptoms. 'When the physician has discovered all the observable symptoms of the disease that exist', he wrote, 'he has discovered the disease itself . . .' He then proceeded to classify disease states in terms of medicines that could be used to treat them.

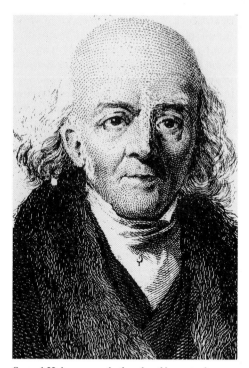

Samuel Hahnemann, the founder of homeopathy

However, Hahnemann's idea of a symptom was much broader than that recognised in orthodox medicine. Symptoms could be mental as well as physical, and each treatment would therefore be highly individualised to accommodate the specific range of symptoms in each case. Practitioners of homeopathy reject the idea of disease entities underlying symptoms, and instead regard symptoms as an expression of the body's intent to rid itself of disease.

Hahnemann advocated three basic principles and these have become basic to homeopathic practice: *Prescription by the law of similars, minimum dose* and *single remedy*.

In the first of these, the homeopath uses the concept of 'like treating like' and compares the specific symptoms presented with a detailed list of 'provings' (a proving is a remedy that has been proved to correspond to a given set of symptoms). The second principle refers to the idea that when a dilution of a 'like' substance is introduced to a diseased body it stimulates a natural healing response. The minimum dose is thus defined as the lowest potency required to provoke this reaction, and homeopathic remedies are invariably diluted for this reason. The third principle requires that the homeopath administer 1 remedy at a time, since 'provings' are of 1 substance only. If one were to prescribe 2 substances apparently amounting to the manifested symptoms, the cumulative effect could be quite different from the effects of the 2 substances individually.

Hahnemann's main works are *The Organon of Medicine* (1810) and *Chronic Diseases* (1828); they remain in print today. There is still widespread interest in homeopathy, especially in India and in Britain, where it enjoys royal patronage. There are also signs of a revival in the United States following the influence there of the Greek-born homeopath George Vithoulkas.

HOT PACK

A treatment utilising a woollen blanket wrung from water heated to 230°C (110°F). The patient lies on the wet blanket — which in turn rests on a dry one, and also on a rubber sheet — and the wet blanket is wrapped around the patient like an embalmed Egyptian mummy. The dry blanket and rubber sheet are then lifted up at the edges and also wrapped around the patient, who remains in the pack for up to 2 hours.

HUMAN POTENTIAL MOVEMENT

A term given to a movement, involving social scientists, health educators and psychologists, which is concerned with research into the potential of human consciousness. This includes such areas as the mind–body relationship, the study of left and right brain hemisphere functions, and techniques facilitating 'peak' and mystical experiences.

Influenced strongly by the work of Abraham Maslow (1908–70), the human potential movement has been associated with the rise of transpersonal psychology

since the late 1960s, and is represented by personal growth centres like the Esalen Institute in California, and similar organisations around the world. *See also Transpersonal psychology, Personal growth.*

HYDROCHLORIC ACID THERAPY

A therapy advocated by Dr Burr Ferguson and Dr Walter Guy in the 1930s, as a treatment for some cancers, anaemia, angina pectoris and pancreatic cell failure.

According to Ferguson and Guy, hypochlorhydria — a condition leading to hydrochloric acid deficiency — is the principal cause of potassium deficiency and this in turn causes widespread functional loss, especially in relation to cellular reproduction. Their approach, therefore, was to supply potassium in a hydrochloric acid solution, thereby enhancing the proper absorption of mineral salts in the digestive process and enhancing cell-life function.

HYDROTHERAPY

A health treatment in which water is employed in the healing process. Hydrotherapy was popularised by Father Sebastian Kneipp (1821–97), who maintained that the purpose of treatment was to 'dissolve, remove and strengthen'. This entailed dissolving the germs of matter containing disease, removing the diseased matter from the system, and then restoring the pure blood to maximal circulation so the body could return to a strengthened state.

Hydrotherapy makes use of 3 basic baths: cold, hot, and alternate hot and cold. Hot water draws blood to the surface, has an enervating effect, and increases sweat gland efficiency. Cold water drives blood away from the surface because the small blood vessels contract, and it also has an invigorating effect on the body. Alternate hot and cold baths reduce inflammation in congested areas, stimulate blood flow, and improve lymphatic drainage.

HYPERICUM

A homeopathic remedy for soothing and strengthening damaged nerve endings resulting from grazes or minor injuries. It can be taken internally for cuts from nails or barbed wire that could cause tetanus infection, or may be used as a tincture on the wound itself. Hypericum also soothes pain resulting from pinched nerves and displaced vertebrae.

HYPNOSIS

From the Greek word *hypnos*, meaning 'sleep', an altered state of consciousness which combines relaxation and enhanced awareness. When hypnosis is used in a clinical situation it is known as hypnotherapy. *See also Hypnotherapy, Auto-suggestion, Guided imagery.*

HYPNOTHERAPY

The clinical use of hypnosis, in which the subject's powers of concentration are mobilised and subconscious memories and perceptions brought into consciousness. Hypnotherapists usually relax their patients progressively, often by using a countdown procedure or relaxing the body limb by limb from the feet to the head.

Once the subject has entered an altered state of consciousness — in effect a light state of trance — the practitioner then provides cues which allow the subject to overcome personal barriers and emotional blockages, and to bring into awareness faculties and abilities which had been formerly neglected.

Hypnotherapy can be used to treat a wide range of conditions, including migraine, obesity, alcoholism, problems resulting from heavy smoking, phobias, low self-esteem, and psychosomatic skin disorders. *See also Auto-suggestion, Guided imagery.*

I

IATROGENIC DISEASE

From the Greek *iatros*, meaning 'physician', any disease condition caused by a doctor or by the medical treatment itself; for example, an allergic response or side-effect caused by a synthetic drug, or infection following surgery. Many homeopaths believe that modern drugs could have unforeseen impact on the human organism, and that while a given drug could repress one set of disease symptoms, it might also stimulate other forms of health imbalance at the same time. This situation arises because allopathic doctors do not seek 'provings' for their synthetic treatments. *See also Homeopathy, Allopathic medicine.*

INDICATOR MUSCLE

In Touch for health, a muscle in the arm or leg used to test for muscle weakness, and by inference, energy imbalance. In this particular therapy, muscle testing is linked to the flow of energy through acupuncture meridians. *See Touch for health.*

INNER GUIDE

The personification of inner wisdom, a figure often visualised in meditation or guided imagery sessions to serve as a friend or counsellor. Figures of this sort, even though 'imaginary', serve to focus one's own inner energies and provide confidence and reassurance in therapy sessions requiring recourse to a spiritual authority figure. Occasionally archetypal inner guides appear spontaneously in altered states of consciousness (trance states, dreams, etc.). Carl Jung's encounter with the spiritual sage Philemon is an example (details are included in Jung's autobiography *Memories, Dreams, Reflections*).

INSUFFLATION

A form of medical treatment in which air, gas or powder is blown into a cavity in the human body, such as the nose or throat. The medical instrument used for this purpose is called an insufflator.

INTUITIVE CHANNEL

— *see Healing channel*

IRIDOLOGY

Also known as iris diagnosis or iridiagnosis, iridology is an alternative health therapy based on the idea that the eyes provide a map of personal health. Derived initially from research by Hungarian surgeon Ignatz von Peckzely and Swedish homeopath Nils Liljequist, modern iridology has been substantially influenced by American therapist Dr Bernard Jensen and the Australian naturopath Dorothy Hall.

Dr Jensen divided the iris into 96 components and identified different organs of the body with specific zones on the 'clockface' of the iris. This work has been developed by Dorothy Hall, who published her book *Iridology* in 1980. For example, in the right iris the liver is located at 37–40 minutes around the dial, the lungs between 45 and 50 minutes, and the oesophagus at 15 minutes. In the left iris, the spleen is located at 22 minutes, the kidneys at 32 minutes and the thyroid gland at 47 minutes.

Iridologists also divide the iris into 3 concentric zones, each equal in size. The first contains the organs of digestion (stomach, intestine, etc.), the second the organs of transportation, utilisation and elimination through the kidneys, blood and lymph vessels, and the third the organs for body support, including the skeleton and skin.

According to the principles of iridology, it is possible to distinguish textures in the iris fibres, for the iris density reflects organic changes in the body. Iridologists also believe that pigment hues change to indicate the presence of toxins in the body. The iris zone where these pigment changes occur provides the key to the affected body organ.

Iridology remains unproven scientifically, but theories have been advanced to explain how it might work. The American pioneer of 'nature cure', Dr

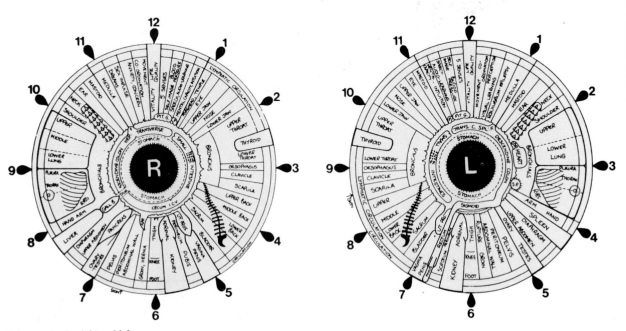

Iris zones in the right and left eye

Henry Lindlahr, believed that the fine nerve filaments of the iris receive impressions from the nervous system, and in this way are linked to every organ in the body. Other therapists maintain that the eye also records indicators of negative emotions and stress.

According to the precepts of iridology, the eye reflects different stages of disease — acute, chronic and destructive. In the first stage, grey-white lines appear in relevant zones of the iris, while in the second, the iris tissues begin to shrivel and turn black — intermingling with the grey-white lines of the acute stage. In the advanced, destructive phases of disease, tissues in the particular iris zones are destroyed, leaving a black spot.

Iridologists use a small penlight and a 10x magnifying lens to assist their analysis. It is generally considered that iris diagnosis is much more effective with the blue or light hazel Caucasian iris than with the non-Caucasian iris which is usually dark brown. *See also Sodium ring, Lymphatic rosary, Nerve rings, Radii solaris, Psoric spots.*

ISOMETRICS

A form of exercise which involves exerting the pressure of one muscle, or muscle group, against another. The technique may also be used against an immovable object, like a bar or wall. Isometric exercises tone and build the muscles. *See also Fitness.*

IYENGAR YOGA

A school of physical yoga developed by B. K. S. Iyengar, a contemporary Indian practitioner. Iyengar's classic work *Light on Yoga* contains over 200 yoga postures, and his emphasis is to extend the body to its limits, using the breath to obtain greater self-control. This increases mind–body coordination and helps tap the inner sources of vitality. Iyengar yoga also strengthens the muscular system and helps improve the respiratory system. *See also Yoga, Pranayama, Asanas, 'Lotus' posture.*

J

JOGGING

The act of running for fitness, an approach designed to enhance cardiovascular health. Joggers usually run along sidewalks or through parks, on a pre-determined route, although others prefer to jog on a treadmill in a gymnasium, thereby allowing stress tests to be conducted via electrodes fixed on the chest. These monitor how the heart, its valves and arteries are performing under pressure.

Jogging is not without its critics. Some health authorities maintain that jogging often causes foot injuries and bone displacements, and that many joggers exceed the recommended distance of 20 kilometres a week — becoming 'addicted' to the endorphins, or natural opiates, which are released in the body to counteract pain.

The jogging movement received a setback in 1984 with the premature death of its 'guru' James Fixx, author of *The Complete Book of Running*. Fixx died of a heart attack, aged 52, while running in Vermont; however, his family had a history of heart disease and defenders of jogging have been quick to point out that it was this, and not exercise itself, which led to his demise.

Statistically it does appear that jogging is beneficial if pursued in moderation. In recent years the number of adult Americans exercising regularly has increased substantially (from 24 per cent of the population in 1960 to 59 per cent in 1984), and the number of deaths from cardiovascular disease per 100 000 people has fallen from 511.6 in 1961 to 424.2 in 1981. This fall is not attributed solely to exercise — other factors such as diet are also involved — but the results are encouraging.

K

KATA

Physical forms or movements which aid self-knowledge and which are utilised in Japanese bodywork practices. Examples include *eiko dai* and *tenshingoso*, which are a feature of shintaido — *see Shintaido.*

KIRLIAN DIAGNOSIS

The interpretation of the so-called Kirlian 'corona', the energy field surrounding an organism, to evaluate patterns of health and disease. The Kirlian effect was discovered by Russian electrician Semyon Kirlian, who observed a person undergoing electrotherapy while he was visiting a research institute. There seemed to be flashes of light between the electrodes and the skin, and Kirlian later proceeded to photograph this effect with special apparatus. On the photographs, an impression of luminescence appeared around Kirlian's fingers.

Modern Kirlian cameras make use of 2 glass sheets between which pass transparent conductive liquid and a silver conductor wire. The object to be photographed (a leaf, a hand, etc.) is placed on the insulated glass plate and an image is recorded on sensitised paper as a high-frequency current passes through the conductor wire. Kirlian photographs are strikingly beautiful and some naturopathic researchers have claimed that they record the degree of life-force or 'bioplasmic energy' present in the object being photographed.

The Romanian scientist Dr Ion Dumitrescu investigated the Kirlian process for 15 years and found that healthy tissue appeared dark when photographed by the Kirlian process, while unhealthy tissue radiated a bright aura. However, American therapist James Knightlinger, who investigated Kirlian patterns and acupuncture meridians, found corona blockages between the meridian areas of the feet and hands linked to afflicted organs — an apparently contradictory finding.

There appears to be no specific correlation between colours in the Kirlian corona and states of health. Colour variations seem to derive primarily from emulsion variables, or reflect the weight of the object photographed on the plate. It is also possible that the ionised biological gases around the body — oxygen, nitrogen, hydrogen — contribute to colour changes in the photographic process. Interestingly, inanimate objects like metal earrings and coins also show Kirlian 'auras', thus dispelling the possibility that Kirlian photography measures an innate 'life-force' in living organisms. *See also Aura, Colour breathing.*

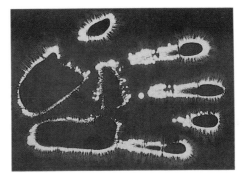

An example of the Kirlian 'aura'

KNEIPP CURE — *see Hydrotherapy*

KUNDALINI

From a Sanskrit term meaning 'coil' or 'spiral', the spiritual and psychic energy which may be aroused systematically by techniques of yoga, and which can be channelled through the chakras from the base of the spine to the crown of the forehead. There are 3 channels associated with kundalini energy. The principal channel is *sushumna*, which corresponds with the central nervous system and connects with the chakras. The *sushumna* is in turn flanked by two other channels, *ida* and *pingala*, representing female lunar energy and male solar energy respectively. *See also Yoga, Chakras.*

L

LAVAGE

The therapeutic treatment in which the stomach is washed in order to remove acids, toxic substances and mucus. A tube approximately 1 metre long is used and is inserted through the mouth and throat. Warm water is introduced through a funnel. The water is later pumped out with a bulb attached to the tube. Lavage should only be performed under medical supervision.

The term 'lavage' is sometimes used with reference to bowel cleansing — *see Colonic irrigation*.

LAVATIO

From the Latin *lavare*, 'to wash', a mouthwash consisting of flavoured essential oils, soap, and three-quarters coloured water. Lavatios are used for cleansing and antiseptic purposes.

LAYING-ON-OF-HANDS

In spiritual healing, a touch-contact between the healer and the afflicted person to effect a cure. The healer believes that in laying-on hands a spiritual energy is transmitted from a divine source to the diseased person, stimulating recovery. A secular explanation of this effect is that the healer appeals to the religious belief system of the patient, producing a psychosomatic, or placebo, response. *See also Spiritual healing, Psychic surgery, Healing channel*.

LEDUM

A homeopathic anti-tetanus remedy especially useful for puncture wounds caused by metal pins, nails or barbs, as well as for bee stings. Ledum is also use-ful to take along on picnics since it can be used for treating mosquito bites and scratches from prickly bushes. It helps relieve deep bruising and is also effective in reducing pain caused by gout.

LOHAN KUNG

A Chinese healing system said to derive from the time of Bodhidharma's meditative retreat in the Songshan mountains, c.527 AD. Bodhidharma, an Indian monk known to the Chinese as Ta Mo, noticed a cumulative effect on his body following long periods of meditation in a windy cave. The symptoms included fatigue, intermittent body aches and pains, and a tendency to fall asleep. He therefore developed a system of 18 movements (known as the Eighteen Lohan Hands) which combined Buddhist yoga techniques, fitness exercises and animal movements. These in turn have influenced the martial arts traditions of aikido, tai chi, wushu, kung fu, taekwondo, etc. Lohan kung seeks to activate the flow of *chi* energy along the meridians of the body, thereby eliminating the 'disharmony' associated with illness.

LOOFAH

The fibrous interior of a gourd plant, which can be used as a body-brush for removing flaky skin — *see Sloughing*.

LOTION

A fluid with healing, antiseptic properties, applied externally to the skin. Examples include arnica, garlic juice, myrhh, eucalyptus and pine. *See also Compress*.

'LOTUS' POSTURE

A classical posture, or asana, in yoga. The practitioner sits on a mat with the left foot over the right thigh and the right foot over the left thigh. The hands may be placed either in the lap or over the knees, palm upwards. The posture is used during meditation, and to raise kundalini energy. *See also Yoga, Meditation, 'Half Lotus' posture, Kundalini.*

LUNAR PHASE CYCLE

A natural birth control method developed by Czechoslovakian psychiatrist and gynaecologist Dr Eugene Jonas. Dr Jonas originally studied Roman Catholic women who were using the 'rhythm method' of birth control, but he became concerned with its limitations — many women in his survey were conceiving on dates outside their expected mid-menstrual cycle ovulation times. Jonas analysed the conception times and found that they fell into a repeating cycle related to the angles between the sun and moon in each woman's birth chart. The women appeared to be fertile when the sun and moon were at the same relative angle as at the precise time of their birth, irrespective of the mid-menstrual ovulation time.

It now appears that a woman is most fertile during the 24 hours preceding the exact recurrence of the sun-moon angle present at the moment of her birth. Since sperms live for 3 days, the fertility period is normally regarded on a broader basis and for contraceptive purposes is taken as a 4-day period repeating every lunar month (12 or 13 times a year).

LYMPHATIC DRAINAGE MASSAGE

A specialised form of face and neck massage often used in conjunction with aromatherapy. The technique involves gentle stroking to help the tender lymph glands shed built-up cellular debris. It also helps recondition the skin. *See also Aromatherapy, Massage.*

LYMPHATIC ROSARY

In iridology, a zone of white beads, resembling pearls, identified around the iris rim. Iridologists believe that this condition indicates slow pituitary and thyroid function. It may also occur in those who are obese. Naturopathic remedies for the 'lymphatic rosary' include herbal remedies rich in iron (nettle, gentian, garlic) and herbs which specifically affect the lymph system (fenugreek and violet leaves) — *see Iridology.*

M

MANTRA

A sacred utterance or sound, often intoned silently as part of one's meditation. Some mantras are given privately by a guru to a disciple, but other mantras have a more general application. The mantra *Om Namah Shivaya*, which forms part of the Siddha Meditation practices developed by the late Swami Muktananda, means simply: 'I honour the inner self'. *See Meditation.*

MASSAGE

The word 'massage' apparently derives either from the Greek word *massein*, 'to knead', or the arabic *mas'h*, 'to press softly'. The idea of the 'healing power of touch' is a very ancient concept and embodies the principle that part of healing is the caring of one person for another. The masseur or masseuse, through stroking and kneading the body, and rubbing in warm soothing oils, not only nurtures the body physically but communicates with the client in a very intimate way.

Massage is recorded in ancient China as early as 3000 BC and was advocated by Hippocrates (c.460–c.375 BC), the famous Greek physician, who noted that 'moderate rubbing' could loosen tight joints. The Greek *gymnasia* were places where the body could be anointed with healing oils and massaged, and the physician Asclepiades (124–56 BC) recommended a blend of massage and physical exercise as part of his treatment.

Massage is an excellent way of stimulating the body's metabolic processes and hastening the reabsorption or release of waste products in the body. By moving blood towards the heart, massage also stimulates blood circulation and enhances the sense of personal vitality. The most common massage movements include kneading the arms and legs, thumping the heels, pulling the joints of the arms and legs, compressing nerve areas, and stroking the back and face. *See also Swedish massage.*

MATERIA MEDICA

Latin for 'medical material', a term used to describe the substances used in the preparation of medicines. The term also refers to the science of medicines and the study of their curative properties, name origins, technical names, natural organic order, physical characteristics, methods of extraction and preparation, active constituents, actions and function, dose and contraindications, etc.

MEDICAL

From the Latin *medicus*, meaning 'physician', that which pertains to the art of healing.

MEDICAMENT

A healing remedy.

MEDICASTER

A second-rate or incompetent doctor: a 'quack'.

MEDICINE

Any subtance used in the treatment or prevention of disease. Naturopaths and homeopaths prefer medicines of natural origin which stimulate the self-healing capacity of the body. They are less inclined to use drugs of synthetic manufacture because of possible unforeseen side-effects.

MEDICINE MAN

In primitive societies, a healer, shaman or priest responsible for divining illness and preparing effective magical remedies. The medicine man protects the community from witchcraft or malevolent forces, and through trance states and incantations holds regular discourse with healing gods and spirits. Cures effected in this way bear some resemblance to faith-healing, in which a supernatural power is summoned to intercede in the healing process. *See also Laying-on-of-hands, Spiritual healing, Healing channel.*

MEDITATION

A technique of mind control that often leads to a feeling of inner calm and peacefulness, and may result in profound experiences of self-realisation and transcendental awareness. Meditation is a discipline found in many of the world's major religions, including Buddhism, Hinduism, Islam and Christianity, but it is also advocated by many practitioners of holistic health for its impact on stress-related disease.

There are 2 broad approaches to meditation. The first focuses on the powers of concentration and requires that one's attentions be fixed on a meditative symbol (for example, a mandala), a rhythmic sound or chant (for example, a mantra) or on one's pattern of breathing. The concept here is to turn the processes of thought inwardly until the mind transcends itself.

The second approach focuses more on 'detached awareness' and emphasises the dispassionate observation of what is happening *now*, rather than on attaining a higher state of consciousness. This technique enables the meditator to understand the flux of life, and the ebb and flow of human experience. *See also Yoga, Pranayama, Mental ataraxis, Transpersonal psychology.*

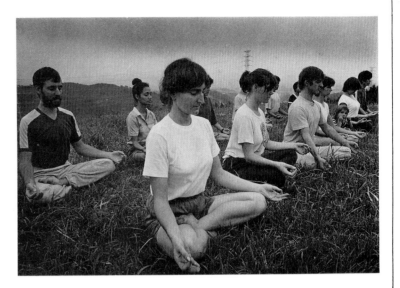

MENTAL ATARAXIS

A term used by psychotherapist Dr Ainslie Meares to describe a meditative method for attaining inner well-being. Derived from a Greek word meaning 'absence of disturbance', the technique involves simple relaxation followed by a state of 'drifting effortlessness' in which the subject, assisted by the therapist, gradually yields all forms of anxiety and stress. Dr Meares believes that this form of meditation produces a specific physiological effect, reducing cortisone levels in the body and enhancing the effectiveness of the immune system. This helps activate the self-regulating functions in the body, fight disease imbalance, and restore the organism to its natural, integrated state. Mental ataraxis is different from guided imagery or self-directed imagery because it does not utilise visualisation images related to disease, preferring instead an abstract meditative approach which undercuts the very basis of stress and anxiety. *See also Meditation.*

MESMERISM

A theory conceived by Austrian physician Anton Mesmer (1733–1815) that a state of trance could be induced in a patient by summoning one's own innate source of 'animal magnetism' and then transferring it at will to the other person. Mesmer graduated in medicine from the University of Vienna in 1766 and began to use

magnetism with his patients. However, he was driven from Vienna by the police and settled in Paris in 1778. Here he treated wealthy aristocrats in a lavish salon. Mesmer wore a shirt of leather lined with silk to contain his magnetic fluid, and his patients sat in a circle around a tub filled with water and iron filings. Iron rod conductors protruded from the tub and patients held these while also bound by a cord to 'close the force'. Mesmer would wave his finger or a wand in front of his patients, fix his gaze on them, and diffuse his 'magnetism' into the air. This, coupled with the magnetism from the tub, was supposed to transfer to the patients, making them well.

Mesmer's theory of animal magnetism is a quaint precursor of modern hypnotism. However, modern hypnotherapists have long since discarded the notion that some form of magnetic impulse passes between the hypnotist and subject. Modern hypnotherapy relies instead on suggestions from the practitioner which enables the subject to discover latent possibilities deep within the psyche. *See Hypnotherapy.*

MIASM

In homeopathy and psionic medicine, a disruptive factor affecting the body's natural curative capacity and the flow of

Meditation — a path to increased self-awareness

vital energy in the organism. Some miasms are considered to be hereditary, so that, according to Dr George Laurence — the founder of psionic medicine — syphilis and TB are the main hereditary miasms, while measles, chickenpox and whooping cough are the dominant acquired ones. Dr Aubrey Westlake, also a practitioner of psionic medicine, believes the hereditary TB miasm underlies many cases of asthma, hay fever and sinus complaints, and may be connected in some cases with leukaemia and diabetes. *See Homeopathy, Psionic medicine.*

MINERAL HAIR ANALYSIS

A naturopathic technique for determining the level of mineral nutrients and toxic metals in the body. Regarded by many practitioners as an alternative to blood serum analysis, mineral hair analysis involves tests on the mineral content of the hair, which are then interpreted as an indicator of body levels as a whole. Hair tests may reveal, for example, a high level of calcium (a sign of possible arteriosclerosis since this is associated with hardening of the arteries through calcium plaques), or a low calcium level (a possible indicator of osteoporosis), a zinc deficiency (associated with growth problems) or other factors which may be used for preventive health. Determining the presence of toxic metals in the body is one of the technique's most useful applications, since even small amounts of such toxins as lead, mercury, arsenic, cadmium and aluminium pose a health threat. Mineral hair analysis measures minerals which have been bound into the hair shaft for some time, and the analysis is therefore also a useful guide to nutritional imbalances which may be occurring on an ongoing basis.

MIRACLE CURE

A seemingly miraculous or sudden remission from disease. Miracle cures have been reported at sacred locations like Lourdes, France, and by spiritual healers who perform laying-on-of-hands, claiming intervention from a divine source. Some cases of cancer involving 'spontaneous remissions' are also claimed as miracles.

A more feasible explanation, especially in relation to diseases of psychosomatic origin, is that the healing treatment causes a placebo response, stimulating the belief system of the patient and in turn the immunological defence mechanisms in the body. *See also Spiritual healing, Psychic surgery, Laying-on-of-hands, Healing channel.*

MOXIBUSTION

A technique used as an adjunct to acupuncture and shiatsu, as a means of stimulating vital acu-points or *tsubo*. Moxa is a dried pulp produced from the herb mugwort. The moxa stick is lit at one end and the other end is applied to the specific acu-points appropriate in the treatment. Moxa works by diffusing a gentle heat and tonifying the point through a transfer of energy. It is ideal for asthma, fatigue, chills and a variety of rheumatoid and arthritic conditions. *See also Acupuncture, Shiatsu.*

MUD BATH

A covering of hot moist clay or peat earth (heated to around 38°C or 100°F) applied to the body for therapeutic purposes. The patient lies on a canvas sheet and the body is covered with mud. The canvas is then wrapped over the body. The patient then rests for up to an hour, and the mud is removed in a shower. Mud baths are used to treat inflammatory skin conditions like boils, sores and bites.

MULL

A suet or lard-based ointment spread onto soft Indian muslin and used in medical treatment.

MUSCLE TEST — *see Applied kinesiology, Touch for health, Food allergy muscle test* (Part 3)

MUSIC THERAPY

The use of music to aid processes of communication and the development of self-awareness. Because music can produce a strong emotional response, it is often used with handicapped children to try to overcome personal barriers and disabilities, and to bring a new sense of order and meaning into their lives. It may also be useful to help children express a wide range of moods and feelings.

Music also has other therapeutic applications in the field of holistic self-development. Ambient music, a form of 'non-intrusive' New Age music, is now being used as an adjunct to meditation, and to enhance guided imagery exercises. Music of this type has been correlated by Steven Halpern with the yoga *chakra* system, and by Nevill Drury with the 5 elements: Earth, Water, Fire, Air, and Spirit — in both cases to enhance visualisation and to lead to the experience of transpersonal states. *See Ambient music.*

N

NAPRAPATHY

A bodywork technique developed by American naturopath Oakley Smith (1880–1970). Naprapathy is a manipulative approach in which shrunken ligament tissue is stretched to help blood and nerve flow return to a normal state. It focuses primarily on the spine and supporting muscles and also utilises heat therapy and dietary supplementation. Naprapathy is not widely practised, even within the United States. *Compare with Rolfing, Osteopathy, Chiropractic.*

NATURAL BIRTH CONTROL

Any method of birth control which does not utilise artificial or chemical means. The latter category includes the contraceptive pill, which suppresses the natural menstrual cycle and may cause blood-clotting in women over 35 years of age. Other 'unnatural' forms of contraception include IUDs which are often uncomfortable and can cause infection, and inserted pessaries which are rather unreliable.

Among the most reliable natural methods of birth control are the lunar phase cycle method — a development of the 'rhythm method' — and the Billings Method, which monitors changes in the vaginal mucus. *See Lunar phase cycle, Billings Method.*

NATURAL CHILDBIRTH

An arrangement whereby the birth of a child takes place in a 'natural' setting, such as in the home, rather than in the 'artificial' or clinical setting of a hospital. Supporters of home births argue that it is relatively rare for circumstances to arise during labour and birth that would demand hospital treatment, and over 90 per cent of these factors could be medically determined. It is also claimed that the home has advantages over the hospital in terms of the familiar people generally present — especially close relatives and friends — who are able to offer support during the labour, birth and post-birth phases. Ideally, home births should be attended by an experienced midwife. *See also Underwater births.*

NATUROPATHY

The philosophy and practice of treating disease by following the principles and laws of Nature, rather than utilising chemicals, drugs, surgery or other 'artificial' or 'intrusive' methods. Naturopaths endeavour to stimulate the innate healing resources of the body itself, through a variety of methods. These include fasting to eliminate toxins, physical manipulative therapies like osteopathy and chiropractic, techniques like acupuncture and shiatsu which stimulate energy flow, and approaches like hypnosis and biofeedback which tap the 'inner potential'. Herbal remedies, mineral and vitamin supplements, and homeopathic treatments are frequently employed, and some naturopaths also practise iridology, a technique of identifying disease symptoms through the different zones of the iris.

The term 'naturopathy' was first used by German homeopath John Scheel, but the underlying concept is best summed up by nature-cure pioneer Henry Lindlahr who stated simply that disease derives from 'improper eating, thinking and living'.

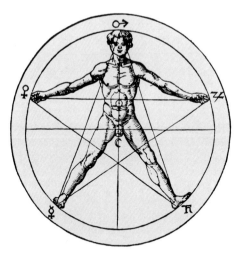

NEGATIVE ION GENERATOR

An electrical device designed to produce negative ions in a home or office environment. Negative ion generators typically work from a 240-volt AC, 50 Hz power source, generating about 300 billion small air ions per second. Smaller versions, working from a 12-volt DC power source, are available for use in a car.

Negative ion generators are used therapeutically for people suffering from bronchial complaints, influenza, hay fever, migraines and sleeplessness. Dr Milos Nedved of the Western Australia Institute of Technology also advocates the use of negative ion generators in hospitals. He believes, for example, that viruses like Legionnaires disease can spread undetected through air-conditioned units in hospitals because of the lack of negative ions in the air. Negative-ion depleted atmospheres are a breeding ground for bacteria. Viruses and microbes can only be transmitted by attaching themselves to positively charged airborne particles; so, in Dr Nedved's view, the introduction of negative ions into the air through a generator would help prevent the germs from travelling.

The North Eastern Hospital in Philadelphia and several Californian hospitals have already introduced negative ion generators in wards for patients suffering from burns, and this has led to considerable relief from pain. However, the National Health and Medical Research Council of Australia has recently confirmed its view, held for 24 years, that there is no reliable evidence that negative ions promote health, and some generators produce unacceptable levels of ozone, thus leading to the risk of respiratory diseases. The debate on the value of negative ion generators is still continuing. *See Negative ions.*

NEGATIVE IONS

Negatively charged molecules which are said to provide a vibrant, healing quality to the air. Negative ions are formed by an intense electrical discharge which frees electrons from atoms of gas. They occur abundantly in the atmosphere near the sea shore (when waves break upon rocks), near waterfalls, or following storms. However, in cities the balance of ions in the air is 5:4 in favour of positive ions and as a result the air often seems flat and lifeless.

In 1969 Dr Felix Sulman, of the Department of Applied Pharmacology at the Hebrew University in Jerusalem, made a special study of the effects of ion-imbalance on human emotions and health. He conducted an experiment in which 2 groups of men and women between the ages of 20 and 65 were confined in rooms containing first a positive-ion excess and then a negative-ion excess. In the first instance the subjects became irritable and fatigued after an hour's confinement. In the second test, however, the subjects all exhibited stronger alpha brain waves (associated with inner peace and well-being) and slow firm pulse. Psychological tests also showed increased alertness and work capacity.

Negative ions can be generated in an office environment by a small compact unit called a negative ion generator. *See Negative ion generator.*

NERVE RINGS

In iridology, the circular patterns in the iris which are regarded as being characteristic of persistent muscular tension. They often manifest in the iris zones for the kidneys, uterus or liver, and — in the case of asthmatics — in the chest and bronchial regions. Naturopathic remedies for 'nerve rings' include magnesium, calcium and potassium phosphates to reduce spasm, and herbal teas like chamomile and valerian to induce relaxation. *See Iridology.*

NEURO-LINGUISTIC PROGRAMMING (NLP)

A therapeutic system developed by linguist Dr John Grinder and mathematician Richard Bandler, who later became a Gestalt therapist. The term derives from the Greek word *neuron*, 'nerve', and the Latin *lingua*, 'language', and indicates that there is a sensory factor in all forms of behaviour which in turn affects the structure and sequence of different forms of communication. The programming

factor relates to habitual thought and behaviour patterns which affect certain outcomes.

Many forms of behaviour do not produce satisfactory outcomes and may lead to psychosomatic disease, aberrant perceptions of life, or states of being well below optimal levels of functioning. The NLP therapist observes the client's behavioural and linguistic patterns, and seeks to guide him beyond personal limitations to new levels of awareness and personal effectiveness.

NEW AGE MUSIC — *see Ambient music*

NOSODES

In homeopathy, potentised preparations of diseased substances used in a medicinal capacity to stimulate the body's immunological defence system. Examples include pertussin (whooping cough), tetanus toxin (tetanus), diphtherium (diphtheria), morbillinum (measles) and parotidinum (mumps). *See also Dilutions, homeopathic.*

O

OCULAR SEGMENT

One of the 7 body segments in Reichian therapy. The ocular segment includes the eyes, ears and nose, and according to Reich 'armouring' can build up at birth, especially if the baby is delivered in an intense and bright environment. Symptoms as far-ranging as dizziness and schizophrenia have been attributed to ocular segment armouring. *See Reichian therapy.*

OINTMENT

A soft fatty substance used as a preparation for healing, or to beautify the skin. Ointments are also known as unguents.

OKI YOGA

A rigorous form of yoga developed by Korean-born practitioner Dr Masahiro Oki, who founded the largest yoga institute in Japan (the *dojo* at Mishima). Oki yoga emphasises balance as the natural condition of physical and mental activity, and the approach incorporates a healthy wholefoods diet, meditation, breathing techniques and vigorous strengthening exercises known as *khoka-ho*. These often draw on practices also found in judo, aikido and karate. Classic Indian asanas like the 'cobra' and 'bow' poses are also employed. *See Yoga, Asanas.*

Oki yoga in action

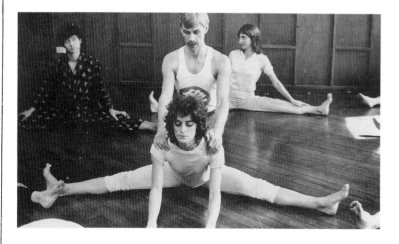

OM NAMAH SHIVAYA

An Indian mantra widely used to focus the mind in meditation. It translates as 'I honour the inner self'. *See Meditation.*

ONE-TO-ONE THERAPY

Any therapy in which the practitioner and subject interrelate on a one-to-one basis, as distinct from a group or workshop situation. Examples include acupuncture, chiropractic, osteopathy, massage, Rolfing and the Alexander Technique. *Compare with Encounter therapy.*

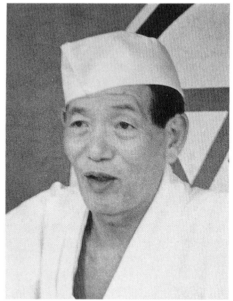

Dr Masahiro Oki

ORAL SEGMENT

One of the 7 body segments in Reichian therapy. The oral segment includes the muscles affecting the chin and throat, the occiput and the annular muscles at the mouth. The tongue, however, is not included. Oral segment armouring may manifest as tight or constricted facial expressions, a habitually open mouth, or a dropped jaw. Voice tone and the rapidity of speech are also key 'oral' factors, and some who are armoured in this segment may require therapy to compensate for deprivation on the mother's breast. *See Reichian therapy.*

ORGONE

Wilhelm Reich's term for *prana*, or life-force, also known to the Chinese as *chi*. Reich believed that orgone has bio-electrical properties. In particular, organic materials absorbed orgone energy, metallic substances reflected it, and blockage of orgone energy led to a rise in temperature. He also believed that the energy could be accumulated, and to demonstrate this he built an 'orgone accumulator' — a cabinet with walls consisting of alternating layers of organic and inorganic substances, and which had an inner lining of sheet iron. The early models had a flexible tube attached which allowed the patient to breathe in the orgone energy. Reich and his followers used orgone accumulators to treat a variety of diseases until the American Federal Food and Drugs Administration declared the equipment fraudulent.

Orgone therapy is now sometimes referred to as 'ionisation therapy'. It is possible to construct a cabinet large enough for a patient to sit in. American novelist William Burroughs attributes his long life to the use of an orgone accumulator. *See also Reichian therapy.*

ORTHOMOLECULAR MEDICINE

The term 'orthomolecular' was coined by Nobel Prize-winning chemist Dr Linus Pauling, and refers to a therapeutic approach in which the enrivonment of cells in the body is adjusted to facilitate their maximum effectiveness. Dr Pauling describes the process as 'the preservation of good health and the treatment of disease by varying the concentrations in the human body of substances that are normally present in the body and required for health'.

Orthomolecular nutritionists assess dietary intake in order to enhance absorption of positive nutrients and remove foreign substances, drugs, chemicals and other toxins from the system. Some orthomolecular practitioners are also concerned with the effects of nutrients on brain function and ways in which vitamin and mineral supplements may be used to treat mental disorders like schizophrenia. Orthomolecular nutrition is closely related to the concept of megavitamin therapy developed by Dr Abram Hoffer and others.

ORTHOPATHY

From the Greek *orthos* 'correct' and *pathos* 'suffering', any treatment which restores health and well-being through the correct intake of food and other healing substances.

OSTEOPATHY

A physical manipulative technique; the name is derived from two Greek words, *osteo* ('bone') and *pathos* ('disease'). Osteopathy was developed by Dr Andrew Taylor Still (1828–1917), a physician who for many years lived in Kirksville, Missouri. Regarded in his own lifetime as a 'lightning bone-setter' and as a quack doctor, Dr Still was a religious man and believed that illness derived from deviations from God's plan in Nature. Convinced of man's self-healing capacity, Dr Still studied the human anatomy and discovered that he could diagnose medical ailments by touching the body and assessing the speed, heat and quality of blood flowing to any given area. He came to believe that mechanical changes to the musculo-skeletal system could result in an abnormal response of both nerve and blood supply to the organs of the body. Osteopathy therefore utilises both massage — to stimulate blood flow to the body tissue — and physical manipulation to correct postural misalignments. Osteopathy resembles chiropractic but places more emphasis on blood circulation than on the nervous system. However, practitioners of these two healing arts treat similar complaints — especially lower back pain, restricted joints and muscle spasm.

OTHER-DIRECTED IMAGERY — *see Guided imagery*

OVULATION METHOD OF BIRTH CONTROL
— *see Billings Method*

P

PALPATION

In osteopathy, a term used by founder Dr Andrew Still to describe the characteristic speed, heat and quality of blood flow to a specific region of the body. This is diagnosed by touch — *see Osteopathy.*

PANACEA

From the Greek *panakeia*, 'universal remedy or cure for all diseases'. The well-known herb ginseng (genus *Panax*), the root of which has medicinal properties and appears to stimulate the body's immune system, is widely regarded in the Orient as a general panacea.

PAST-LIVES THERAPY

A technique of hypnotic regression in which a subject is led back to the experience of 'previous lifetimes' in which major traumas apparently occurred. The traumas are believed to have a continuing effect in the present lifetime, manifesting as disease or mental imbalance.

The direct hypnotic encounter with past-life events provides an emotional release from their impact at a subconscious level, and helps free the subject, in this lifetime, from the psychosomatic stress factors impinging on daily life. Many past-lives therapists accept reincarnation as a fact, but others maintain that it is not necessary for them to actually believe in the concept for the therapy to be effective. The subject may be simply imagining the past-life persona in response to wish-fulfilment, fantasy etc., but this image still provides a context for therapeutic treatment, enabling the therapist to help the subject overcome various fears, anxieties and traumas. The fact that a second 'personality' is involved helps in fact to make the treatment more palatable, since there is a sense of distance between the trauma and its effect, even though the 2 figures are seen as being linked in destiny.

PATIENT'S WITNESS

A patient's blood sample used in dowsing practices, counterposed against a 'diagnostic witness' which contains diseased material. The patient's witness is used, for example, by practitioners of psionic medicine who utilise a W. O. Wood chart. The patient's witness is placed in the right-hand corner of the chart, directly opposite the diagnostic witness on the left, and a pendulum is then used to take a reading. *See also W. O. Wood chart, Psionic medicine, Diagnostic witness, Dowsing, Radiesthesia, medical.*

PELVIC SEGMENT

One of the 7 body segments in Reichian therapy. The pelvic segment includes the legs, pelvis and genitals. Fear or repression expressed in this segment may manifest as a pulled-back pelvis or in tightly muscled buttocks. Treatment may include pelvic thrusting accompanied by shouting to release anger locked into this body segment. The pelvic region is especially sensitive and is usually the last body segment treated — *see Reichian therapy.*

PERSONAL GROWTH

A concept central to the idea of holistic health and self-actualisation. Personal growth refers to the idea that subjects can explore the personal boundaries of their being and develop due potentialities, talents and creative endeavours. This may involve the physical, mental and spiritual aspects of one's being and lead to increased fulfilment and a sense of personal enrichment in one's day-to-day life.

Personal growth is developed in an experiential setting so that the subject has direct involvement in the processes which lead to greater self-awareness. This may include workshop experiences or one-to-one therapy with a health practitioner. *See also Self-actualisation, Transpersonal psychology, Human potential movement.*

PESSARY

A medication which is applied by insertion through the vagina. Certain types of 'foaming pessaries' are used as a form of contraception.

PETRISSAGE

In massage, kneading and squeezing movements designed to soften and stretch hardened and contracted muscles. Petrissage also draws blood to the region being worked on, and improves the tone of the skin. The movements employed in petrissage may prove useful in restoring defective circulation.

PHRENOLOGY

The art of reading the 'bumps' on a person's skull in order to demonstrate a relationship between skull conformations and characteristics of mind and body. Widely dismissed as a superstition, phrenology is nevertheless defended by those who maintain that certain regions of the brain can be 'developed' in the same way that an athlete develops muscles. Traditional phrenological associations are shown in the accompanying diagram.

PINE-NEEDLE BATH

A remedial bath in which extract of pine-needles is added to the hot water, producing a vapour which is soothing for the air passages in the lungs. This type of bath is also suitable for those suffering from rheumatism, nervous conditions and renal or heart disorders.

PLACEBO

The word 'placebo' comes from the Latin for 'I will please' and refers to the original function of placebo tablets, which were given by the doctor to please the patient. The placebo made the patient feel he or she had taken something tangible to help overcome the illness or complaint.

A placebo is strictly a treatment which is prescribed for a complaint but which does not intrinsically affect the nature of the illness. It is now recognised, however, that placebos play a valuable psychological role in the treatment of disease, and may help to mobilise the self-healing capacity of the body. It is vitally important that the patient believes in the value of the placebo for it to be 'effective'.

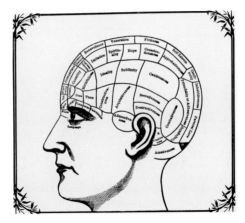

Phrenological divisions of the brain

PLACENTAL EXTRACTS

Extracts used in cosmetic preparations. Liquid placental extracts are removed from unborn animal placentas, usually those of cattle, during the third and fourth months of pregnancy. Placental extract contains DNA and alkaline phosphatase, and is believed to stimulate cell respiration within the skin. It also increases blood circulation in the vessels, revitalising the tissue. Some placental extract cosmetics may contain albumin, oestrogen, progesterone and pregnenolone acetate to smooth out wrinkles.

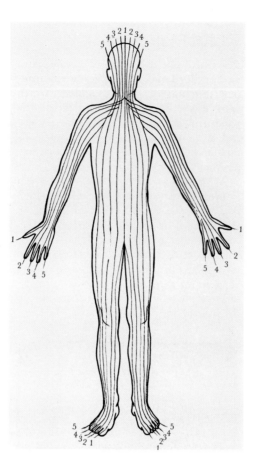

Polarity balancing encompasses chi *channels in the body*

POLARITY BALANCING

A technique developed by Austrian-born American naturopath Dr Randolph Stone. Stone integrated occult theories, acupuncture, shiatsu, ayurvedic medicine and herbalism to produce a conceptual framework which emphasises 'energy-flow' in the body, and resembles both Wilhelm Reich's notion of orgone and the Chinese idea of *chi*.

Polarity therapists endeavour to locate areas in the body where the flow of energy has become blocked or impeded, causing emotional tension and pain. As the therapist stimulates energy-flow in the body, through pressure or touch, the blockages break down and the toxins are eventually eliminated — through the breath, sweat, faeces, urine or emotions.

Stone accepted the idea that the central axis of the body is neutral, the right-hand side positive and the left-hand side nega-tive. In his book *Health Building*, Stone wrote:

An excess amount of the positive current produces irritation, pain, swelling and heat in the tissues, organs and areas of the body, due to excess amounts of blood in that area, and the opposite or negative pole energy is required to balance it. The positive current is the sun energy of fire and radiant warmth in normal amounts. The right hand is the conductor of this energy. For negative tension, congestion, spasm and stasis, the right hand contains the antidote, the positive polarity current . . .

The left hand is the conductor of the negative or moon current, which is cooling, soothing, refreshing and toning. Place it over the seat of pain, where the positive currents are in excess, giving the above-mentioned symptoms. Wherever the pain is, that excess calls for release of irritation, heat, swelling . . . which the negative current can provide.

Dr Stone also recommended a two-fold dietary cycle, to cleanse and then build the body. The cleansing diet, or 'liver flush' includes a drinking mixture containing olive or almond oil, lemon and orange juice, garlic and pepper, followed by a herbal tea and fruit or vegetable salads for lunch and dinner. Meat, milk, eggs, coffee, alcohol and carbohydrate foods are excluded.

Dr Stone followed this diet with what he called the 'maintenance diet'. In the morning hot water with lemon juice is taken, followed half an hour (or more) later with a non-citrus fruit salad or whole-grain porridge. The main meal of the day is lunch and it should include fresh fruits and vegetables, sprouting grains, beans and seeds. Stone warned that typically the Western diet contains too much rich food and substances which are almost indigestible, quite apart from the fact that most of us eat too much anyway!

POTENCIES

In homeopathy, the dilutions or 'strengths' of different remedies. Tinctures diluted in a ratio of 1 part to 100 parts of water and alcohol are 1c dilutions or potencies, and a solution made of 1 part of a 1c dilution and diluted a further 100 times would be 2c. The most common potencies used in a homeopathic treatment are 6, 12 and 30 centesimal — *see Homeopathy.*

POULTICE

A bag containing linseed meal and other medicaments, dipped into boiling water for a few minutes, squeezed to remove excess water, and then laid on an inflamed area of the body. A bandage is used to retain the poultice in position.

PRANA

A Sanskrit word usually translated as 'life-force' and used by practitioners of breath-related therapies like yoga and rebirthing. The term is used to describe specific vital energies in the body and can also be used in a more general and all-encompassing way to denote the principle of life itself.

PRANAYAMA

In yoga, the science of breath control. Pranayama involves cycles of rhythmic breathing which may be used to raise kundalini energy or stabilise the flow of prana (life-energy) in the body. *See Prana, Kundalini, Yoga, Rebirthing.*

PREVENTIVE MEDICINE

That branch of health care which specialises in steps which can be taken to prevent the onset of illness and disease. Of special importance among the preventive modalities are sound diet and nutrition (especially in relation to cholesterol in the diet), stress management therapies, and the different forms of exercise which improve cardiovascular efficiency (jogging, rebounding swimming, aerobics, etc.).

PRIMAL SCREAM

In primal therapy the subject is guided gradually towards the experience of 'primal pain' — deep-seated pain which has been repressed. As realisation of this 'pain' floods increasingly into consciousness, the subject's awareness builds to a peak and this expresses itself through the 'primal scream' — a direct encounter with the inner self. The primal scream is followed by a profound sense of relief because conflicting facets of the self have been acknowledged and integrated — *see Primal Therapy.*

PRIMAL THERAPY

According to the founder of primal therapy, Arthur Janov, mental illness has its origins in primal pain, which has been carried around since childhood. This 'pain' is of a deeper nature than superficial pain and derives from such causes as serious humiliation, rejection by a parent, or terrifying isolation. The events then built up to an overload stage where they became unconscious, and at this point the pain became blocked.

The repression of pain leads to the formation of an 'unreal self', and according to Janov the new persona engages in a smothering process, increasingly shielding out the pain and refusing to acknowledge its existence. Janov believes that the 'unreal self' begins to form from the age of 6, and by the teen years the character is fairly fixed — neuroses expressing themselves through emotional and intellectual patterns.

Primal therapy seeks to dismantle the barrier of neurotic defence patterns built by the unreal self to shield the person from the experience of pain. Primal therapy endeavours to tap the deepest emotions beyond the defences and guide the subject towards the experience of primal pain, for as Janov says, 'Until we feel the pain, we suffer'.

The process of guidance is, however, a sensitive one, and the therapist has to be careful not to plunge the patient in too quickly. Healing finally takes place in the 'primal zone' — an area of consciousness where feelings are accepted and integrated. *See also Primal scream.*

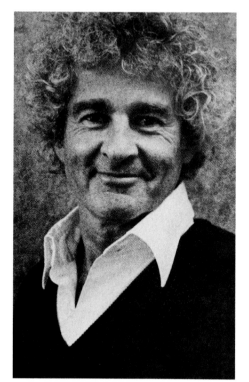

Arthur Janov, the founder of primal therapy

PRIMARY CONTROL

In the Alexander Technique, the relationship of head, neck and back required for good posture. When this relationship is in a state of balance the subject exhibits a relaxed, poised style of posture which is in contrast to unbalanced, tense styles of posture reflecting stress and contraction — *see Alexander Technique.*

PROGRESSIVE RELAXATION

A relaxation technique which involves relaxing different parts of the body in turn. Usually one begins with the feet and ankles and then progresses to the calves, knees, thighs, buttocks, abdomen, chest and arms — relaxing each of these in sequence.

PSIONIC MEDICINE

A development from medical radiesthesia utilising dowsing, aspects of homeopathy, and the concept of energy flow. Conceived by Dr George Laurence, psionic medicine seeks to diagnose body imbalance by focusing on the original and basic cause of disease, not its symptoms. Dr Laurence borrowed Samuel Hahnemann's idea of miasms — disruptive factors affecting the body's inherent self-healing capacity and the flow of life-energy. According to Dr Laurence, a high proportion of mental illness derives from inherited miasms in conjunction with acquired toxins. Syphilis and TB are the main hereditary miasms, and measles, chickenpox and whooping cough the main acquired ones. Another member of the Psionic Medical Society, Dr Aubrey Westlake, believes the hereditary TB miasm underlies many cases of asthma, hay fever and sinus complaints, and may also be connected to leukaemia and diabetes.

Psionic medical practitioners make use of a W. O. Wood chart to register pendulum readings which reflect the balance of health to disease in the body and endeavour to detect patterns of potential disease which could be transmitted as miasms from one generation to another. *See also Radiesthesia, medical, Dowsing, W. O. Wood chart.*

PSORIC SPOTS

In iridology, brownish-black pigment flecks in the iris tissue which appear to 'float' between the iris and the corneal layer covering it. Iridologists believe that the zone in which these flecks occur is significant, and that it can highlight potential deficiencies or points of vulnerability in the organ or organs concerned. *See Iridology.*

PSYCHIC MASSAGE

A massage in which the practitioner responds to healing energies and magnetic currents perceived around the patient's body (that is, the 'psychic energy field'), rather than utilising techniques of direct physical contact. The masseur or masseuse believes that the patient's etheric, or spiritual body is being massaged, rather than the physical organism. This practice is also known as 'spiritual massage'. *See also Aura.*

PSYCHIC SURGERY

A healing practice, found mainly in the Philippines and Brazil, in which the practitioner appears to penetrate the patient's skin and withdraw tissue, clots, cysts, etc. that are causing ill-health. There are over 30 Filipino healers who specialise in psychic surgery, and there have been many cases of claimed miraculous cures. However, there is also documented evidence of fraudulence and deception in which the practitioners utilise concealed mica flecks to make incisions, substitute betel-nut juice for blood, and employ advanced techniques of sleight-of-hand to simulate 'psychic surgery'. The tumours allegedly removed from patients' bodies have frequently been found to be animal fat or vegetable matter.

Critics of psychic surgery have been outspoken in branding the practitioners as frauds, and an American judge, Daniel H. Hanscom — who convened a lengthy investigation of the practice in 1974 — described psychic surgery as 'pure and unmitigated fakery'. However, these criticisms overlook the fact that psychic surgery can have a powerful placebo effect on the patient, stimulating the self-healing capacity of the body by mobilising the patient's belief that an effective cure has occurred. 'Exposure' of sleight-of-hand practices undermines the placebo value of this healing tradition which, by its very nature, supplies 'evidence' to the patient that a dramatic operation has taken place.

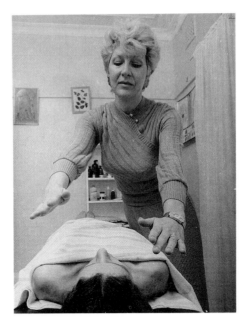

Psychic massage — healing through the aura

PSYCHOCYBERNETICS

A concept developed by Dr Maxwell Maltz, drawing on research by Norbert Wiener. According to the principles of psychocybernetics, the mind and brain function inter-dependently and the brain must transmit the concept of health into the body's cell tissues before any state of disease can be eliminated. This means that a patient has to be convinced that the healing of disease is a practical and worthwhile possibility.

Maltz's concept is focused in the power of positive thinking and emphasises that a positive state of mind is vital for healing to occur.

PSYCHOMETRY

A diagnostic technique used by spiritual healers to determine the characteristics, circumstances and state of well-being of people who are not present, but using objects that have been in their possession. The practitioner might use a personal object like a watch, a ring, or other piece of jewellery, and then hold the object with the eyes closed in order to receive 'psychic impressions' from its owner. The term 'psychometry' itself was coined by psychic researcher Dr J. R. Buchanan, and comes from the Greek words *psyche* ('soul') and *metron* ('measure'). *See also Healing channel.*

PSYCHOPERISTALSIS

A concept developed by Norwegian psychotherapist Gerda Boyesen and her colleagues Dr Trygve Braatoy and Dr Aadel Bulow-Hansen, concerning the function of intestinal peristalsis to 'dissolve and discharge residual metabolic waste products of psychosomatic origin'. Following in the Reichian tradition that the body reflects the mental condition and that effective bodywork therapy can in turn cause emotional release, the technique of psychoperistalsis involves influencing the intestines by massaging the hypertonic flexor muscles which 'hold' the feelings of anxiety. The Boyesen method includes administering a small tactile shock-impulse to eliminate the 'startle reflex' pattern in the muscles. The therapist then places a stethoscope on the patient's abdomen and listens to the internal rumblings which follow. In successful psychoperistalsis, release of this particular type of body armour is characterised by extended peristaltic sounds, 'as if a chain reaction had been initiated'. Psychoperistalsis can lead to a state of abreaction (the release of repressed emotion). *See also Reichian therapy, Body armour.*

PSYCHOSYNTHESIS

A comprehensive approach to human development and personality integration formulated by Italian psychiatrist Dr Roberto Assagioli (1888–1974) from 1911 onwards.

Assagioli was a colleague of Freud and Jung, but believed that psychoanalysis did not pay sufficient attention to the 'higher' aspects of man — specifically those regions of the psyche now known as 'transpersonal'. Psychosynthesis emphasises the integration of energies relating to the centre of awareness and the will.

Initially these are thought of as the 'I', or personal self, but this subsequently develops towards knowledge of the transpersonal self.

Psychosynthesis is not identified with a single technique or practice, and in fact encompasses a variety of approaches and modalities. Use is often made of guided imagery and visualisation exercises. Overall, psychosynthesis functions in 5 main fields: the *therapeutic* (psychotherapy, doctor–patient relationships); *personal integration and actualisation* (self-realisation of personal potential); *education* (involving parents and educators in schools); *interpersonal relationships* (between couples, partners, family members, etc.) and *social relationships* (between and within groups). *See also Transpersonal psychology, Self-actualisation, Guided imagery.*

PYRAMID ENERGY

In the 1930s a French explorer named Antoine Bovis took refuge from the sun in the pharoah's chamber of the Great Pyramid at Giza, Egypt, which is located at the centre of the structure, one-third of the way up from the base. Bovis found it very humid, but was surprised to find that the bodies of a dead cat and some other desert animals had not decayed there but had simply dehydrated. Bovis wondered whether the structure of the pyramid itself had something to do with this effect, so he later made an exact model of the pyramid, aligned it north-south and east-west, and placed a dead cat inside it in a comparable position to the central chamber. He found that once again the body dried out but did not decay.

Following on this theme, some alternative health practitioners have suggested that 'pyramid energy' can be used to enhance the flavour and storage-life of food and drink. Typically a 9-inch (23 cm) pyramid frame is used; it is placed, with vortex up, over vegetables, fruit, meat, fish and beverages. According to Australian naturopathic researcher Graydon Rixon, pyramid models:

• arrest the bacterial breakdown in meat

and can be used to dehydrate vegetables and fruit without diminishing their flavour;

- help cheap wines become milder and more palatable after a night in the frame;
- stimulate plant growth;
- increase the potency of vitamin supplements.

English researcher Alan Geffin, who uses pyramid frames to enhance the taste and quality of tap water, also agrees that 'pyramid energy' can improve the taste of wine, and claims that he has been able to store small pieces of meat and fish for up to a month under a pyramid.

Large open pyramid frames are used by some practitioners for meditation — specifically to enhance connection with the universal life-force.

R

RADIESTHESIA, MEDICAL

Form of dowsing in which the practitioner uses a pendulum to diagnose disease. Usually a geometric chart, scale or rule is also used, and this indicates different categories of disease. A specific point on the scale indicates maximum vitality. In addition, various 'witnesses' are positioned on the chart. These represent diseases or organs of the body on the one hand, and the patient on the other (in the form of hair, nail clippings or a sample of blood). Practitioners of medical radiesthesia believe that all matter has innate energy fields and that the human body can tune in to these fields through the dowsing instrument. The movement of the pendulum is therefore crucial in the diagnosis. If it swings in a clockwise or anticlockwise direction

before reaching the 'optimal' point on the scale, this indicates a point of lowered vitality. *See also Dowsing, Diagnostic witness, Patient's witness, W. O. Wood chart, Psionic medicine.*

RADII SOLARIS

In iridology, dark 'wheel spokes' in the iris which present a distinctive contrast to the raised white fibres. Iridologists believe that radii solaris indicate the presence of infection and inflammation, and that they often result from toxic waste residues. They can also be caused by stress. Naturopathic treatment includes the use of holly as a purgative herb, and implementation of a revised lifestyle pattern in which stress factors are acknowledged and rectified — *see Iridology.*

RADIONICS

A system of medical diagnosis devised by American doctor Albert Abrams. In 1910, while Abrams was examining a patient's ulcer, he noticed that a small area of the abdomen produced a dull note when it was percussed, or tapped. In due course, Abrams came to believe that different diseases produced different areas of dullness in the body, and diseased tissue could be diagnosed using electronic equipment — specifically, a variable resistance box. Abrams found that cancer produced dullness with 50 ohm resistance, while syphilis did so with 55 ohm resistance. Abrams later changed his approach, replacing the diseased tissue samples with a drop of the patient's blood.

Abrams' radionics equipment was later modified by Dr Ruth Drown in the United States and George de la Warr in Britain, but charges of fraud were brought against both of them. This form of diagnosis is rarely practised today.

RADIX

A one-to-one neo-Reichian therapy developed by health educator Chuck Kelley. In Reichian terms, radix works from the ocular through to the pelvic segments of the body and utilises bioenergetic techniques to overcome pain, anger and fear. The experience resolves itself in abreaction. *See also Bioenergy, Reichian therapy, Abreaction.*

REBIRTHING

A bodywork technique utilising hyperventilation breathing to induce a state of emotional climax and catharsis. Based on the Indian science of breath, pranayama, the rebirthing technique has been developed by Leonard Orr and Dr Stanislav Grof.

In a rebirthing session the patient relaxes and uses a 'connected breathing' rhythm in which there is no pause between the in-breath and the out-breath.

The therapist monitors this breathing as it produces a state of hyperventilation and leads the patient into an altered state of consciousness. The basic idea is for the patient to develop an inner vibrational state (known medically as 'tetany') and to then build this to a peak — passing through emotional blockages or overcoming traumatic memories which rise into consciousness.

In many people rebirthing produces a feeling of spiritual renewal. As Orr comments: 'You merge with your breath, flowing, glowing, soaring, relaxing profoundly, your mind melting into your spirit, surging, awakening your inner being and the quiet sounds of your soul.'

Rebirthing is usually done with the subject resting on a mat ('dry rebirthing') and may be accompanied by peaceful or intense music, depending on appropriateness (the latter is used by Dr Grof in his special approach which he now calls 'Grof breathing'). It is also possible to apply the techniques of rebirthing in a hot-tub ('wet rebirthing'). *See also Pranayama, Wet rebirthing.*

REFLEXOLOGY

A natural health therapy which focuses on the reflex points of the feet. There are approximately 72 000 nerve endings in each foot, which in turn connect to other parts of the body. Practitioners maintain that by applying massage to those nerve endings, an impulse is conveyed to the other organs. Different regions of the sole connect with such organs as the pituitary glands, lungs, bladder, kidneys, stomach and spleen, and the impulse transmitted to each of these organs causes a reflex response, stimulating the organ to return to its optimal body function.

The reflexologist applies firm pressure with the thumb, focusing in each case on specific pressure points. Reflexology not only stimulates nerve endings but is also effective in crushing crystalline deposits — mostly of uric acid and excess calcium — which form around the nerve endings of the feet.

Reflexology is sometimes referred to as 'zone therapy'.

Zones on the sole, utilised in reflexology

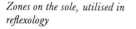

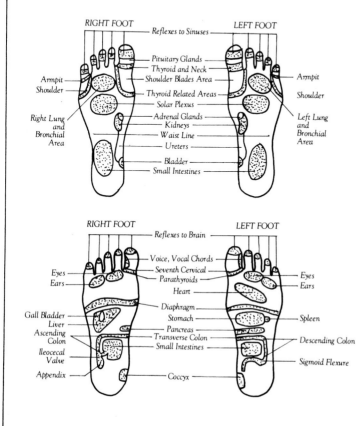

RIGHT FOOT LEFT FOOT

Reflexes to Sinuses
Pituitary Glands
Thyroid and Neck
Armpit
Shoulder
Shoulder Blades Area
Thyroid Related Areas
Armpit
Shoulder
Solar Plexus
Right Lung and Bronchial Area
Adrenal Glands
Kidneys
Left Lung and Bronchial Area
Waist Line
Ureters
Bladder
Small Intestines

RIGHT FOOT LEFT FOOT

Reflexes to Brain
Voice, Vocal Chords
Seventh Cervical
Eyes
Ears
Parathyroids
Eyes
Ears
Heart
Diaphragm
Gall Bladder
Liver
Ascending Colon
Stomach
Pancreas
Spleen
Transverse Colon
Ileocecal Valve
Small Intestines
Descending Colon
Appendix
Sigmoid Flexure
Coccyx

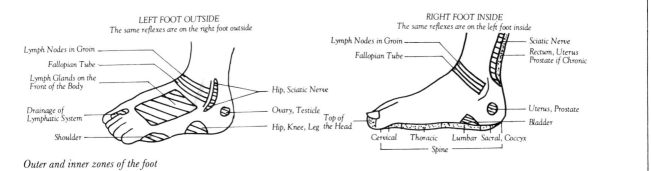

LEFT FOOT OUTSIDE
The same reflexes are on the right foot outside

Lymph Nodes in Groin
Fallopian Tube
Lymph Glands on the Front of the Body
Drainage of Lymphatic System
Shoulder

Hip, Sciatic Nerve
Ovary, Testicle
Hip, Knee, Leg

RIGHT FOOT INSIDE
The same reflexes are on the left foot inside

Lymph Nodes in Groin
Fallopian Tube

Sciatic Nerve
Rectum, Uterus Prostate if Chronic

Top of the Head

Uterus, Prostate
Bladder

Cervical   Thoracic   Lumbar Sacral, Coccyx
Spine

Outer and inner zones of the foot

REICHIAN THERAPY

Bodywork therapy derived from Wilhelm Reich's concept of character and body armouring. Reich trained in medicine at the University of Vienna and later worked with Sigmund Freud. Like Freud, Reich was interested in the sexual aspects of personality and he came to the view that repression of the emotions and sexual instincts could lead to blockages resulting in rigid patterns of behaviour (character armour) and the tightening of specific muscle groups (body armour). As such blockages increased, the energy flow through the body would be impeded and in chronic instances could lead to a marked deterioration of health.

For Reich the climax of sexual orgasm was a satisfying release from tension that allowed sexual energy to be discharged in the context of both the physical embrace and love between partners. By contrast, people who felt guilty or inadequate in terms of sexual expression often repressed their emotions, resulting in the neurotic, negative behaviour patterns Reich termed 'character armouring'.

Reichian therapy involves the dismantling of the layers of pent-up emotion through 7 different zones of the body. These body segments are the ocular, oral, cervical, thoracic, diaphragmatic, abdominal and pelvic *(see separate listings)*.

RHUS TOX

A homeopathic remedy used for rheumatism, stiff joints and arthritis. Rhus tox (from the plant *Rhus toxicodendron*) eases muscular pain and stiffness, and helps minimise acid deposits in the joints and muscles. It is also useful for skin allergies and hay fever. It is normally used as Rhus tox 6 potency.

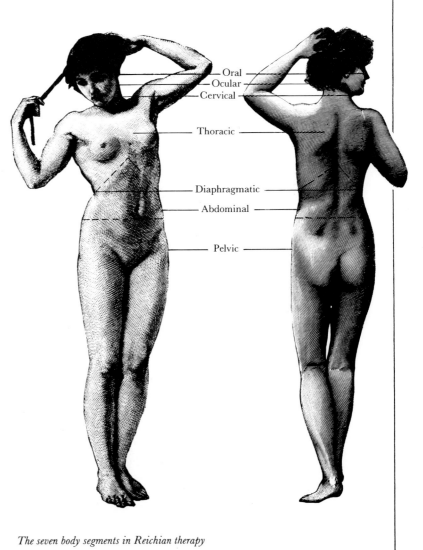

Oral
Ocular
Cervical
Thoracic
Diaphragmatic
Abdominal
Pelvic

The seven body segments in Reichian therapy

ROLFING

A bodywork approach developed by Swiss-born American biochemist Dr Ida Rolf. The aim of Rolfing is to re-order the major segments of the body — head, shoulders, thorax, pelvis and legs — into a vertical alignment. According to Rolf, any distortions in man's posture are accentuated by gravity. Rolfing utilises a deep massage technique which at times can be painful: pressure is applied with the knuckles to loosen the fascia and muscles and allow the fibres to return to their proper position.

After Rolfing sessions the body acquires a new sense of lightness, the head and chest are lifted, and the trunk is lengthened. The body joints tend to have more freedom, and the body movement is more fluid. Rolfing seems to allow more efficient use of the muscles with less expended energy.

Rolfing usually requires 10 sessions spaced over 5–10 weeks.

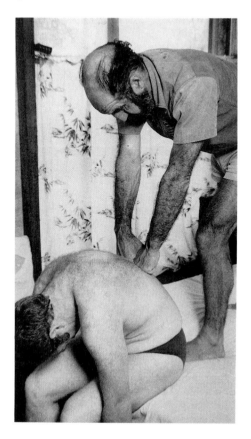

In Rolfing, pressure is applied with the knuckles

RUTA GRAVEOLENS

A homeopathic remedy from the rue plant, *Ruta graveolens*, used to strengthen and tone ligaments and tendons and to ease pain and stiffness following physical exertion or manipulation. Ideal for sporting injuries (ligament strain, bruised knees, etc.), it can also be used to relieve pain from 'slipped discs'. It is normally used as Ruta graveolens 6 or 12 potency.

S

SAMADHI TANK

A sensory isolation tank used for relaxation. The tank is constructed from fibreglass and eliminates external sounds and light. It also contains heavily salinated water heated to 'ambient skin temperature' (approximately 35.2°C) and has a sliding door which can easily be folded back from the inside.

The subject floats naked inside the tank for around 45 minutes, learning gradually, over a number of 'floats', to surrender personal stress, tensions and anxieties. Some people may experience claustrophobia on the first occasion, but during subsequent sessions these fears tend to dissipate. The samadhi tank concept derives from original prototypes developed by Dr John Lilly while he was undertaking brain research for the National Institute of Mental Health in the United States. 'Float to Relax' centres may now be found in many countries of the world. *See also Float to Relax.*

SAUNA BATH

A Finnish therapeutic treatment, now popular in many countries, in which one sits in a steam-saturated room specially constructed for the purpose of containing heat. The sauna temperatures range from 100–120°C (212–250°F) and a session generally lasts from 5–20 minutes. Sauna baths are followed by a plunge into cold water — usually a shower or swimming pool.

SCANNING

In the Bates Method, a natural treatment for vision improvement in which the eyes are moved rapidly from one small spot of focus to the next — *see Bates Method.*

SEIZA

A Japanese term, used by practitioners of Oriental bodywork therapies. It describes the act of sitting in a kneeling position while keeping the back straight.

SELF-ACTUALISATION

An expression used by American psychologist Abraham Maslow to describe 'the full use and exploitation of talents, capacities, potentialities . . .' Maslow was interested in discussing the creative and intellectual capacities of healthy people, rather than those suffering from disease or neurosis, and his thinking is central to the rise of transpersonal psychology and the human potential movement — *see Transpersonal psychology, Human potential movement.*

SELF-DIRECTED IMAGERY

A visualisation method used in self-hypnosis to enable subjects to control their own healing processes. For example, in learning pain control a subject might visualise an image epitomising the pain and then a second image to counteract it, or drain it of potency. In some forms of cancer therapy, for example the visualisation techniques pioneered by Dr Carl Simonton and Dr David Bresler in the United States, subjects visualise the source of their cancers in the body and then use other positive images to erode and finally overcome the disease-image. *See also Auto-suggestion, Guided imagery.*

SELF-REALISATION

A term used in different schools of meditation and yoga, to denote knowledge of one's true, inner self or spiritual enlightenment.

SENSORY ISOLATION TANK — *see Samadhi tank*

SENTIC CYCLES

A system of classifying the emotions, developed by Viennese-born physiologist and musician Dr Manfred Clynes. According to Dr Clynes each emotion has a specific dynamic form of expression and these are coded into the central nervous system of each human being. Clynes' so-called 'Standard Cycle' consists of 7 emotions — anger, hate, grief, love, sex, joy and reverence — and in a therapeutic application, subjects are taught to express these emotions in sequence while listening to a guidance tape. According to Dr Clynes, different emotions have a characteristic time span for their expression, ranging from 4.8 seconds for anger to 9.8 for reverence.

SEXUAL THERAPY

Any therapy designed to enhance the quality of sexual expression and fulfilment, either as a means of personal self-development or to improve relations with one's partner. Wilhelm Reich encouraged his patients to develop what he called 'orgastic potency' — 'the capacity for surrender to the flow of biological energy without any inhibition, the capacity for complete discharge of all dammed-up sexual excitation through involuntary pleasurable contractions of the body . . .' Reich discovered that as a result of such self-expression his patients also learned to develop tenderness and sensitivity in their sexual relationships.

As several specialists have indicated, however, sexual therapy should also emphasise the capacity for love as well as sexual release. Psychiatrist Thomas Szasz has made the point that 'love . . . so transcends the physiological need for tension-relief that it can be spiritually satisfying even in the absence of providing relief from sexual tension . . . love is a profoundly personal experience'. Dr James Lynch, an authority on human relationships, also confirms this view. 'Human love involves much more than an orgasm . . . one of the agendas is companionship.'

Sexual therapies therefore vary across a wide spectrum from those emphasising the physical release of pent-up or repressed sexual energies to those which regard friendship, love and caring as the most important aspects of a sexual relationship. *See also Reichian therapy.*

SHAMAN

In primitive societies, a medicine man, priest or sorcerer who is able to enter a trance state at will and who serves as an intermediary between the people and the realm of gods and spirits. Shamans may be required to banish the spirits of disease or recover the lost soul of a sick or dispirited person. *See also Medicine man, Spiritual healing.*

SHIATSU

A Japanese bodywork technique utilising traditional acupuncture points, but employing manipulation and pressure from the thumbs, fingers and palms rather than needles or mechanical instruments. Shiatsu reinforces joints and muscles, and focuses on the efficient flow of energy throughout the meridians and autonomic nervous system. Often referred to as a 'one-point' pressure system, shiatsu has an advantage over acupuncture in that it can be self-administered — the subject simply has to know which of the 365 *tsubos* requires pressure in order to treat the specific complaint. Thumb pressure is the most common form, and is applied for around 2–7 seconds to the body surface. Shiatsu is also known as *acupressure. See also Acupuncture.*

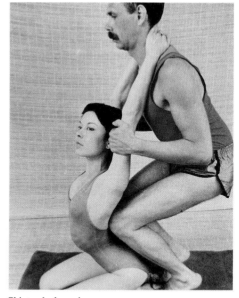

Shiatsu bodywork

SHINTAIDO

An approach to human movement and expression formulated by Japanese educator Hiroyuki Aoki. Drawing on Japanese martial arts traditions, Aoki developed shintaido as a 'body way' that would utilise physical movement to express the inner spirit of man and eliminate superfluous action.

There are several shintaido 'forms', among them *eiko dai*, which includes 'embracing the world' and then running as freely as possible, and *tenshingoso*, designed to express the idea of tapping inner peace and creating one's own world. Shintaido emphasises the interrelatedness of body, mind and spirit, and combines physical exercise with poetic physical expression. Shintaido, as one writer has said, 'gives us a glimpse of worlds that are bigger than our imagination'.

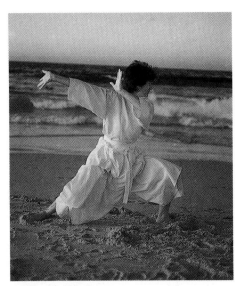

A shintaido 'form'

SITZ BATH

In hydrotherapy, a bath designed in 2 sections so that the hips and feet can be immersed at different temperatures. The person sits in the larger bath with the lower abdomen covered by water and the knees raised so that the feet extend into the second, smaller, adjoining bath. Sitz baths are useful for treating illnesses of the lower abdomen — especially genital, urinary and intestinal disorders — and may also be suitable for inducing sweating in elderly patients. The person sitting in the sitz bath can be covered with a blanket and the bath itself provides safe support.

SLOUGHING

A cosmetic technique of removing flaky skin, or dead tissue cells, from the body using a loofah. Vigorous massage of the thighs may help reduce pockets of cellulite. *See also Loofah, Cellulite* (Part 3).

SODIUM RING

In iridology, a dense white narrow band identified around the outside rim of the iris. Iridologists maintain that this condition often correlates with stiffness in the joints and recommend natural forms of sodium, like vegetable salt, as a curative agent. The sodium ring is sometimes known as the calcium ring because it correlates with calcium deposits on the walls of both major and minor blood vessels. *See Iridology.*

SPECIFIC POINT PRESSURE

In massage, pressure applied to a specific point on the body, such as an acupressure point (as in shiatsu) or a particular point on the foot (as in reflexology). This may be achieved by overlapping the thumbs and applying pressure on the point in question.

SPIRITUAL HEALING

An ancient healing tradition in which an appeal is made to a spiritual being — usually a god or spirit — to participate in healing the sick. Sometimes the god is believed to manifest as a divine presence; on other occasions the healing 'energy' is transmitted through a medium (the spiritual healer) to the patient, and a cure effected. The technique of laying-on-of-hands is a common form of spiritual healing.

Christianity has a strong healing tradition and has its very foundations in Jesus Christ's spiritual powers. During his lifetime around 40 healing miracles were recorded, and in the Middle Ages, the Church encouraged recognition of the shrines of saints and claimed that their relics could also transmit a healing power. Several denominations of the Christian Church today hold regular healing services where the sick can receive laying-on-of-hands, anointing with oil, and prayer.

Spiritual healing is not confined to the Christian tradition. It was practised in ancient Egypt and Greece, and today many alternative healers who practise as psychometrists and 'intuitive' or healing channels perform essentially the same task — of transmitting a healing energy to those who are sick. *See also Psychic massage, Miracle cures, Placebo, Psychometry.*

SPIRITUAL MASSAGE —
see Psychic massage

STANDARD CYCLE

A term used in sentics to describe 7 basic emotions, considered in sequence — *see Sentic Cycles.*

STARTLE RESPONSE

In bioenergetics, an inhibitory muscular pattern in which flexor muscles hold themselves in a stress position. This response may also be accompanied by inhibited breathing patterns and deformed posture. If the flexor muscles can be released by therapeutic massage or other bodywork techniques, the startle response and the state of anxiety associated with it, can be eliminated. *See also Body armour, Bioenergetics, Reichian therapy.*

STARTLE RESPONSE

In the Alexander Technique, the body's response to a sudden noise or action. The startle response distorts the shoulders and arms, shortens the length of the torso, and increases tension in the legs. On an extended basis the response can lead to different forms of postural imbalance; for example, lordosis, kyphosis or scoliosis.

STEAM BOWL

Steam bowls are used in natural cosmetic health care. The bowl is filled with boiling water and herbs like rosemary, thyme or lavender, and a towel is draped over the head and bowl, producing a 'canopy' effect. A shallow breath pattern is then used, the head is lowered over the bowl, and the steam is absorbed into the pores of the skin (any make-up should be removed first). The resulting perspiration clears out tissue wastes and after approximately 2 minutes the face should be splashed with herbal toner or cool water. *See also Facial steambath.*

STRUCTURAL REINTEGRATION

A term used by Ida Rolf to define the principal aim in Rolfing. This therapy seeks to restore the body to its normal vertical alignment through a technique of deep massage and physical manipulation. In Rolfing the body is 're-ordered' through its major segments: the head, shoulders, thorax, pelvis and legs — *see Rolfing.*

SUBLUXATION

In chiropractic, an incomplete dislocation of a bone or vertebra — *see Chiropractic.*

SULPHUR BATH

A remedial bath used to treat rheumatism, skin complaints and various nervous disorders. The solution consists of 60 g (2 oz) of potassium sulphide dissolved in approximately 68 litres (15 gallons) of water.

SUPPOSITORY

A medication which is applied by insertion into the rectum or vagina. The medication may be intended to treat a local condition or be absorbed into the body system as a whole.

SWEDISH MASSAGE

A form of vigorous massage which stimulates the circulation of blood through the soft tissues of the body. Swedish massage utilises rubbing and stroking actions, kneading, squeezing, slapping and pounding. Deep massage is sometimes also employed. Swedish massage probably derives its name from Peter Ling (1776–1839), a Swedish pioneer of massage.

SWINGING

In the Bates Method, the act of turning the head from side to side to loosen tense neck muscles. Swinging is designed to relax the eyes and is performed in conjunction with palming — *see Bates Method, Palming.*

T

TAI CHI

A Chinese form of self-expression resembling slow, graceful dance but intended primarily as a means of surrendering to the natural flow of energy in the universe. The words *tai chi* translate as 'supreme ultimate' and reflect the idea of a universal life-force which sustains each individual and unites him with all other forms of manifestation. Tai chi is linked historically to oriental martial arts like kung-fu and karate, but it is more contemplative — replacing aggression and hostility with sensitivity and the capacity to yield to an overriding calm.

Some tai chi movements are said to derive from the motion of birds and animals, and all are designed to complement each other. They begin with stillness and produce a sense of revitalisation as well as a profound feeling of serenity and well-being.

There are different forms of tai chi. Some traditions require strict adherence to specific movements, while others are more free-form, placing greater emphasis on spontaneous self-expression. As well-known contemporary exponent of tai chi, Al Chung Liang Huang, writes in his book *Embrace Tiger, Return to Mountain*, 'Tai Chi is to help you get acquainted with your own sense of potential growth, the creative process of just being you'.

TAPOTEMENT

In massage, movements which 'strike' at the body, for example, hacking, cupping or flicking. These movements bring the blood to the surface, stimulate weak muscles and the nervous system, and help break down adhesions around the joints. Tapotement should not be applied to the kidney region. *See also Massage, Hacking, Cupping, Flicking.*

THALASSOTHERAPY

From the Greek *thalassa*, meaning 'the sea', a therapeutic approach based on the concept that seawater and the plant life within it can assist a variety of ailments, ranging from arthritis and rheumatism to weight and skin complaints. This type of therapy may also include flexing and toning exercises performed while swimming.

Thalassotherapists maintain that the body fluids have a natural affinity with seawater because of mankind's aquatic evolutionary origins. Blood plasma is in fact reasonably similar to seawater in composition.

THORACIC SEGMENT

One of the 7 body segments in Reichian therapy. The thoracic segment includes the chest and chest cage, the hands, arms, intercostal muscles, pectorals and deltoids, as well as the scapular and spinal muscles. Thoracic segment armouring may manifest as a tight rib-cage or depression of the sternum. Blocked emotions associated with this segment of the body include anger, pain, fear and love. Some armouring, for example, may result from a lack of parental nurturing. Babies separated from their mothers for lengthy periods following a difficult birth may also suffer armouring in this segment. *See Reichian therapy.*

TINCTURE

A dilute solution of a substance in alcohol, used as a medicament; for example, tincture of iodine.

TONING

A meditative technique developed by American healer Laurel Elizabeth Keyes. Toning evolved as a means of releasing meditative energy through sound — an expression of the energy Laurel Keyes believes lies dormant in everyone, awaiting release.

In toning the subject stands erect with the feet apart and the shoulders evenly aligned. The eyes are closed and the body is allowed to sway slightly from side to side, inviting the life-rhythms to manifest. The 'tone' comes up from the earth through the feet, rather than emanating from the mind, and as the voice responds to this influx of energy there is an accompanying feeling of release. The voice is toned low from the earth, but gradually rises in exultation to the sky. As Laurel Keyes has said, 'Let the body be free, let the voice be free, let health emerge'.

The natural range of toning seems to be from A to A, above and below Middle C. Toning blends naturally with medi-

tation and slow, rhythmic breathing, and ideally any toning session should conclude with a visualisation in which one feels filled with pure, cleansing light. Laurel Keyes believes toning to be effective because it releases tensions, pressures and blockages. As she has said, 'Once you feel energetic and alive, you *are*!'

TOUCH FOR HEALTH

A modified form of applied kinesiology developed by Dr John Thie in the early 1970s. Touch for Health is a holistic health therapy which draws on Dr George Goodheart's notion that most forms of muscle spasm are 'secondary' rather than 'primary'. Essentially, Touch for Health shows how to release energies in the body and enable it to regain health and balance.

Touch for Health emphasises that changes in body posture and the tone of certain muscles affect the position and function of the internal organs and the energy available to them. The Touch for Health practitioner utilises acupuncture meridians as 'channels of energy' and relates each meridian to an 'indicator muscle' — usually in the arm or leg. The practitioner then tests for muscle weakness — not in a specific, localised sense, but as an indicator of an energy pattern occurring within the body as a whole. All aspects of mind and body are interrelated, so anxieties, stresses and even nutritional factors reveal themselves in posture and muscle patterns.

The Touch for Health approach is both diagnostic and preventive in its emphasis, showing the subject in each case how to identify energy imbalances and prevent their recurrence in the future. *See also Applied kinesiology.*

TRAGER THERAPY

A bodywork therapy developed by American medical practitioner Dr Milton Trager. The Trager practitioner makes extensive use of touch-contact with the patient's body, and endeavours to encourage the patient to experience the 'freeing-up' of different parts of the body. The idea is to use motion in the muscles and joints to produce positive sensory feelings which are then fed back into the central nervous system. The end result is a feeling of lightness, freedom and flexibility. As Dr Trager has said: 'When the body *feels* lighter, it begins to move as though it *were* lighter'. Each session of Trager therapy lasts for around 1–1½ hours.

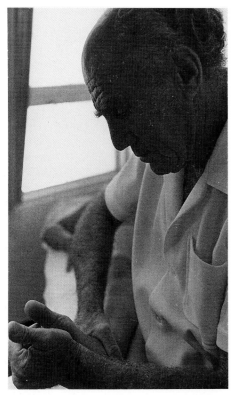

Dr Milton Trager

TRANCE, HYPNOTIC

An altered state of consciousness in which a subject's powers of concentration are mobilised and subconscious memories and perceptions allowed to rise into consciousness. Hypnotherapists relax their subjects progressively, often by using a countdown procedure or by progressively relaxing the body limb by limb from

the feet to the head. The pioneering European hypnotherapists recognised the value of imagination for therapeutic purposes, and combined relaxation techniques with guided imagery. For example, Alfred Binet encouraged his patients to 'talk' to the visual images that arose in what he called 'provoked introspection' and Wolfgang Kretschmer described the process in 1922 as *bilderstreifendenken* — 'thinking in the form of a movie'. For Kretschmer, and for other therapists since, hypnotic trance could be used to 'expose internal psychic problems' that presented themselves in the consciousness of the subject. *See also Hypnosis, Guided imagery.*

TRANSCENDENTAL MEDITATION (TM)

A form of meditation advocated by the Indian spiritual teacher Maharishi Mahesh Yogi. TM requires that the person meditating relax totally and concentrate on repeating an individual, secret mantra. The Maharishi believes that when the mind is attuned to the mantra, it acquires a more profound and transcendental power, helping the person attain true self-knowledge. In due course, the mind is emptied of its contents and the experience of 'Pure Being' remains. This is the true nature of the mind, and attaining this transcendent state enhances one's sense of happiness and unity with life.

Transcental meditation has over 6 million adherents in the United States and is also popular in Britain, Europe and Australia. *See also Meditation.*

TRANSPERSONAL PSYCHOLOGY

A name given to the so-called 'fourth force' in psychology. Transpersonal psychology follows on from 'first force' classical psychoanalytical theory, 'second force' behaviourist psychology and 'third force' humanistic psychology. It deals with such areas of human consciousness as self-transcendence, peak experience, and ultimate values, as well as focusing more on health and well-being than neurosis and disease.

The term 'transpersonal' itself refers to that which transcends the ego. The term was first used in 1967 in a lecture by Dr Stanislav Grof, the psychiatrist who helped develop rebirthing, and it became the title of a new movement in psychology.

The rise of interest in transpersonal psychology is closely associated with the human potential movement and such personal growth centres as the Esalen Institute in California.

TRICHOLOGY

A branch of natural health care specialising in treatment for thinning hair, hair loss and scalp problems. Thinning hair and hair loss can be due to hereditary factors, but may also result from problems associated with the adrenal or pituitary glands, blood sugar imbalances and anaemia. Some trichologists are exploring the use of nutritional supplements for hair and scalp problems, focusing especially on the vitamins A, C, B complex and E, as well as the amino acid tyrosine and zinc. However specific, scientifically validated findings have not yet been presented.

TRITURATION

In homeopathy, the act of grinding together 1 part of finely divided, otherwise insoluble materials (for example, gold, copper, quartz, vegetable carbon) with 100 parts of lactose, to form a 1c potency. This process is then continued to the 6c dilution. At this stage the solution is dissolved in water to arrive at standard potencies. Through trituration the founder of homeopathy, Dr Samuel Hahnemann, extended the range of homeopathic remedies available.

TSUBO

Also known as acu-points, the specific points on different meridian channels utilised in acupuncture and shiatsu.

TURKISH BATH

A type of remedial bath which produces profuse perspiration. Hot dry air (approximately 60°C or 140°F) is applied to the body for around 20 minutes, followed by a rubdown, massage and cold water douche. Turkish baths stimulate the skin and may be used to treat such conditions as rheumatism, eczema and malaria. *See also Douche, Hydrotherapy.*

U

UNDERWATER BIRTH

A technique of birth delivery, supported by Jacque Mayol, Michel Odent and Igor Charkovsky, among others, in which the mother delivers the newborn child in a bath, attended by a doctor and midwife. Advocates of this method maintain that it is a 'non-violent' type of birth for the child and provides a relaxing and sensual environment for the mother. For many it simply extends the view of Leboyer, who believed that newborn babies should be immersed briefly in water.

Michel Odent has delivered more than 100 'water babies' in his clinic in France and uses the term *Homo delphinus* to describe them — they are, he believes, 'human dolphins'.

UNGUENT — *see Ointment*

V

VEGETATIVE NERVOUS SYSTEM

An expression used in bioenergetics, especially with reference to psychoperistalsis. It refers to the nervous impulse responses which correspond to the functions of the abdomen and intestines. *See Psychoperistalsis.*

VIBRATION

In massage, a movement in which the practitioner holds the arm rigid and applies pressure with the fingertips or the flat surface of the hand. Vibration massage is useful as a means of relieving pain and tension, and can also be used to disperse flatulence and loosen stiff joints.

VOICE DIALOGUE

A therapy created by Jungian analysts Dr Harold Stone and Dr Sidra Winkelman to uncover 'sub-personalities' within the individual consciousness. According to Stone and Winkelman, the most important aspect of the current evolution of human consciousness is to become aware that the mind consists of many different parts. These include archetypes, energy patterns and 'sub-personalities' — each a different but coherent way of thinking, feeling, behaving and perceiving. Each of these constituent forces is capable of acting autonomously and directing one's life in unique and specific ways.

In voice dialogue workshops the subject sits in a chair surrounded by other empty chairs representing different 'sub-personalities'. The subject moves to these other chairs when he or she feels inclined to become *that* aspect of the self only. At the same time the person keeps up a voice dialogue pertaining to the different facets represented by each move, speaking from the viewpoint, for example, of a 'mother', a 'child', a 'victim', a 'warrior' or a 'self-critic', and so on.

These movements are watched and evaluated by a 'facilitator' (or listener) who remains calm and objective, offering only subtle suggestions and noting unnoticed moves occurring between one sub-personality and another.

Voice dialogue is best known in the United States— with centres in several cities — but it is now gaining recognition in Europe and Australia.

W

WET REBIRTHING

A type of rebirthing technique where the patient floats naked, face down, in warm water wearing a snorkel and nose-clip, while maintaining the connected breath cycle. The patient is supported by a therapist during the float, which is often conducted in a hot-tub.

The basic idea is that the patient should surrender his ego to the surroundings, thereby allowing for an experience resembling that of a foetus in the womb. The patient is then lifted by the therapist out of the tub onto a nearby mat and covered with blankets, so that an extended period of rest or meditation is then possible. *See Rebirthing, Connected breath cycle.*

W. O. WOOD CHART

Named after a prominent dowser, the W. O. Wood chart is used by practitioners of psionic medicine to register pendulum readings which determine degrees of balance and imbalance in treating disease. Health is represented as zero on the chart *(see diagram)*, and deviations are marked as 'plus' or 'minus' readings. A threefold variable applies because different factors are brought to bear at each point of the triangle. A sample of the patient's blood (known as the patient's witness) is placed in the right-hand corner and a selection of disease entities in homeopathic potency (the diagnostic witness) in the left-hand corner. Proposed homeopathic remedies are placed at the apex. When the appropriate treatment is correctly established, the dowser's pendulum should swing up and down the zero line without deviation. *See also Homeopathy, Dowsing, Radiesthesia, medical, Diagnostic witness, Patient's witness.*

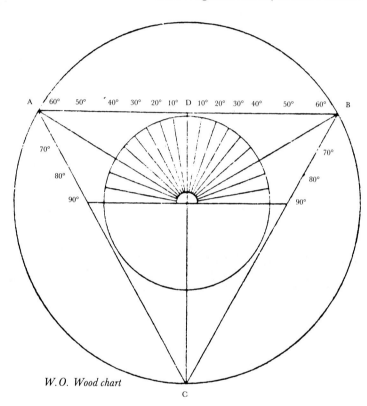

W.O. Wood chart

WUSHU

Chinese aerobic exercises, ancient in origin, including aerial leaps, turns, slaps, kicks and lunges. Like ballet, wushu features fluid coordinated movements and emphasises a straight spine, with energy perceived as radiating forth from the limbs. Although wushu evolved from Stone Age hunting skills, it is not combat-oriented and focuses on graceful flowing movements. It is popular in China today, both as a performance sport and as a type of exercise.

Y

YIN AND YANG

In Chinese medicine *yin* and *yang* represent the two different polarities of life-energy in the universe. *Yin* refers to that which is passive, negative and inward-looking, and is designated as feminine. *Yang* is active, positive and outward-looking and is designated as masculine.

The *yin* organs of the body are the hollow organs related to absorption and discharge: the large and small intestines, the gall and urinary bladders, and the stomach.

The *yang* organs are the denser organs with a regulatory function, and these include the heart, liver, spleen, kidney and lungs.

The balance of *yin* and *yang* energy is considered integral to the maintenance of good health, and practitioners of Chinese medicine test for imbalances of *chi* through pulse diagnosis and personal observation of the patient. Energy imbalance may then be rectified through the techniques of acupuncture or acupressure (shiatsu), both of which stimulate an energy response in different meridians (energy channels) of the body. *See also Acupuncture, Shiatsu.*

YOGA

From the Sanskrit *yuj* 'to bind together', Hindu spiritual teachings and techniques related to the attainment of self-realisation and union with Brahman. Yoga is popular in the West both for its physical applications in yoga postures, or asanas, and for its spiritual and mental discipline.

The 4 main concepts in yoga are *karma*, the law of cause and effect which links people to the universe; *maya*, the illusion of the manifested world; *nirvana*, the absolute reality beyond illusion, and the techniques and principles of yoga itself, which enable practitioners to gain liberation from their senses. Yoga is considered to be a way of training to see things as they *are*, rather than as they *seem*. One of the basic techniques in yoga is therefore meditation, since this turns one's consciousness toward the inner reality, bringing it finally to the transcendence of illusory perceptions.

In order that the mind be calmed, a certain number of obstacles *(klesas)* have to be overcome. Basically, these are ignorance, the sense of ego and identification with the body, attention to pleasure, repulsion from pain, and the desire for life. From the yogic viewpoint, people are trapped in a world clouded by impure perceptions and preconceived ideas. It is this false reality that has to be transcended. According to the important yogic philosopher Patanjali, there are 4 basic processes: withdrawal of attention from the external world; concentration of energy in a definite direction; the subsequent spontaneous flow of consciousness, and finally unity of consciousness with the godhead *(samadhi)*.

In kundalini yoga, psychic energy is raised through the channel known as *sushumna*, which corresponds to the spinal cord, and *ida* and *pingala*, which intercoil around it, corresponding to the sympathetic nerve ganglion on either side of the spine. The *kundalini* energy is aroused from the base of the spine and passes through 7 energy centres or *chakras*.

As a *yogi* (male) or *yogini* (female) practitioner of yoga finds unity of mind and body, he or she merges with the object of perceptions and loses all sense of duality, finally perceiving the 'Supreme Reality' beyond the limitations of the senses. *See also Asanas, Chakras, Kundalini, Meditation, Iyengar yoga.*

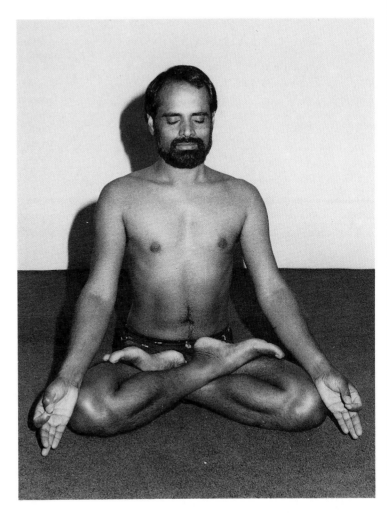

clasped in a vertical position behind and above the head. Yoga mudra stretches the lumbar region of the back and compresses the organs of the abdomen. It enhances body mobility and helps maintain the body in good shape. *See also Yoga, Asanas, Iyengar yoga*

In kundalini yoga psychic energy is raised through the sushumna

YOGA MUDRA

A yoga exercise in which, after taking the 'lotus' position *(padmasana)*, the subject intensifies the pressure on the ankle and knee joints. This is done by bending forward so that the face touches the ground while at the same time the hands are

Z

ZONE THERAPY — *see Reflexology*

TREATMENTS USING ALTERNATIVE HEALTH THERAPIES

A

ACNE

There is a huge range of suggested treatments for this unsightly skin disease which affects so many adolescents. Most of them are concerned with changes of diet or with ointments or herbal preparations to soothe and cleanse the skin. Some also advocate vitamin and mineral supplements. However there are some cases of acne which do not respond to any of these traditional treatments and patients have turned to more unusual remedies. Some have found their condition improves with the application of acupressure. Points commonly used are at the inside of the elbow, above the knee, the thumb and in the hollow under the collarbone. Homeopathic practitioners have had good results by treating acne with substances such as *rhus tox, sulphur,* and the mineral tissue salts *kali sulph.* and *calc sulph.* depending on the particular type of acne. Sometimes the condition seems to get much worse in the initial stages of treatment but this is part of the cure.

ARTHRITIS

Arthritis is a very painful disease for which orthodox medicine has found no really effective cure. There are a number of herbal remedies and many people have found relief by making changes to their diet, by fasting or by taking vitamin and mineral supplements. However there are other patients who have found relief in different ways. There are a number of homeopathic remedies including *rhus tox, belladonna, mercurius* and *ledum* but since there are so many different types of arthritis it is best to consult a qualified homeopathic practitioner.

Acupressure and massage give relief to some patients. The appropriate acupressure points should be pressed 3 times for 10 to 15 seconds, then the whole area should be massaged gently using peanut oil.

Sometimes the condition responds to a change in climate or to regular swimming, especially in seawater. A very old but sometimes effective remedy is to bury the patient in warm, moist sand right up to the neck for about half an hour every day for 2 weeks. Arthritic hands or feet can be placed in a warm paraffin bath for half an hour three times a week. Hot or cold compresses can also give relief from the pain though they will not cure the complaint. For some patients the traditional copper bracelet worn around the wrist or ankle is very effective.

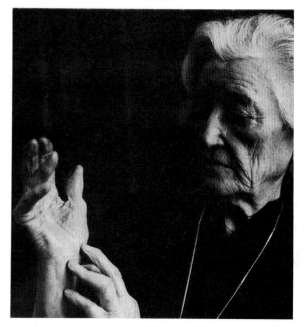

Arthritic joints can be treated with homeopathic remedies

ASTHMA

Asthma is caused by a combination of factors including stress, allergies and heredity. It needs treatment both in the obvious acute stage while the patient is having difficulty breathing and also in the periods of respite. There are a number of homeopathic pills which can be used during an attack. They include *aconite, arsenicum, phosphorus, spongia* and *lachesis.* A qualified practitioner should be consulted to find the appropriate one.

The application of acupressure to specific points such as that at the inner hollow of the elbow or in the centre of the chest can be surprisingly effective in bringing immediate relief. Massage of the abdomen and solar plexus area and of the back and neck and even the hands and feet has been recommended during an attack. In the period between attacks many asthmatics are helped by following a special diet and by taking vitamin and mineral supplements. Special breathing exercises, such as the programme devised by Dr Ernesto Escudero in Buenos Aires, have helped many asthmatics. The patient should sit in a relaxed position by an open window and inhale in short gasping breaths about 25 times. Other exercises require the patient to breathe in and out slowly using the muscles of the abdomen. Many children are helped by learning to play a wind instrument or by regular swimming training. The disciplined exercise involved in tai chi and yoga are helpful for many asthmatics.

B

BED WETTING

Bed wetting is often a nervous habit which a child will eventually outgrow but which causes great social embarrassment and inconvenience. Occasionally it is caused by some physical defect or by a chronic kidney problem so the child's general health does need to be checked. Besides the many herbal remedies there are several homeopathic pills available including *causticum*, *pulsatilla* and *equisetum*.

A soothing massage of the lower abdomen and buttocks is recommended by some people. This can be followed by stimulation of the acupressure points below the navel, in the hollows at the back of the neck or in the hollow below the anklebone. Sometimes simple remedies such as snug warm pyjamas, a hot water bottle and the avoidance of excitement before bedtime will be sufficient. Regular doses of magnesium have also been recommended.

BRONCHITIS

For many years orthodox doctors prescribed antibiotics for bronchitis though it is now generally accepted that they have no real affect on the bronchitis itself. There are several herbal treatments and many people advise dietary supplements, especially vitamins, as well as the elimination of certain foods. Homeopathic pills such as *aconite*, *bryonia*, *hepar sulph*, *ambra grisea* and *rumex crispus* are often prescribed. It is widely agreed that the patient should avoid smoking or close contact with smokers, especially in areas where air pollution is already high. Breathing exercises can be very helpful and many people benefit from regular yoga exercises because of the special breathing and postural change involved. Relaxation techniques such as meditation, autogenics and auto-suggestion have had very good results. The coughing associated with bronchitis can be relieved by acupressure. Many people recommend the practice of lying flat on the stomach with the head hanging over the side of the bed for about 5 minutes to allow the mucus to drain. This is then blown out through the nose. The use of humidifiers in the bedroom is coming back into favour, especially for young children, and some people recommend the traditional hot mustard foot bath as well as the method of wrapping the chest in hot towels which are changed regularly. A hot drink, particularly lemon juice and honey, is very comforting.

C

CANCER

Dietary approaches to reducing cancer-risk are summarised elsewhere in this book but there are also other factors to be considered in combating this multi-factorial disease. Although mainstream medicine considers cancer substantially in physical terms — as an abnormal proliferation of cells resulting in tumours which may be treated with various forms of surgery, radiotherapy and drugs — there does seem to be growing evidence that certain types of cancer are directly related to extreme stress.

Dr Paul Roesch, professor of medicine at New York Medical College, maintains that stress inhibits the immune system and that while any given individual may develop millions of cancer cells many times during his or her lifetime, under normal circumstances a healthy immune system can destroy these abnormal cells. This viewpoint was also shared by the renowned authority on stress, the late Dr Hans Selye, who noted that 'the interrelation of mind and body is deeper and more complex than we thought it to be . . . As long as the immune system is functioning and functioning efficiently, the growth of cancer will usually be suppressed. But even a slight shift in cellular balance can produce a malignant growth . . . We must clearly realise that stress is a condition, a state of body and mind, but it manifests itself by measurable chemical changes in the organs of the body.' (Quoted from 'Stress, the basis of Illness' in E. M. Goldwag (ed.), *Inner Balance*, New Jersey 1979.)

An important approach to combating cancer-risk is therefore to reduce the stress factors in one's daily life — in addition to maintaining a healthy diet and reducing wherever possible the various environmental and lifestyle practices linked to cancer (e.g. smoking, living in areas affected by high radioactivity etc.).

Stress can be reduced by many varied techniques of relaxation and meditation including those derived from the Hindu and Buddhist mystical traditions. It also helps if one learns to develop a positive attitude to life itself, since invariably visualising positive outcomes has a distinct bearing on health and on overcoming disease. It needs to be emphasised, however, that cancer is an extremely complicated disease and there are no simple solutions. Readers are advised to study a broad range of diagnostic and preventive approaches, both orthodox and 'alternative', and to seek perspectives which throw light on their own particular line of enquiry. *(See also Stress.)*

COLDS AND FLU

Although these are the commonest of all ailments, orthodox doctors freely admit they have found no cure. Even the controversial flu vaccine is of limited value as it is directed only to specific strains of the flu virus. There are an enormous number of natural remedies for colds and many of these will lessen the severity of the symptoms and shorten the duration of the disease.

The many herbal treatments and dietary supplements have been discussed in other sections. Homeopaths prescribe a number of different pills including *arsenicum*, *pulsatilla*, *mercurius*, *ferrum phos.* and *nux vomica*.

Acupressure can be used to soothe specific symptoms. For instance, the running nose can be dried up by pressing at the outer base of both nostrils then massaging all along the sides of the nose. The spot between the eyebrows is then pressed several times and the cheek bone and eye socket area gently massaged with the flat of the hand.

Practitioners of hydrotherapy advocate sitting for several minutes in a cold bath before going to sleep in a warm bed. For those who feel this method is too painful, a hot bath or shower can be followed by a cool shower.

Deep yogic breathing is sometimes recommended to increase the amount of oxygen in the body and aid the healing process. For a cold accompanied by chest congestion, heated oils can be rubbed onto the chest or hot towels wrapped round as a poultice.

Recent research has suggested that people who are suffering from stress and anxiety are likely to have more frequent and more severe colds. Any relaxation techniques such as meditation, autogenics, yoga or autosuggestion can be used to prevent the occurrence of colds.

CONSTIPATION

This is a complaint which causes many people unnecessary worry because they have been conditioned to place great importance on the regularity of their bowel movements. Occasional constipation can be caused by a number of factors including stress, illness, change of diet or daily routine and will soon correct itself, particularly if plenty of fruits and vegetables are eaten. There is a general view that the diet of many western people contains insufficient fibre and that we should all make a conscious effort to eat more whole grains and fruits and vegetables. If constipation causes discomfort, especially in elderly people or invalids it can be treated by various homeopathic pills including *lycopodium*, *nux vomica* and *plumbum*.

Acupressure points include the tip of the coccyx, the sole of the foot or the nail of the big toe. This is usually followed by massage of the bottom of the spine and the lower abdomen. This can be done every morning using a lubricant of olive oil or crushed garlic. Hand and foot reflex point stimulation is another technique which has been used with

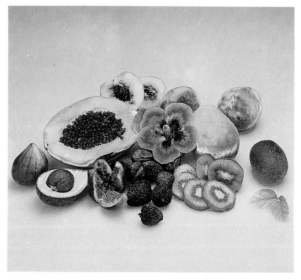

Eating fresh fruits is an ideal way to treat constipation

some success. Regular exercise of any kind is beneficial and there are several exercises devised especially by chiropractors and osteopaths to help release nerve interference affecting the colon and stomach. There are numerous herbal remedies and foods such as prunes or olive oil which have laxative properties. Some people recommend a cold hip bath or a hot compress or both used alternately. Any technique which promotes relaxation or stress control can have a very beneficial effect on constipation.

CROUP

This condition tends to affect children under 3 years of age and is characterised by a harsh 'barking' cough and difficult breathing patterns. Prior to the development of croup it is not unusual for the child to suffer from a sore throat and bloodshot eyes.

Croup results from a viral infection which causes the larynx and trachea to become inflamed and partly blocked. The blockage itself results from swelling in the lining of the windpipe and this is exacerbated by thick mucus which sticks to the walls of the trachea.

The best treatment for croup is to use a humidifier to release steam into the air around the sleeping child. The wet, steamy air loosens the secretions caused by the viral infection and enables the child to clear his or her air passages by occasional coughing. The moist air also soothes the lining of the trachea. If the child continues to breathe with difficulty or becomes cyanosed (blue) or pale after a coughing spell, seek medical advice.

D

DIARRHOEA

Diarrhoea is usually only a minor disorder caused by bacterial infection, stress, or food poisoning but it can be a symptom of a more serious complaint, so persistent diarrhoea should not be ignored. It is particularly serious in small children. Many people recommend fasting as the best treatment and this can be accompanied by herbal teas. When the worst symptoms are over the patient should eat only a light diet of foods such as rice, apples and yoghurt and avoid all rich, fatty or highly spiced foods. It is important to drink as much water as possible to replace lost body fluids. Some people recommend vitamin and

mineral supplements especially the vitamins A, B complex, pantothenic acid, and magnesium.

Homeopaths offer a number of pills including *veratrum album*, *aconite* and *chamomilla* while some naturopaths advocate placing ice packs on the lower part of the spine to stimulate the nerves responsible for the excretory functions.

In Oriental medicine digestive disorders are taken very seriously. There are a number of acupressure points which can be stimulated including the inside of the elbow and the point below the nail of the middle finger.

Massage and relaxation can also be used very effectively. The Oriental technique of moxibustion can be used with surprisingly good results.

E

EARACHE

General advice is to keep the ear warm (perhaps with a hot water bottle) and to avoid cold winds. Homeopathic pills include *ferrum phosphoricum*, *pulsatilla*, *arsenicum* and *belladonna*. A compress of heated salt is sometimes recommended as is a boiled clove of garlic placed outside the ear. There are several herbal remedies which can be used. Sometimes the condition will respond to gentle massage of the ear, neck and temples.

ECZEMA

Eczema, with its characteristic painful rash, dry skin and intense itchiness, is a complaint which affects a considerable number of people, particularly young children. Many people grow out of the condition completely, some find they have periods of respite and for others the affliction is constant. It is not a disease which is well understood and, perhaps because it is not life threatening and often disappears of its own accord, many patients feel that orthodox doctors do not take it sufficiently seriously. The most common treatment is to prescribe a steroid ointment such as hydrocortisone. Eczema is often thought to be associated with stress or with food allergies so the usual treatments are to prescribe tranquillisers and to eliminate certain foods, especially eggs and milk products. Many people find that they are allergic to certain soaps or cosmetics or to synthetic clothing.

It is not always realised that there are about 14 different types of eczema, each of which occurs with varying intensity, so it is a disease with enormous individual differences and it is by no means possible to prescribe a universal cure.

There is a growing body of evidence from eczema sufferers who have found relief from one of a variety of 'alternative' therapies. The naturopathic approach is to make a detailed examination of all aspects of the patient's life style and then to prescribe a combination of treatments which will include advice on diet, exercise and relaxation.

In many cases treatment by an osteopath or by a chiropractor is also suggested, as it has been found that some slight spinal problem can interfere with the blood supply and this in turn can affect the condition of the skin. Hydrotherapy is often advised to cleanse the pores and improve the circulation and muscle tone.

There are a number of homeopathic remedies, the most common of which are *graphites*, *sulphur*, *mezareum*, *psorinum* and *rhus tox* but it is important to have an experienced practitioner give an individual diagnosis.

Mineral supplements have been found to give relief to some patients, and so too have acupuncture and acupressure though these are not always acceptable to young children.

Patients whose condition is made much worse by anxiety have found the finger pressure of shiatsu very helpful. Others have turned to reflexology or to Touch for health. A few have had quite spectacular results from hypnotherapy. Because of the psychological effects of this unsightly disease a great many patients find they feel much better after joining some kind of group which offers supportive counselling and helps them to accept their condition.

H

HEADACHE

This is an extremely common complaint and one which takes a number of different forms. It can be a symptom of a more serious disease, it can be the intense and incapacitating pain of migraine, or it can be a minor temporary complaint due to stress, eyestrain, sinus congestion, air pollution, constipation, low blood sugar or any of a number of other causes. Frequent and severe headaches should always be taken seriously and investigated by a competent medical practitioner.

Ordinary headaches can often be relieved by a very simple remedy — a good sleep, a warm bath, relaxation, fresh air or a cup of tea and something to eat. There are a number of herbal teas which are often very effective. Headaches are believed to be caused by contraction of the muscles of the scalp so gentle massage is often a good remedy. Different types of headache can be relieved by acupressure applied to the appropriate points. So a headache behind the eyes can often be helped by pressure to the lower edge of the back of the skull and one at the front of the head may respond to pressure on the series of points down the centre of the forehead. A general headache may be relieved by pressure applied by the thumb to the index finger.

Homeopathic remedies include *gelsemium sempervirens*, *allium cepa*, *nux vomica* and *bryonia*.

Some people find breathing and relaxation exercises extremely helpful. So too is self-hypnosis, using any technique which works for the subject, such as visualising the painful area as growing smaller and smaller or by imagining a healing blue light round the head.

Migraine headaches are often brought on by certain foods, particularly chocolate, so these should of course be avoided. Sometimes a headache which fails to respond to any other treatment will be found to be due to pressure on the spinal nerve and can be relieved by treatment from a chiropractor.

HEART DISEASE

Obviously diet plays a large part in whether we are vulnerable to heart attacks and it is wise as a preventive measure to reduce high fat and sugary foods, drink less alcohol and eat a variety of healthy foods, including wholegrain bread and cereals, fresh vegetables and fruit. In addition to this, regular physical exercise will certainly help to alleviate a potential heart disease condition.

The heart is a muscle, and muscles become bigger and stronger when exercised. Nevertheless, recent studies show that fitness exercises like jogging, swimming and aerobic dancing mainly benefit the muscles in the limbs rather than the heart itself. Where these aerobic activities do have a benefit, however, is in lowering the heart-rate and easing blood pressure.

The heart of a person in good condition beats around 45–50 times a minute, whereas an unconditioned person requires 70–75 heart-beats to pump the same amount of blood around the body.

When the heart-rate is lower the heart muscle can rest between heart-beats.

Exercise will enlarge the heart's main pumping chamber and make the heart-beat more efficient, and there is also a positive effect on breathing patterns. A person who exercises regularly needs fewer breaths to sustain a given activity and the conditioned heart transmits more oxygen-rich blood to the muscular tissues with comparatively less effort. Finally, exercise raises the number of protective high-density lipoproteins (HDLs) in the blood — these help to remove cholesterol from the blood vessels — and also helps reduce levels of triglycerides, another form of blood fat potentially damaging to the arteries.

Obviously there are precautions you can take prior to or during exercise. If you favour jogging, choose comfortable running shoes, especially designed for this purpose. Run on grass rather than hard surfaces whenever possible and avoid running in a lop-sided, unbalanced way. In general, do not continue to exercise if it is painful — the pain is the body's way of telling you you have gone too far.

HIGH BLOOD PRESSURE (HYPERTENSION)

There are several ways of reducing high blood pressure so that it returns to the normal healthy range of 100–130 (systolic) and 60–80 (diastolic). Dietary means of treating hypertension are summarised in *Treatments: Part 3* and include reducing kilojoule (calorie) and salt intake. However there are other factors which may cause hypertension and these can be eliminated systematically.

Obesity An overweight condition is often linked to a rise in blood pressure because of added strain on the heart. It is also significant that blood volume increases with body weight, and in overweight people the heart therefore has to pump more blood through the blood vessels to nourish the tissues. Cutting down on calorie intake and exercising regularly will help to reduce obesity.

Exercise Hypertension will benefit from regular jogging, running, cycling, swimming and aerobic exercise. A conditioned heart can pump more oxygen-rich blood to working muscles, and can do this with less effort. Vigorous exercise enables people to sustain intensive activity over an extended period. However it may be wise to consult a doctor or naturopath before undertaking vigorous forms of exercise too soon. In the case of James Fixx — the noted jogger who died while exercising — his genetic risk of cardiovascular disease was high and jogging apparently placed excessive strain on his heart. In normal circumstances, though, blood pressure rises less during exercise than it would otherwise.

Emotional Factors Emotional stress should be minimised whenever possible so that life takes on an easier pace and worries become less paramount. Changes can be made in one's lifestyle and behaviour so that more time is put aside for rest and relaxation. Rest takes the strain off the arteries and heart, and regular sessions of relaxation (e.g. for 20 minutes a day) will help to lower the blood pressure gradually.

Cigarettes Death from heart attack is twice as common in cigarette smokers than in non-smokers and hypertension can itself lead to heart attack. Cigarette smoking aggravates the effect of high blood pressure on the arteries and may substantially increase the risk of heart attack. For this reason, those who have high blood pressure and who also smoke should endeavour to minimise or eliminate smoking altogether (if necessary, with the aid of sessions of hypnosis).

I

INDIGESTION

This is a common complaint which is particularly likely to affect those who lead a stressful life and rapidly consume rich, fatty foods, especially 'takeaways'. It is easier to prevent than to cure. Small amounts of sensible foods chewed well and eaten slowly in a relaxed atmosphere are unlikely to cause indigestion. Smoking before a meal or drinking cold fizzy drinks with it are both habits which tend to cause indigestion.

Many dietitians pay considerable attention to the combinations of foods which are most suitable to be eaten together and to foods such as yoghurt and pawpaw which actually help the digestive process. Some recommend supplements of vitamin B and niacin.

Perhaps because the complaint is so common there are a large number of herbal remedies recommended. Homeopathic pills include *carbo vegetabilis*, *arsenicum album* and *nux vomica*. Massage of the abdominal area for several minutes while lying on the back will often relieve the worst symptoms. There are several acupressure points which can be stimulated to aid digestion. These include the corners of the mouth and the point on the abdomen about 4 centimetres below the navel. Practitioners of reflexology massage the instep of the foot for about five minutes twice a day and then pull on the middle toe for at least a minute. Regular yoga exercises will often improve stomach and digestive problems.

M

MENSTRUAL DISORDERS

There are a number of problems which can be experienced by women around the time of menstruation. These include missed or irregular periods (amenorrhoea), excessive bleeding (menorrhagia), painful periods (dysmenorrhoea) and premenstrual tension (PMT). Orthodox doctors tend to prescribe diuretics and tranquillisers though some recommend hormone therapies. Vitamin B6 supplements have been very effective for PMT and supplements of niacin have been shown to relieve menstrual cramps, especially when taken in combination with rutin and vitamin C.

Herbalists offer a variety of remedies for 'women's complaints'. Homeopathic pills vary according to the type of complaint and to the emotional condition of the patient but include *arsenicum*, *chamomilla*, *cimicifuga* and *belladonna*.

Many naturopaths feel PMT is caused by toxic accumulations in the body so their treatment is concerned with changes to the diet and periodic cleansings. The traditional method of bringing on menstruation by hot baths or placing hot towels over the lower back can often be effective. So too is the method of relieving menstrual pains by alternating an ice pack on the lower back for 10 minutes with a hot water bottle on the lower abdomen for about an hour. There are several acupressure points which can be stimulated to bring relief from menstrual irregularities. These include the point about 3 centimetres below the navel and the skin between the big toe and the second toe.

Specific exercises have been devised to strengthen and tone the abdominal muscles. If practised regularly they can be very effective in correcting menstrual problems. Emotional and psychological factors are thought to play a large part in causing menstrual disorders. Many women have found their problems are cured after they have taken a course in hypnotherapy, autosuggestion, biofeedback or any similar therapy.

O

OSTEOPOROSIS

Osteoporosis is associated primarily with women who have passed through menopause. When the ovaries no longer produce the protective hormone oestrogen, the loss of bone density is accelerated, and between the ages of 45 and 75 many women may lose 30% of their skeletal structure — twice as much as men, who have substantially greater bone density to begin with.

The strength of the skeleton is directly related to adequate amounts of calcium and one preventive measure is to ensure appropriate intakes of calcium-rich dairy products from the mid-20s through to older age (see *Treatments: Part 3*). However various forms of exercise can also be useful as a preventive measure against osteoporosis.

According to Dr Morris Notelovitz, professor of obstetrics and gynaecology at the University of Florida College of Medicine, exercises like bicycling, jogging and brisk walking actually stimulate the formation of new bone. Tennis may also be a suitable form of exercise. A recent study undertaken at the University of North Carolina showed that a group of 300 active older women had forearm bones 15–20% denser than comparable inactive women, and tennis players are known to have thicker bones than those who do not play the sport. However other types of exercise like swimming — which does not force the bones to work against gravity — do not lead to increased bone mass. Specialists in osteoporosis recommend that bone-forming types of exercise should be undertaken prior to the age of 35 in order to achieve high peak bone-mass, and such exercises should be continued after menopause.

P

PAIN CONTROL

Muscular aches and pains can derive from a variety of causes — postural, functional and emotional. The most obvious forms of physical pain — caused, for example, by displaced vertebrae or bones impinging onto nerves — can be treated by a variety of specialist manipulative techniques, especially those employed in osteopathy and chiropractic. Various

ge may also be applied.
a functional or emotional
nore elusive.

...on may suffer from a persistent
...at chiropractic, orthopaedic sur-
...e of eye specialists prove to no

...ase the subject visited a Feldenkrais
practi... ...d was advised that the left shoulder
hung lowe... ...nan the other and as a result the head
was tilted to the left to compensate. This effect was
causing the headache. Using the Feldenkrais System,
which emphasises efficient body function and freer
movement, the subject was able to learn to hold his
head in a way that caused no pain. The Feldenkrais
approach has also been found to be valuable in cases
of repetitive strain injury (RSI) and back pain.

Other forms of pain — sometimes called 'psycho-
genic' — occur as a result of psychological disturbances. In these cases the pain has an unconscious
origin and may require some form of psychotherapy
employing healing imagery that accesses pain on the
inner level.

Utilised in such modalities as hypnotherapy and
psychosynthesis, images used as visualisations may
help to promote the release of pain-killing endorphins
in the brain, producing a direct effect on the pain-
receptors in the nervous system. Certain imagery
techniques help to reduce the sensation of pain —
distancing it from the subject or reducing its impact
in specific regions of the body.

Roberto Assagioli, founder of psychosynthesis,
also believed it was especially useful to use mental
substitution — transferring the attention towards
pleasure and away from pain as part of the psychotherapeutic process. In some types of therapy
patients may also be asked to establish an imaginary
dialogue with the pain and seek advice from the 'pain
entity' on how to eliminate it. These methods
endeavour to reduce the pain to a manageable perspective, especially if it is caused by substantially
unconscious emotional factors.

POSTURAL PROBLEMS

Postural abnormalities like lordosis, kyphosis and
scoliosis are typically caused by muscular holding
patterns which move the vertebrae out of their normal alignment. The vertebral muscles themselves
may be at fault but the abdominal muscles and diaphragm — which influence spinal stabilisation and
pelvic balance — may also be a contributing cause.

Postural problems of this type can be treated by
osteopathy and chiropractic and specific forms of
physical therapy like Rolfing — which emphasises
correct 'gravitational alignment' of the body
segments.

Another approach is that of the Alexander Technique. Practitioners of this method often claim that
postural abnormalities result from the so-called
'startle pattern' which distorts the shoulders and
arms, shortens the length of the torso, and causes
increased tension in the legs. The startle pattern itself
derives from the physical response to stress and
manifests specially in the tendency to pull the head
back from the neck. This pattern can become habitual whether we are standing, walking or sitting. The
Alexander Technique endeavours to identify postural
abnormalities and to teach the subjects being treated
how to re-learn correct patterns of body usage.

It may also be the case that the postural problems
are associated with muscular contractions in the body
which result from 'emotional blockages'. The various
types of Reichian therapy and such cathartic forms of
bodywork as deep tissue muscle therapy seek to
release the negative holding patterns underlying the
physical symptoms by eliminating the unconscious,
negative emotions associated with them.

R

REPETITIVE STRAIN INJURY (RSI)

Although RSI may simply be caused by repeated patterns of excessive physical exertion — especially in
manual labour or repetitive keyboard functions —
there may be psychological correlates to RSI as well.
According to a study conducted by Judith Wall of the
Australian National University, victims of RSI are
often tense worriers who appear to have more personal 'crises' than non-sufferers. Also they are often
heavy smokers. In a survey of 144 public servants
who suffered from RSI, Ms Wall found that typically
RSI sufferers had antagonistic relations with their
superiors and found their work more stressful than
those who did not have a problem with RSI. Treatments for stress-control may therefore be of benefit to
some RSI sufferers (see Stress).

Many cases of RSI are, however, purely physical
and one of the alternative therapies which is
especially useful is the Feldenkrais System of body

awareness. This method uses various techniques to develop increased freedom of body movement and it is possible to educate workers to learn how to move efficiently, even when sitting in front of a VDT screen, rather than adopting 'frozen' posture patterns.

RHEUMATISM

The traditional belief that copper bracelets ease the pain of rheumatism and some forms of arthritis may have a scientific basis after all. Professor Ray Walker, Associate Professor of Chemistry, Newcastle University, has researched the absorption of copper into the body for 10 years, and undertook a study on 240 subjects who were willing to co-operate in tests on copper bracelets. He divided the 240 subjects into 3 groups of equal numbers of those who had worn copper bracelets before and those who had not. One group wore copper bracelets for a month and then imitation copper bracelets for a subsequent month. The second group wore imitation copper bracelets for the first month and genuine ones for the second month, while the third group wore no bracelets at all.

Professor Walker's research showed that previous users of copper bracelets were significantly worse off when not wearing their bracelets and his chemical analysis showed that minute quantities of copper were dissolved by the perspiration and absorbed through the skin. The exact mechanism by which copper eases rheumatic pain is still not known.

S

SORE THROAT

Some people suffer repeatedly from sore throats which occur whenever they are particularly tired or their general health is not good. The general treatments advised are rest, lots of liquids (particularly hot lemon drinks), and a mild, light diet. There are numerous herbal remedies which will bring some relief and one of the most popular folk remedies is apple cider vinegar. Another traditional remedy is a salt-water gargle. Homeopathic pills include *belladonna*, *mercurius*, *phosphorus* and *aconite*. Acupressure can be applied to the points below the anklebone or at the outside lower corner of the thumbnail. Some

people recommend exercising the tongue by sticking it out as far as possible for about 30 seconds then relaxing it. This exercise should be repeated 4 or 5 times and is said to increase the blood circulation to the throat, thus aiding the healing process.

STRESS

Normal levels of stress stimulate positive action — for example in crises at work or, say to escape an attacker in a dark alley. The endocrine glands release adrenalin, the heart and breathing rates increase, and oxygenated blood is directed towards the brain and skeletal muscles. After the stress stage passes, the body recuperates and returns to the normal state of relaxed alertness. Negative stress, or stress overloading, can lead to a variety of symptoms including continuing high blood pressure, headaches, backaches and insomnia. Extreme stress may also be a contributing cause to such multifactorial diseases as heart disease and cancer.

The following tips are worth pursuing to reduce stress:

- Reassess and adjust your schedules to remove some of the urgency in your day-to-day life.
- Eat your meals, talk and drive your car at a less frenetic pace.
- Learn more about your inner self, especially your mind and feelings and develop an awareness of how these aspects of your self influence your behaviour.
- Exercise regularly, whether with brisk walks, jogging, swimming or aerobic sports.
- Improve your nutrition so that your diet is more balanced (this will mean reducing high salt, fat and protein intake, and focusing more on fresh fruit and vegetables).
- Learn to release your emotions in a positive way, rather than bottling up anger and resentment.
- Learn to relax, and try to keep aside a special time for this practice, for example 15–20 minutes each day.

Choose a quiet, cool room free from distractions and sit in a comfortable, relaxed posture (a semi-reclining position is ideal; if you lie down you may go to sleep). Now imagine a soothing, relaxing wave flowing through the soles of your feet, up to your ankles, calves and thighs, and then passing into your abdomen, chest and arms. Feel that you are shedding your pent-up stress and tension with each deep breath that you release.

Some people find it relaxing to listen to specific styles of soothing music (see *Ambient music*) while others may be drawn to techniques like mantra yoga (where the meditator focuses on specific sacred or personal sounds) or Float to Relax (where the meditator floats in darkness in a tank containing a solution of water and epsom salts).

These are individual choices and an ideal prelude to any of these is to learn first how to relax at home and work in the more obvious and accessible ways described above.

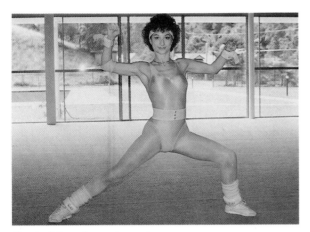

Exercise helps reduce varicose veins

T

TOOTHACHE

Unfortunately this is usually a sign of some underlying problem which will require a visit to the dentist. However there are several methods which can give temporary relief from the pain. Some herbal remedies are recommended, particularly oil of cloves or a piece of garlic placed directly onto the tooth. Alcohol rubbed onto the tooth will deaden the pain for a while as will a piece of ice or a hot salt-water gargle. Perhaps surprisingly, a cold foot bath or a hot water bottle placed on the feet can often bring relief from toothache. Acupressure points which may be stimulated include those at the temples, just in front of the angle of the jawbone, and between the second and third toes and at the corner of the fingernail of the index finger. Massage applied at the hollow at the base of the skull will often soothe the pain.

Homeopathic remedies include *mag. phos.*, *chamomilla*, *coffea* and *magnesia carbonica*. There is some evidence that thiamine pills, taken in 10 mg doses every day for a week, will reduce the pain experienced during a visit to the dentist.

V

VARICOSE VEINS

Varicose veins are unsightly, painful and potentially dangerous as they can lead to leg ulcers and blood clots. Orthodox doctors sometimes treat very serious cases with surgery but this is often not satisfactory as the recovery period is long and the cure is often only temporary. There is a strong hereditary factor in determining those who are likely to develop varicose veins and women who have had several pregnancies or who spend a lot of time on their feet are particularly at risk. Many women wear elastic support stockings or pantihose every day and find these help to stop their legs from aching. It is a good idea, too, to elevate the feet whenever possible, both when sitting down and when lying in bed. A simple footstool and a pillow under the foot of the bed will suffice.

Exercise, particularly bike-riding, is usually very beneficial and, if it is necessary to spend a long time standing, try to move the feet and legs as much as possible — just shaking, raising and lowering your heels and bending and stretching the knees will help stimulate the blood circulation. For those who like a more structured approach there are several yoga exercises which can be helpful.

Herbalists offer a variety of treatments for varicose veins and it is worthwhile consulting a dietitian who will provide information about appropriate foods, stressing particularly those full of fibre. Some practitioners advocate supplements of vitamin E to help all problems related to poor circulation. Other supplements sometimes recommended include calcium lactate, rutin, pantothenic acid and vitamin C. A rather messy but sometimes effective remedy is to soak bath towels in white oak bark or hay flowers, wrap them round the legs and leave them on all night. This should be done twice a week initially and then weekly. Hydrotherapy can also be very beneficial for varicose vein sufferers. The best treatment is to walk in waist-high seawater for about 15 minutes, then rest with the feet up, then repeat the process. If this is not possible, a swimming pool will do.

PART 3

DIET, NUTRITION AND BODY FUNCTION

A

A, VITAMIN — *see Vitamin A*

ABRASION

The removal of superficial layers of the skin by scraping. This may result in raw bleeding areas which become vulnerable to infection.

ABSCESS

A localised accretion of pus in any part of the body, formed by the disintegration of tissues.

ABSORPTION

The ability to take substances — such as food, nutrients and medicines — into the human system.

ACETYLCHOLINE

A chemical released from nerve-endings and used as a neurotransmitter — relaying nerve impulses to the muscles and glands. Acetylcholine plays an important role in memory recall and control of muscular and sensory signals.

ACID- AND ALKALI-FORMING FOODS

Following the absorption of food in the body, a residue remains which may be either acidic or alkaline. Increased acidity is associated with many disease symptoms in the body and it is considered helpful to orientate the diet substantially towards alkali-producing foods as a general preventive health-care measure. The accompanying table compares acid and alkali-forming foods.

Acid-forming foods: Meat, fish, poultry; eggs; cheese; grains, bread and cereals; cranberries, prunes and plums.
Alkali-forming foods: Milk and yoghurt; vegetables; fruits (other than acid-forming fruits).

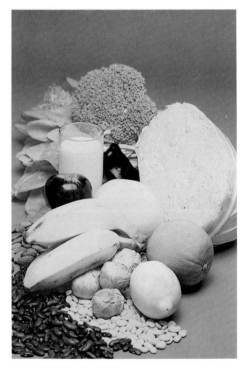

Some alkali-forming foods

ACIDOSIS

A condition of excessive acidity in the body. Respiratory acidosis results from changes in breathing patterns, which in turn produce carbon dioxide pressure changes in the blood. Metabolic acidosis develops following intake of acids, alkalis and other substances which are metabolised, altering the hydrogen ion concentration.

ACUTE

A term used to describe a disease condition which is short in duration but comparatively severe. *See also Chronic.*

ACYLTRANSFERASE

An enzyme which serves as one of the body's natural mechanisms to prevent blood cholesterol from building up on the artery walls. Those who lack this enzyme develop hardened arteries. Lecithin is required for the synthesis of this enzyme. *See also Lecithin.*

ADENOIDS

Small areas of tissue at the back of the nose. The adenoids form part of the body's defence against germs which enter through the nose. In some children the adenoids swell and obstruct nose breathing.

ADHESIONS

Scar tissues that can arise in any section of the body following surgery, or as a result of infection or bleeding. Adhesions do not necessarily cause pain.

ADRENAL GLANDS

Two small glands located above the kidneys. These glands produce hormones which pass into the blood and assist in regulating body function. One of these is adrenalin, which increases heart rate and enables the body to respond quickly in an emergency.

ADRENALIN

A hormone secreted by the inner part, or medulla, of the adrenal glands — which are located in the upper poles of the kidneys. Adrenalin constricts the blood vessels of the stomach, lungs and skin, making more blood available to the heart, lungs and voluntary muscles. It therefore facilitates emergency situations characterised by the 'fight or flight' response.

ADUKI BEAN *(Phaseolus angularis)*

A reddish-brown seed found in the bean pods of a bushy Japanese plant widely grown also in Korea and China. Aduki beans form an important part of the macrobiotic diet and are now available in Western health food stores. Chinese and Japanese herbalists traditionally made a juice from boiled aduki beans which is prescribed to help kidney complaints.

AEROBICS

Vigorous exercise, often accompanied by music and characterised by continuous movement. The practice of aerobics is designed to tone large muscle groups in the legs and back, stimulate the heart and lung activity, and thereby increase the demand for, and intake of, oxygen. Jogging, swimming and cycling are examples of aerobic exercises. *See also Fitness, Jogging, Anaerobics.*

AGAR-AGAR

An organic substance obtained from the *Gelidium* species of red algae and used as an ingredient in various Oriental and macrobiotic cuisines. Agar-agar is usually presented in the form of straw-coloured powder or pale strips which dissolve in hot water and produce a jelly when cool.

ALANINE

A non-essential amino acid of the neutral class. It is important for healthy functioning of the skin and adrenal glands. Food sources include alfalfa, carrot, lettuce, cucumber, spinach, watercress, apples, apricots, grapes, oranges and almonds.

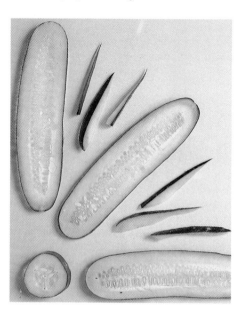

Alanine is found in cucumbers

ALBUMIN

The major protein in blood plasma. Excretion of albumin in the urine can be an indicator of kidney damage.

ALGAE

Primitive plants of the thallophyte group, but distinguished from other members in this category (for example, fungi) because they contain chlorophyll. Algae may be unicellular and microscopic, or multicellular in form, and are found both in fresh and saltwater, as well as on land. Many types of sea algae, for example agar-agar, kombu and nori, are popular foods in macrobiotic and wholefood cuisine.

ALIMENTARY CANAL

In the human body, the passage from the mouth to the anus through which food passes and is in turn absorbed and digested. The alimentary canal includes the mouth, the oesophagus, the stomach, the duodenum, the small and large intestines, and the anus. It is also known as the gastrointestinal tract.

ALKALOID

A physiologically active substance which forms salts when combined with acids and, when soluble, produces alkaline solutions. Alkaloids are often poisonous and are found in several plants which have a physiological effect on the body. Well-known examples include morphine, cocaine, quinine, strychnine, nicotine, caffeine, and atropine.

ALLANTOIN

An astringent ingredient used in cosmetic creams and lotions to regenerate the skin and stimulate cell renewal.

ALLERGEN

Any substance which produces an allergic response — *see Allergy*.

ALLERGY

A state of physical hypersensitivity to substances which, for most people, are harmless. Allergies can be caused by house dust, pollen, food, fruits and even temperature changes, and may manifest in a variety of disease symptoms — including asthma, arthritis, Crohn's disease, hay fever, migraines and various skin complaints. Allergies may also be less obvious, producing feelings of tension, depression, insomnia and forgetfulness.

Naturopaths treat allergies by endeavouring, through a process of careful elimination, to isolate the dietary or environmental component which triggers the response. For example, partially digested proteins from wheat and milk absorbed systemically can cause migraines, while certain food peptides may induce the organism to produce antibodies causing inflammation and joint degeneration. Toxic metals, food preservatives and colourings, cow's milk, wheat products and yeast-containing foods have all been linked to allergic responses.

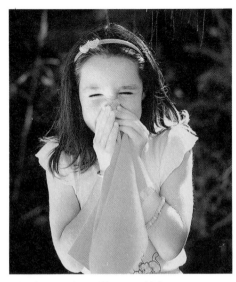

Allergies are a form of hypersensitivity

ALMOND *(Prunus amygdalus)*

There are two kinds of almonds: the sweet almond, a pink-flowering tree grown commercially for its nuts, which are eaten raw or used in cooking, and the bitter almond, which is often grown as an ornamental tree and produces white flowers and nuts which are crushed for their bitter oil. The latter is sometimes used in flavouring but is poisonous in large amounts. Almond oil of either type is used widely in cosmetics to soften and whiten the skin and keep it free from wrinkles. Almonds are rich in protein and natural fats. They provide a balanced source of magnesium, calcium and phosphorus, and contain a significant amount of vitamins B and F.

ALOPECIA

A skin disease causing loss of hair.

ALPHA-TOCOPHEROL
— *see Vitamin E, Tocopherols*

ALUMINIUM

A common toxin in foods cooked in aluminium utensils. During the cooking process, fine particles of aluminium may dissolve, enter the bloodstream, and be deposited in the body organs, muscles and tissues. Aluminium poisoning can manifest in the form of irritation of the gastrointestinal tract, pains in the lower abdomen, constipation, eczema and skin rashes, and in aching muscles. It also affects the brain chemistry producing depression, loss of memory and — in extreme cases — senile dementia.

Stainless steel and enamel pots are preferred to aluminium utensils for these reasons.

ALVEOLI

Small air sacs in the lungs. Here carbon dioxide is exchanged for oxygen during the breathing process.

AMENORRHOEA

The absence of menstruation for more than 3 cycles. Amenorrhoea may be caused by a variety of factors: heavy exercise, sickness, conditions of over- or under-weight, and fluctuating oestrogen levels. Natural hormone treatments can restore periods to their normal cycle. *See also Menstruation.*

AMINO ACIDS

These are groups of organic compounds, each containing an amino group and a carboxyl group. The alpha-amino acids are the building blocks from which pro-

THE Irish priest at the centre of the Aids revenge scare was facing mounting criticism yesterday over his role in bringing the scandal to light. 14/9/95

Father Michael Kennedy was accused of failing to ask vital questions which could have quickly established the validity of claims

By PAUL HARRIS and TONY GALLAGHER

men with the HIV virus. The priest, a third cousin of assassinated President John F. Kennedy, said on Sunday that a 25-year-old tattooed redhead had been seeking 'terrible revenge' on the opposite sex. Five

claimed. On T Kennedy insisted which can increas infection, were alert.

Early yesterday had never occurre tion the men abou or about whether homosexual. He

teins are formed. There are over 20 different amino acids and these are combined in various ways to form different proteins. The protein in the food we eat is not the same as that in our bodies, and some food proteins are more suitable for human consumption than others. Some amino acids can be made by the body from other amino acids, but others cannot and so must be supplied by the food we eat. These are called the essential amino acids and include lysine, tryptophan, methionine, leucine, isoleucine, valine, threonine, arginine and histidine. Eggs contain all the essential amino acids in the correct proportions. Generally animal proteins such as milk and meat provide more useable protein than plant foods, but this is compensated to some extent by the fact that we tend to eat a greater bulk of plant food. Plant foods which are exceptionally high in protein are soya beans, oatmeal and mung beans. It is important to eat a mixture of proteins at each meal so that any deficiencies in one food are balanced by the others. Vegan diets which exclude meat, milk and eggs should be very carefully planned to ensure that they contain a balance of all essential amino acids.

ANAEMIA

A deficiency of red blood cells, or the oxygen-carrying substance haemoglobin. This condition results in a reduction in the oxygen-carrying capacity of the blood. Anaemia is characterised by pallor of the skin and may be accompanied by headaches, a feeling of weakness, and breathlessness.

ANAEROBICS

Strenuous exercise in which the body quickly becomes depleted of oxygen. In this form of exercise the body becomes more quickly exhausted and less body fat is burned than in aerobic exercise. An example of anaerobics is sprint running. *See also Aerobics, Fitness.*

ANAESTHESIA

A state in which there is an absence of awareness of external impressions, especially loss of feeling and sensation.

ANALGESIA

The absence of pain sensation in which there is no loss of consciousness: all tactile senses remain active.

ANDROGENS

Hormones secreted by the testes which control protein build-up and male sex characteristics (deeper voice, hair distribution). If synthetic androgens are given to women in substantial quantities they produce 'masculine' qualities.

ANEURYSM

A weakening in the wall of an artery or vein. This causes a bulging effect, and the increased pressure of the blood may lead to a risk of rupture.

ANGINA PECTORIS

A type of heart condition in which the blood supply to the heart is no longer adequate. This may be caused by hardening or thickening of the coronary arteries, and can result in chest pain after too much physical exertion.

ANKYLOSIS

Loss of normal movement in the bones of a joint.

ANOREXIA NERVOSA

A frequently psychosomatic condition in which a person has such an extreme fear of gaining weight that very little food is eaten and there is a compulsive desire to exercise. Typically, anorexic patients are underweight women in their teen years or early 20s, with low self-esteem and a distorted perception of their physical size. The usual treatment is psychological counselling.

ANTACIDS

Substances which reduce fluid acidity in the digestive system. Examples include aluminium hydroxide and magnesium oxide. Antacids are used to treat indigestion and peptic ulcers.

ANTIBIOTICS

A large group of chemical substances which are used predominantly to treat infectious diseases, because of their destructive effect on invading bacteria or disease entities. Common examples include penicillin and streptomycin.

ANTIBODIES

Substances in the blood which produce immunity to germs and viruses. *See Immune system.*

ANTI-EMETIC

A substance used to stop vomiting.

ANTIOXIDANTS

Substances which protect the cells of the body against the oxidising process, and which are believed to help slow down the ageing process. Antioxidants also support the immune system by reducing the impact of stress, whether physical or mental. The primary antioxidants include the following:

Vitamin A: When humans and animals consume plants containing beta-carotene this converts to vitamin A. This nutrient protects the skin, mucous membranes and the linings of the stomach and lungs. It also acts as a 'scavenger' of the free radicals produced by cigarette smoke, chemical fumes and urban air pollution. Because most cancers are malignancies of epithelial tissue, vitamin A is also an important nutrient in diets protecting against cancer.

Vitamin C: An immune system stimulant which helps manufacture white blood cells, adrenal hormones, antibodies and interferon. The immune system deteriorates with age, rendering the body more susceptible to the onset of degenerative diseases, and for this reason the need for vitamin C increases as one gets older. Vitamin C is also essential for the synthesis of collagen, the inter-cellular 'cement' that bonds tissues together and allows for the healing of wounds.

Vitamin E: A nutrient which promotes oxygenation — the healthy use of oxygen for respiration — while also restricting oxidation caused by free radicals. The life-span of red blood cells is substantially extended by optimal levels of vitamin E.

Selenium: A trace mineral, the absence of which is linked with cancer, heart degeneration and allergies. Selenium can replace and enhance the function of vitamin E to some extent, and is vital for the body's manufacture of an enzyme to disarm free radicals.

Vitamin B-complex: The B vitamins protect the tissues against the destructive aspects of hormones like cortisone and adrenalin which reduce the body's immune response, although they also ensure that they can be generated when required, as a response to stress.

Antioxidants are also used as food additives to control deterioration caused by oxidation of fats and oils. Oxygen causes rancidity, discolouration and loss of nutritive value. Vitamin C, in the form of ascorbic acid, prevents the browning effect in canned peaches and other fruits.

ANTIPRURITIC

A substance used to reduce or prevent itching.

ANTIPYRETIC

A substance used to lower the body temperature in cases of fever.

ANTITUSSIVE

A substance used for the relief or prevention of coughing.

AORTA

The main trunk of the arterial system, conveying blood from the heart to all regions of the body, with the exception of the lungs.

APPETITE

The desire to consume food. Appetite varies with metabolism and occupation relating to factors such as energy output, and can also be influenced by psychological factors (as in anorexia nervosa and bulimia). Pregnant women usually eat more food than normal, as do children during peak periods of growth.

APRICOT *(Prunus armeniaca)*

Particularly when dried, apricots are a good source of carbohydrate and dietary fibre, and contain a small amount of protein. They are a very good source of vitamin A and also of iron, as research has shown that the iron in apricots is especially easily assimilated by the body. Apricots also contain significant amounts of other minerals such as calcium, potassium and phosphorus, and some vitamin B and C.

The ash of apricot kernels contains a substance called amygdalin which has been used to treat skin tumours and is thought by some to slow down the development of cancer. The oil from apricot kernels is a good source of vitamin E, and is used in cosmetic creams to soften and moisturise the skin and reduce signs of ageing.

ARGININE

An essential amino acid of the basic class. It is important for building cartilage, controlling muscle contractions and cell breakdown, and for the reproductive organs. It is found in most green vegetables and in carrots, radishes, potatoes and parsnips.

ARTERIOSCLEROSIS

A hardening of the walls of the coronary arteries, making them thick and less elastic. This condition adversely affects blood flow in the arteries concerned and causes angina. It is most common in those who smoke or who have a high serum cholesterol level. *See also Atherosclerosis.*

ARTERY

A vessel in the body which carries blood from the heart to the tissues. Arterialisation is a process in which venous blood is changed into arterial blood through oxygenisation.

ARTHRITIS

Inflammation of the joints, leading to swelling, pain and immobilisation of the area affected — *see Joints.*

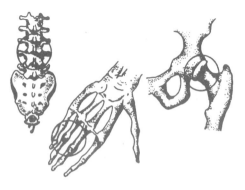

The joints most commonly affected by arthritis include the vertebrae of the lower back (left), the knuckles (middle) and the hip (right)

ASCORBIC ACID — *see*
Vitamin C

ASPARAGUS *(Asparagus officinalis)*

A well-known vegetable which, in earlier times, was reputed to stir up 'bodily lust in man or woman'. It is used by modern homeopaths to treat rheumatism and oedema, and is known to have laxative and diuretic properties. The crushed seeds can relieve nausea.

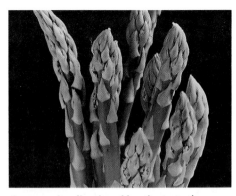

Asparagus has diuretic and laxative properties

ASPARTIC ACID

A non-essential amino acid of the acidic class. It is important for controlling heart and respiratory functions, and for slowing down the destruction of bones and teeth. It is found in most salad vegetables such as celery, cucumber, carrot and tomato, and in apples, lemons, apricots, pineapples and almonds.

ASTHMA

The periodic constriction of the breathing tubes, resulting in wheezing and difficult breathing. Asthma is sometimes hereditary, but may also be due to an allergic response to house dust, mites or animal fur, etc. Inhalers, special breathing exercises, swimming and allergy tests may all be of benefit to asthmatics.

ATHEROSCLEROSIS

From the ancient Greek, *athere* ('gruel') and *skleros* ('hard') a disease popularly known as 'hardening of the arteries'. Atherosclerosis is a type of arteriosclerosis characterised by the thickening and hardening of the artery walls as a result of fatty deposits. These deposits appear to be related to high cholesterol levels in the blood. They increase the likelihood of heart attack because the narrowing of the affected blood vessels impedes the flow of oxygen-rich blood to the heart.

Chest pains (angina) are an initial sign that the heart is not receiving sufficient oxygen from its blood supply. During extended periods of oxygen loss (more than 10 minutes), sections of the heart muscle actually die. The severity of the heart attack depends on the amount of muscle affected.

ATHLETE'S FOOT

An itchy fungal infection of the skin between the toes, especially common in those involved in swimming at public baths or barefoot activities. A variety of creams and disinfectant powders are available as treatments.

ATROPHIC VAGINITIS

Thinning and drying of the vaginal walls following menopause. Caused by a lack of the oestrogen hormone, the condition is characterised by itching and often results in painful sexual intercourse. Oestrogen creams, lubricants and regular sexual intercourse diminish the problem.

ATROPHY

Any decrease in tissue in a specific part of the body. Atrophies can be both normal and abnormal (or pathological).

AUTONOMIC NERVOUS SYSTEM

The nerve system controlling the involuntary functions of the body, which are normally beyond conscious control; for example, peristaltic action and the beating of the heart. Research in biofeedback (at the Menninger Institute in Kansas, as well as at several universities and medical centres) indicates that some autonomic nervous system functions can be brought under conscious control. *See also Central nervous system.*

AUTO-TOXAEMIA

A naturopathic concept that disease results from an imbalance of natural functions and that man as a species appears to have an ongoing capacity for 'self-poisoning' the system. Many factors of ill-health are substantially self-determined and include the production of toxins from improperly metabolised proteins, partially destroyed hormones resulting from liver malfunction, and the absorption of toxins from the colon. The naturopathic concept of preventive health care flows from careful attention to dietary intake, nutritional balance and, where required, vitamin and mineral supplementation.

B

BACTERIA

Single-celled organisms, several of which produce a state of ill-health in the body. The harmful effects of bacteria can be countered by antiseptics or antibiotics.

BARLEY (*Hordeum* species)

A cereal food cultivated since earliest times in ancient China, Egypt, Greece and Rome. Young barley leaves include in their juice an extraordinary range of nutrients including calcium, magnesium and iron, and an excellent balance of the vitamins B1, B2, B6, B12, C and E. Barley juice also contains polypeptides which promote cellular metabolism and neutralise heavy metals like mercury into insoluble salts. *See also Green magma* (Part 1).

BASAL BODY TEMPERATURE

The temperature of the body when at rest, recorded before a person rises from bed in the morning. It can be used as a method of natural birth control to check for ovulation (the temperature drops after ovulation and then rises and stays up until menstruation). This method of birth control is estimated to be 75–80 per cent effective.

BASAL METABOLISM

The energy used by the body to maintain such functions as circulation, muscle tone and body temperature. Basal metabolism can vary, for example, in pregnant women where there are increases in body weight and protein-tissue formation.

B-COMPLEX VITAMINS

So called because B vitamins do not occur singly but in combinations. They include biotin, choline, folic acid and inositol. When used as food supplements, individual B vitamins should be taken together with B-complex vitamins, brewer's yeast, wholegrains or wheatgerm. *See Vitamins listings.*

BEE POLLEN

Male flower spores gathered by bees and mixed with nectar to form granules which are then fed to young bees. Bee pollen contains a number of proteins, enzymes, vitamins and minerals, and is used by some athletes as an energy booster. Those who suffer from hay fever may also find that a course of bee pollen can alleviate symptoms. Pollen may be mixed with honey, yoghurt or fruit juices. The usual daily intake is 1–3 teaspoons.

BENIGN

A term used to describe a condition of ill-health or disease which is not malignant or potentially fatal. It is commonly used with reference to cancerous growths.

BILE

A secretion of the gall bladder which enters the gastrointestinal tract and assists in the digestion and absorption of fats. Bile contains 97.7 per cent water and small amounts of sodium glycocholate, various inorganic salts, lecithin, cholesterol and organic pigments.

BIOCHEMIC TISSUE SALTS — *see Schuessler tissue salts*

BIODEGRADABLE

Any substance which can be microbiologically broken down and absorbed into the atmosphere or ground.

BIOFLAVONOIDS

A group of naturally occurring water-soluble compounds sometimes referred to collectively as vitamin P, but the true status of these compounds as vitamins has not yet been confirmed. The group includes citrin, rutin and hesperidin.

Bioflavonoids often work in association with vitamin C, and have several functions in the body. They help strengthen weakened blood vessel walls, reduce heavy bleeding and bruising, and enhance the action of adrenalin and noradrenalin. They also tone the body muscles, and in the form of methylated bioflavonoid derivatives work against bacteria and influenza virus A. Bioflavonoids also act as antihistamines and antioxidants, protecting vitamin C and adrenalin from oxidation and decreasing levels of copper in the blood.

Bioflavonoids occur naturally in buckwheat, red peppers, blackcurrants, rosehips and in the white pith of citrus fruits. Foods rich in vitamin C are usually rich in the bioflavonoids as well. Bioflavonoids are used therapeutically to treat high blood pressure, tissue inflammation, varicose veins, respiratory infections, oedema and bleeding gums, as well as certain allergic reactions. RDA: not established.

BIOTIN

A vitamin of the B complex which helps the body to use other vitamins of the B group. It regulates cell growth and metabolism, and the production of fatty acids, as well as helping to maintain the proper functioning of the thyroid and adrenal glands. Prolonged use of antibiotics may cause deficiencies of biotin in the body. Symptoms include drastic hair loss, skin inflammation and dryness, fatigue, depression, muscle cramps and nausea, loss of appetite and anaemia. Good sources of biotin include brewer's yeast, whole grains, liver, legumes, molasses, soya beans and spinach.

BIRCHER-BRENNER SYSTEM

Nutritional principles established by Dr Bircher-Brenner, founder in 1902 of the now famous Zurich clinic. Dr Bircher-Brenner's system emphasises raw food and 6 basic principles:

- Half the daily food intake should consist of fresh raw plant food grown in healthy soil.
- One should start a meal with raw food and, where applicable, then proceed to cooked food.
- Green leafy vegetables containing chlorophyll should be eaten daily.
- Eggs and cheese are preferred to meat as a source of protein.
- Common salt, vinegar and pepper should be avoided and, if required, herbs, biochemic salt, yeast products and honey may take their place as flavourings.
- Wholegrain cereals (including the germ) are preferred to processed varieties.

BLACKMORE'S CELLOIDS

Mineral remedies developed by Australian naturopath Maurice Blackmore (1906–77) as a refinement of the Schuessler tissue salts. Schuessler believed that disease could be treated by rectifying mineral deficiencies, but according to Blackmore it was difficult to prove scientifically that Schuessler's minute homeopathic mineral doses could have any tangible effect on the living organism. The celloids included much more substantial content. Aware of the excess salt in the common diet, Blackmore also discarded sodium chloride from Schuessler's list, reducing his own range to 11 key mineral compounds.

In his work *Celloids: A Text Book for Physicians*, Blackmore made the following comparison:

The Schuessler Remedies consist of a very minute dosage of crude mineral, averaging to one part per million, or one molecule in six or a dozen tablets, and it is possible that because they are crude mineral that this is the only method of application that could be adopted and may be successful.

The Celloids, on the other hand, have a content of active micro-nutrients nearly equivalent to half the weight of the tablet, and if this quantity of crude mineral were prescribed it could constitute a poisonous dosage. Thus one has only

one part per million and the other 400,000 parts per million, making it obvious that there is no basis for comparison of the active ingredient.

Blackmore's assessment of the celloid mineral treatments is outlined in the table opposite.

BLADDER

A hollow organ in the body, the function of which is to store and secrete liquids. The principal bladders in the body are the gall bladder, a sac which is located under the liver and stores bile, and the urinary bladder which stores and excretes urine.

BLOOD CHOLESTEROL LEVEL — *see Serum cholesterol level*

BLOOD CLOT

A semi-solid accretion of blood cells and proteins which forms in the blood vessels.

BLOOD PRESSURE

Two readings are taken by medical practitioners. The *systolic pressure*, or upper reading, registers the amount of force the heart uses to drive the blood through the arteries; the *diastolic pressure*, or lower reading, records the resistance exerted by the artery walls on the blood.

Several factors influence blood pressure, including the strength of the heart, the elasticity or degree of hardness of the artery walls, and the volume of blood. Other factors may be stress-related or involve dietary intake, concerning such factors as excess alcohol or salt.

Naturopaths regulate blood pressure by improving the function of the kidneys (malfunctioning kidneys cause fluid retention in the body, increasing blood volume) and by dietary modifications — using in particular supplements of vitamin C (1–5 g per day) and vitamin E (500–1000 IU). Vitamin B6, garlic and the bioflavonoids may also be recommended in varying doses.

BLACKMORE'S ASSESSMENT OF CELLOID MINERAL TREATMENTS

Celloid mineral	Formula		Signs of possible deficiency	Function
CALCIUM compound	Calcium phosphate Sodium phosphate Iron phosphate	100 mg 200 mg 12 mg	Calcium — the 'skeletal' mineral. Bone and teeth degeneration. Membrane disorder — lungs: chronic cough, asthma, sore throats, sore eyes, sinus, polypi, catarrh, colds. Muscular pain and weakness — painful, delayed childbirth, aching limbs. Circulation and vascular disorders — swollen and varicose veins, cold hands and feet, chilblains. Stomach — tenderness, pain after eating, poor appetite.	The old, the young, and expectant mothers need calcium especially. Predisposition to colds and cold hands and feet indicate the need for calcium Acid-forming foods like white bread, white sugar and vinegar precipitate your calcium. Bone calcium is in the form of calcium phosphate and elemental calcium plays an important role in many cellular functions, especially correcting allergic reactions.
CHLORIDE compound	Potassium chloride Iron phosphate Sodium phosphate	50 mg 12 mg 200 mg	Chlorine — the 'glandular' mineral. Inflammations, infections and congestions — in any tissue. Cysts and swellings — swollen limbs, fibrous lumps or growths, bunions, bruises, sprains and contusions. Skin disorders — itching and rashes, warts, scar tissue, mouth ulcers. Bile disorders — indigestion from fats, sluggish liver. Glands — swelling and malfunction. Female — poor fertility.	Maurice Blackmore observed over decades of naturopathic practice that failure of reproduction in humans and animals because of internal scarring or glandular malfunction often results from potassium chloride deficiency. Potassium chloride is indicated for the second stage of inflammatory conditions and all catarrhal discharges. Because of its importance to the glandular system, potassium chloride is a very important mineral in correcting many hormonal problems in women.
IRON compound	Iron phosphate Potassium chloride Sodium sulphate	15 mg 8 mg 65 mg	Iron — the 'blood' mineral. Blood disorders — anaemia, haemorrhages, nosebleeds, hot flushes. Inflammation — all complaints ending in 'itis', fever, throbbing pains. Infections and congestions — lung, brain together with potassium chloride. Soft tissue damage — strains, sprains, cuts, bruises — checks inflammation and bleeding. Headaches — 'blinding' type of headaches. Female — menstrual disorders.	Iron is essential for the proper function of haem which carries oxygen in the red blood cells. Iron is essential to the body's energy producing functions and according to the principles of celloid mineral therapy, should be employed in all acute inflammatory conditions and fevers. As with calcium, iron supplements are important in pregnant women. The celloid formula is more easily absorbed than many iron supplements composed of metallic iron compounds.
MAGNESIUM compound	Magnesium phosphate Potassium phosphate Sodium sulphate	100 mg 25 mg 200 mg	Magnesium — the 'nerve' mineral. Nervous disorders — tics, spasms and twitchings, trembling, squinting, convulsions, poor coordination, stuttering. Nerve pains — neuralgias, sharp shooting headaches and other pain, night cramps, pains aggravated by cold.	Magnesium combined with phosphorus is the main constituent of the white nerve fibres or controlling nerves, so magnesium phosphate is the remedy for nerve disorders — it is nature's own antispasmodic. The need for magnesium phosphate and calcium phosphate is interrelated. Coffee, tobacco, alcohol and refined sugars appear to adversely affect magnesium metabolism. Whole wheat has eight times the magnesium content of white refined flour.
PHOSPHORUS compound	Sodium phosphate Calcium phosphate Iron phosphate Potassium phosphate Magnesium phosphate	150 mg 25 mg 12 mg 25 mg 25 mg	Phosphorus — the 'mood' mineral. Emotional imbalances — anxiety, gloomy moods, sensitivity, shyness, backwardness. Nervous exhaustion — sleeplessness, weariness, loss of strength, 'noises' in the head. Low resistance — tendency to recurring colds, infections or debility, loss of mental or physical efficiency. Female — post-natal depression.	Phosphorus occurs in the celloid range as the five phosphates of sodium, iron, magnesium, potassium and calcium. A lack in the diet may mean general debility, so supplementation with these phosphates should prove a good general tonic. Phosphorus is a constituent of bone, teeth, brain, hair and nerve tissues. It is a general tonic for the nervous system.
POTASSIUM compound	Potassium phosphate Potassium chloride Potassium sulphate	25 mg 25 mg 25 mg	Potassium — the 'brain' mineral. Mental conditions — depression, irritability, crying bouts, hysteria, sleepwalking, noise sensitivity, excess appetite or eating binges. Physical symptoms — yawning, stretching, 'ball in the throat', offensive breath.	Potassium is the great healing element of the body and combined with phosphorus is the main constituent of the grey nerve fibres and brain matter. Combined with chlorine, it is the glandular element which suspends decomposition. Diets high in salt can produce potassium deficiency. Quite a lot is needed by the body, so nature has provided twice as much in food as any two other elements put together. However the potassium compounds are easily lost in cooking or processing which is part of the modern dietary dilemma.
SILICA compound	Silica Sodium phosphate	25 mg 200 mg	Silica — the 'skin and hair' mineral. Arthritis — nodule and spurs. Skin disease — boils, including gumboils, carbuncles, pustules, abscesses, ulcerations, styes, discharges and pus. Head and scalp — falling or brittle hair, sensitive sore scalp, small lumps or nodules on head, head sweating. Tissues — thickened tissue, brittle nails. Female — mastitis.	Silica promotes elimination of accumulated waste matter and breaks down abnormal growth of tissues, such as arthritic nodules, and abscesses. Its role in the structure of connective tissue indicates its use in arthritic conditions, falling hair and flaking nails. Its metabolic presence appears to preserve the calcium metabolism from distortion or loss from the effect of other chemicals. Silica is also a factor in the preservation of healthy youthful skin. It is required to form and preserve collagen tissues, together with the bioflavonoids, vitamin C and protein.

BLACKMORE'S ASSESSMENT OF CELLOID MINERAL TREATMENTS   continued

Celloid mineral	Formula		Signs of possible deficiency	Function
SODIUM compound	Sodium phosphate Sodium sulphate Potassium chloride	200 mg 200 mg 25 mg	Sodium — the 'fluid' mineral. Stomach disorders — acidity, dyspepsia, heartburn, stomach ulcers, sour vomit. Elimination — frequent urination, kidney stones, offensive perspiration, fluid retention. Annoying habits — anal itching, nasal irritation, teeth grinding. Skin sensitivity — pimples, sensitivity to insect bites. Head — morning headaches, creamy catarrh, diseases of the eye. Female — leucorrhoea — creamy vaginal discharge.	Sodium is important to the digestive processes in the stomach, and then works in the blood to balance viscosity and keep it free from thickening waste material; it keeps calcium in solution so it can reach all tissues. It is synergistic to the effect of all other colloidal minerals and it is therefore included in each celloid mineral formula. Sodium sulphate controls water distribution and keeps bile, pancreatic and intracellular fluids at normal consistency.
SULPHUR compound	Sodium sulphate Potassium sulphate Calcium sulphate	200 mg 25 mg 12 mg	Sulphur — the 'purifying' mineral. Liver ailments — jaundice, yellowish stools or diarrhoea, dropsy, sore liver, biliousness, associated headache, usually top of skull. Skin disease — skin sores, psoriasis, dandruff, carbuncles and boils, acne. Joints and limbs — dropsy, gout. Bladder — frequent urination, cystitis.	The sulphates in combination with sodium regulate intracellular fluid and keep bile and pancreatic fluids at normal consistency — they are the great blood cleaners. Sulphur is higher in concentration in skin, hair, nails and joints. The colloidal sulphates appear to have some relationship with vitamin A, which taken together will improve skin clarity and quality.

BLOOD PRESSURE MEASUREMENTS — *see* *Sphygmomanometry*

BODY SYSTEMS

There are 9 body systems in the human

There are nine body systems in the human organism

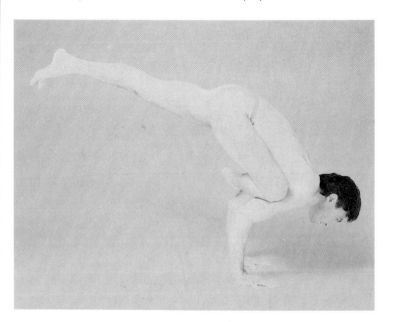

organism, and they comprise the following:

- *the skeletal system*, which includes the bones of the body, held together by ligaments;
- *the muscular system*, including the muscles of the skeleton, the blood vessels and hollow organs;
- *the digestive system*, including the teeth, saliva-producing glands, oesophagus, stomach, liver, gall bladder and the small and large intestines;
- *the respiratory system*, including the nose, pharynx, larynx, trachea, bronchi and lungs;
- *the circulatory system*, including the blood and blood vessels, lymph and lymph vessels and the heart;
- *the excretory system*, including the kidneys, ureters, bladder, liver, urethra, lungs and skin;
- *the nervous system*, including the brain, spinal cord, nerves and ganglia;
- *the reproductive system*, including the testes, vas deferens, prostate, penis and urethra in the male, and the ovaries, vagina, uterus and fallopian tubes in the female;
- *the endocrine system*, including the adrenals, thyroid, thymus and pineal

glands, pituitary body and pancreas; some functions of the ovaries and testes are also included.

BODY TISSUE

Groups of similar cells performing a particular function in the body. There are various types of body tissue:

- *Connective tissue* is found throughout the body and has a binding role. It provides the foundation for nerves, organs and blood vessels.
- *Epithelial tissue* is found in the skin, the digestive system, the nose, throat and lungs, and has the function of protecting and secreting.
- *Muscle tissue* allows for the function of bodily contraction and expansion, both voluntary and involuntary.
- *Nervous tissue* enables nerve impulses to be relayed to different regions of the body.
- *Vascular tissue* carries different substances to different regions of the body, for example, the lymph and blood.

BRAN

The tough outer layer of wheat or other grains which, together with the germ, is removed when the grain is milled to produce white flour. Many nutritionists believe this is actually the best part of the grain. Wheat bran is a rich source of high quality protein, vitamins of the B complex, phosphorus, magnesium, copper and selenium. It is also one of the best sources of dietary fibre and has a laxative effect. It is believed to play a significant role in reducing the risk of many diseases, particularly bowel cancer, and to actually absorb noxious chemicals in the colon.

BRAZIL NUT *(Bertholletia excelsa)*

A hard-shelled nut which is an excellent natural source of protein and the amino acid methionine. Brazil nuts are ideally eaten with other nuts, or with fruits like apples and pears. Naturopaths recommend that, in general, nuts should not be combined with foods consisting of animal protein and concentrated starch.

BREAD

A complex carbohydrate food which, especially in wholemeal varieties, provides an excellent source of nutrients and dietary fibre. The quality of bread depends, of course, on its constituent grains. The whole wheat kernel, for example, consists of 3 edible parts. Bran is the covering of the grain and is rich in carbohydrates, B vitamins, proteins and minerals — especially iron. In the centre of the kernel lies the carbohydrate-rich endosperm. This is the only part of the wheat which is found in refined white flour. At the bottom of the grain is the germ, which is the embryo of the new wheat plant. This contains valuable quantities of B vitamins (particularly thiamine), protein, vitamin E, minerals and carbohydrates.

Despite popular misconceptions, bread is not a fattening food. In addition, there has been a tendency to undervalue carbohydrates in the diet. Medical researchers now recommend that carbohydrates should make up to 50–60 per cent of the kilojoules in the diet — especially in the complex form found in breads, cereals and vegetables. So bread is a worthwhile food, and apart from being low in fat, also contains no sugar and has the advantage of being reasonably low in salt.

Breads with added fibre are suitable for people on slimming diets, and bread is also an appropriate food for athletes, who should ideally obtain around 60 per cent of their energy from carbohydrates.

BREWER'S YEAST

Originally used as a medicine by the ancient Egyptians, brewer's yeast is a very popular nutritional supplement available in health stores everywhere. Today it is available either in tablet form or as a dried powder which can be added to food and drinks. It is a very good source of protein and contains 16 of the 20 amino acids. It is particularly rich in all vitamins of the B group (especially vitamins B1 and B2) and also contains large amounts of phosphorus, iron, potassium, calcium, magnesium and significant amounts of selenium and chromium. Brewer's yeast is an excellent dietary supplement to correct any vitamin B deficiency which may show symptoms such as fatigue, depression, acne, mouth sores and palpitations. It has been used successfully to treat psychiatric patients suffering from nervous illnesses.

BROMIDES

Substances which, in the body, are associated with sedative action, producing mental dullness, apathy, loss of memory or appetite, drowsiness or constipation.

BRONCHI

The large air-conducting tubes in the lungs. These divide into bronchioles within the lung, and the bronchioles in turn open into the alveoli — the actual site where oxygen and carbon dioxide are exchanged between the blood capillaries and the air.

BUCKWHEAT, saracen corn
(Fagopyrum esculentum)

A grain-like plant with pink flowers which are said to be particularly attractive to bees, and from which they make excellent honey. The seeds can be made into a heavy flour which is used in the popular American buckwheat cakes or roasted and added to muesli. Buckwheat is used commercially to make rutin tablets (also referred to as vitamin P) These are often prescribed by naturopathic and homeopathic doctors to reduce high blood pressure, varicose veins, chilblains and other circulatory disorders. Buckwheat is also a valuable source of vitamin B and A, and of phosphorus, magnesium, calcium and iron.

BULIMIA

A health disorder in which a person (usually a young woman) regularly consumes large quantities of high-calorie foods and then either vomits or uses laxatives to avoid gaining weight.

Typical bulimics are of normal weight but suffer from low self-esteem, have a distorted body-image and often feel frustrated in their lives in terms of personal effectiveness. *See also Anorexia nervosa.*

BUNION

An inflamed swelling or bump, especially at the joint of the big toe. A tendency to bunions can be inherited and they can also be a sign of developing arthritis. The best treatment is to wear shoes that do not cramp at the ball-and-toe area of the foot and to periodically soak the feet in warm water.

C

CAFFEINE

A naturally occurring stimulant found in significant quantities in both tea and coffee. Caffeine stimulates the respiratory centre in the brain, usually increasing the rate of breathing. It may also slow the heart (when taken in normal doses), increase this rate (taken in high doses), and can also affect the blood pressure. High doses of caffeine may cause nervousness and irritation, heart palpitations and restlessness. Even in moderate doses it has an habituating effect.

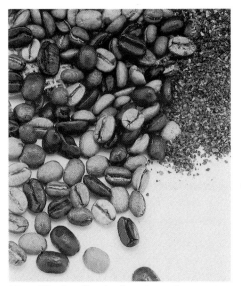

The caffeine in coffee stimulates the respiratory centre in the brain

CALCIFEROLS

Substances which collectively make up vitamin D. The principal calciferols are ergocalciferol, also known as vitamin D2, and cholecalciferol or vitamin D3. Vitamin D2 is made by irradiating ergosterol, present in plants, with sunlight. Vitamin D3 is produced in the body following the action of sunlight on 7-dehydrocholesterol in the skin. This produces cholecalciferol, which is in turn transported to the liver. After further chemical processes, the active form of vitamin D3 emerges from the kidneys. The principal function of vitamin D is calcium metabolism. *See Vitamin D.*

CALCIUM

Calcium is the most important mineral in the body and makes up more than half the total mineral content. The average adult has about 1.2 kg (2½ lb) of calcium, mostly in the bones. Calcium strengthens bones, teeth and cartilage, and helps in blood clotting, conducting impulses between the nerves, stimulating muscle growth, contraction and relaxation, and maintaining normal heart functions. The body must have an adequate supply of vitamin D before calcium can be effectively absorbed from the intestines. The recommended daily intake is 800 mg a day, but many people need more than this, particularly children and adolescents, and also pregnant and lactating women, who may all need up to 1400 mg a day. Post-menopausal women tend to lose calcium from their bones and should be careful to maintain an adequate calcium intake. Deficiency symptoms include osteoporosis (brittle bones), rickets (in children), arthritis, cramps, backache, insomnia, rheumatism, tooth decay, rapid pulse, limb numbness, poor blood clotting, and irritability.

Good sources of calcium are milk and all milk products — particularly cheese, molasses, nuts (especially almonds), bone meal, leafy green vegetables such as broccoli, fish, figs and dates.

CALORIE

A unit of heat, used to describe the amount of energy in food, produced by combustion. When used to measure the food energy level a calorie is in fact a kilocalorie — 1000 times the amount required to raise 1 cc of water by 1°C. It equals 4.2 joules. *See also Kilocalorie.*

CANCER

A malignant tumour, the cells of which grow rapidly, without restraint. This cell multiplication is abnormal and, if it continues, disorganises the normal functioning of the body. Cancer tumours can begin in any tissue or organ in the body and can be effectively treated if all the cells are removed. If the tumour is small when discovered there is more chance of containing it, but cancers spread through the lymph system and the bloodstream. The original tumour is called a primary cancer and the additional cancers, secondaries. When secondaries form, the cancer is much harder to treat.

Figures released in the United States in 1984 (which reflect a pattern followed in other modern industrialised nations) show that the most common cancers in men are cancer of the lung (22%), prostate (18%), colon and rectum (14%), and in women, cancer of the breast (26%), colon and rectum (15%), uterus (12%), lung (10%) and ovary (4%). Leukaemia and lymphomas account for around 7–8% of cancer incidence in both sexes.

The chances of surviving cancer vary with early detection and the particular form of the cancer. If breast cancer is detected while less than 2 cm in size, there is a 90% chance of survival, but lung cancer has a poor outlook, with only 10% of sufferers surviving 5 years. Bowel cancer has a 30–40% survival rate, stomach cancer 13% and pancreatic cancer 4%. Leukaemia treatment is often successful: acute lymphatic leukaemia has a 42% survival rate and chronic lymphatic leukaemia 54%.

CAPILLARIES

The smallest vessels in the body capable of carrying blood cells. Capillary walls are only one cell thick.

CARBOHYDRATES

Food constituents utilised by the body as energy fuel. Carbohydrates include starches, sugars, gums, dextrins and cellulose, and represent around half of the normal food intake.

Approximately 80 per cent of energy from blood sugar contributes to the maintenance of body temperature and 20 per cent contributes to kilocalorie expenditure. Simple sugars—like honey and fruit sugars—are easily absorbed by the body after being converted into glucose, or blood sugar, which provides fuel for energy. Other categories of carbohydrate include the following:

- *Complex carbohydrates*, e.g. white sugar, provide glucose but do not provide the sustained energy levels of simple sugars.
- *Starches* are more complex than simple

sugars and take a longer time to convert into glucose; wholegrain bread is an example.
- *Cellulose* is not absorbed by the body, but plays an important role in the digestive and eliminative process.

Most fruits and vegetables contain carbohydrates in some form, although not all fruits and vegetables are equally starchy. Asparagus, green beans, peas, lettuce, celery and spinach are low in starch, while cane and maple sugar, dates, figs, grapes and bananas are relatively high. Cellulose is found in the skins of fruits and vegetables.

CARCINOGEN

A substance which is considered to stimulate or cause the growth of cancerous tumours. Some of the constituents of cigarette smoke are regarded as potential carcinogens.

CARDIAC OUTPUT

The volume of blood pumped by the heart.

CARDIANT

Any treatment which affects the heart. Cardiants fall into 3 categories:

- *Sedatives* lessen the force of the heart's action and include aconite, antimony and digitalis.
- *Stimulants* increase the pulse and include alcohol, camphor, cocaine, galvanic current and spearmint.
- *Tonics* stimulate the cardiac muscles and include caffeine and valerian.

CARDIOVASCULAR

That which relates to the blood-carrying system in the body: specifically the heart and blood vessels.

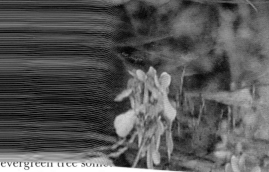

tree. Their sweet flavour is rather similar to chocolate, but they do not have the high levels of caffeine and oxalic acid which are found in cocoa beans. Carob is sometimes prescribed to cure digestive upsets because of the pectin it contains.

Carob is also rich in the B vitamins, thiamine, niacin and riboflavin, and contains vitamins A and D as well as minerals like calcium, magnesium, phosphorus, potassium, iron and silicon. Carob has more fibre than cocoa and its calcium content is 3 times greater than that of milk.

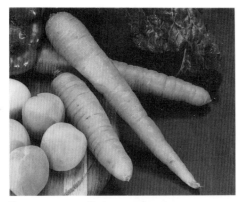

Carrots are an excellent source of carotene

CAROTENE

An important nutrient found especially in fresh carrots. Alpha, beta and gamma carotene are precursors of vitamin A, which is essential for good eyesight (especially night vision) as well as reducing high blood cholesterol levels.

Carotene can be derived in large quantities only through consumptions of raw carrots, or freshly made carrot juice. Cooking, dehydration and heat destroy it immediately.

Carotene is also lost as a result of bacterial fermentation when fresh carrot juice is allowed to stand for too long — it may diminish in nutritional value after 2 or 3 hours. Pasteurisation destroys taste of carrot juice and turns it ...n, so dietitians recommend that car- and carrot juice be consumed fresh never possible.

CARRAGEEN

A vegetable gum extracted from various types of red seaweed. Carrageen is used as a thickener in dairy products, but there are currently doubts about its safety as a food additive.

CARROT *(Daucus carota)*

The cultivated carrot is a nutritious vegetable and is particularly important as a rich source of carotene from which the body manufactures vitamin A. Carrot soup is very easily digestible and is a useful remedy for diarrhoea. Carrot juice reduces stomach acidity and heartburn and, because of the potassium salts it contains, is also a useful diuretic. Two or 3 raw carrots eaten daily for about a week should rid the body of roundworms. The seeds of wild carrots can be made into an infusion to relieve colic, flatulence and fluid retention, and to bring on menstruation. After research showed that people with high levels of vitamin A were less prone to develop certain types of cancer, some people began to consume large quantities of carrot juice every day. This can be a dangerous habit as vitamin A is toxic in large doses.

CARTILAGE

Connective tissue in the body which is comparatively more flexible than bone. Cartilage is the pad of 'gristle' which acts as a buffer between adjoining bones.

CASEIN

The protein of milk.

CASHEW *(Anacardium occidentale)*

A nut of Brazilian origin (its name was originally *acaju*), the cashew has a relatively low fat content and a high concentration of essential amino acids — specifically tryptophan, valine and isoleucine — all of which are supplied in amounts exceeding the RDA per 100 g portion. Combined with brazil nuts or almonds, cashews provide an excellent source of protein and are a fine accompaniment for fresh fruit and vegetables in the vegetarian or vegan diet.

CASTOR OIL

An oil extracted from the seeds of *Ricinus communis* and used as a purgative or cathartic. Castor oil is also used in the manufacture of soap.

CATARACT

A clouding of the lens of the eye so that less light reaches the eye, affecting the vision.

CATARRH

Inflammation of the mucous membranes, particularly of the nose, accompanied by congestion and excessive secretion of mucus.

CATHARSIS

A state of purification or cleansing following the use of a purgative. The term can be used to describe cleansing of the bowels, but it is also used in several psychotherapeutic modalities to refer to a state of emotional release. *See also Rebirthing, Abreaction, Reichian therapy* (Part 2).

CAYENNE, capsicum, cayenne pepper, Hungarian cayenne, paprika, chili pepper, red pepper, bell pepper *(Capsicum* species)

The fruit of any member of *Capsicum*, which includes a wide variety of red, green and yellow peppers of different sizes and tastes — ranging from the sweet bell capsicums which are eaten as a vegetable, to the tiny, hot chili peppers used as very strong spices. They were used as a fruit and a medicine in the West Indies, and were brought back to Europe by Columbus in the fourteenth century. Capsicums are a very good source of vitamin C and may be taken in powdered form, as paprika, to ward off colds and flu. Small quantities of capsicum will stimulate the appetite, and as an infusion they can be taken to ease stomach pains and diarrhoea, and to aid digestion, particularly in old people or invalids. However, they should not be used for long periods. Cayenne is a powerful general stimulant and will act as a catalyst to speed up the absorption of other medicines. It stimulates and regulates blood flow, strengthens the pulse, improves circulation to the hands and feet, and is a useful first-aid remedy. Externally it can be applied in an ointment to relieve rheumatism, bruises and chilblains, and to draw out splinters. It is said that a small amount of cayenne sprinkled inside your socks will keep your feet warm!

CELERY, celeriac *(Apium graveolens)*

A widely cultivated vegetable, considered by the ancient Greeks to be an aphrodisiac. It is very rich in vitamins and minerals, and eating fresh stalks promotes healthy muscle development, is good for the skin and stimulates the appetite. Celery is also said to be helpful for alcoholics, and to bring on menstruation. The stalks, when cooked in milk, assist in the treatment and prevention of arthritis and other muscular pain. The seeds, which can be made into a tea, are also beneficial for arthritis, rheumatism and bronchitis and, when combined with juniper berries, stimulate the kidneys. The tea also has a sedative effect on the nervous system. The oil from the root of the plant is said to restore sexual potency after a debilitating illness.

CELLULITE

A gel-like substance consisting of fat, water and waste substances which become trapped in lumpy, immovable pockets beneath the skin. Cellulite accumulates in the body as a result of several factors, including poor eating and breathing habits, fatigue, sedentary lifestyles, constipation and poor circulation. Cellulite is not the same as ordinary body fat and requires special dietary treatment which helps purify the body of accumulated toxic wastes. Deep breathing coupled with regular exercise, relaxation and massage may also assist.

CENTRAL NERVOUS SYSTEM

The brain and spinal cord in the body. It consists of the nerve cells and fibres of the brain and spinal cord, and is linked to peripheral nerves which affect voluntary actions and sensory awareness.

CEREBRAL

That which relates to the higher functions of the brain; for example, speech and thought.

CEREBROVASCULAR

That which relates to the cerebrum and associated blood vessels.

CERVICAL

That which relates to the neck or cervix.

CERVICAL DILATION

The natural process in which the cervix opens during childbirth and menstruation.

CERVICAL MUCUS

Mucus secreted by the glands of the cervix, and which can be examined periodically during the menstrual cycle to determine the onset of ovulation. *See Billings Method* (Part 2).

CERVIX

The neck of the womb; the area which opens during childbirth. Cancer of the cervix is comparatively common, but is often preventable in women of a young age.

CHELATE

A mineral made available to the body in an organic form, thereby allowing assimilation. The most effective form of chelation occurs when a mineral molecule (for example) is surrounded by a hydrogen-saturated protein from the ingested food.

The term 'chelate' itself derives from the Greek word for 'claw', and in the chelation process the bonded mineral–protein passes through the intercellular spaces in the intestinal tissue, thereby gaining absorption (most inorganic mineral traces would normally pass through the body system unabsorbed).

There are also natural chelates, such as vitamin C, which has a detoxifying effect on certain minerals, and aspirin, which chelates copper from the lining of the stomach.

The chelation effect can also be induced by supplementation with EDTA (ethylenediamine tetra-acetic acid), a synthetic amino acid which 'shovels up' minerals in the system and, like vitamin C, can be used to rid the body of metal toxins. *See Chelation Therapy* (Part 2).

A wild plant also commonly cultivated

people to offset the stimulating effects of caffeine. Chicory is a general tonic with diuretic and laxative effects. It is recommended for a number of digestive problems including lack of appetite and for jaundice, gall bladder problems, gout and rheumatism. It is also helpful for reducing mucus.

CHIVE *(Allium shoenoprasum)*

A culinary herb rich in sulphur, iron and calcium. Chives are not usually used medicinally, but make a tasty appetiser and generally help with digestion, particularly of fatty dishes. They are said to be good for the kidneys and, if eaten regularly, to help guard against anaemia and assist in lowering blood pressure.

CHLOROPHYLL

The green pigment present in the leaves of plants, and produced by photosynthesis. Chlorophyll is rich in iron, magnesium and potassium, and has a blood-building function. It rejuvenates old cells as well as promoting new growth, and stimulates the vascular system, the intestines, the uterus and the lungs. It also inhibits bacterial growth, cleansing the body of pollutants and poisons.

Chlorophyll is a natural deodorant and can be taken for cases of excessive body odour. One of the best sources of chlorophyll is wheatgrass juice — the solid content of which consists of 70 per cent chlorophyll.

CHOLESTEROL

A crystalline, lipid substance found in all tissues of the body, especially the brain,

ons, and is also an important component

In terms of diet, cholesterol is ingested from animal and dairy foods, but the amount of dietary cholesterol in the bloodstream depends on how much saturated fat is consumed in the diet. The more saturated fats, the higher the blood cholesterol is likely to be. Cholesterol is also synthesised in the body (the liver manufactures 600 mg every day) but it is not readily soluble and over the years leaves residues in the arteries. The latter may then become clogged up to such an extent that blood is unable to reach the heart or brain, resulting in a heart attack or stroke.

Extensive scientific research indicates that high blood cholesterol is directly linked to coronary heart disease, and that lowering blood cholesterol levels significantly reduces the incidence of heart attacks. Unfortunately, cholesterol differs from fat in that it cannot be 'burned off' by exercise. At the time of his death while jogging in Vermont, jogging 'guru' James Fixx's cholesterol rating was 250 — 30 points above the Pritikin danger threshold. So how can the cholesterol level be reduced? Most nutritionists advise reducing fat intake by minimising the amounts of fatty meats and dairy products consumed. The accompanying table indicates the fat content of popular foods. *See also LDL and HDL cholesterol, Pritikin Diet.*

							82%
							80%
							50%
...sage	27%	Steamed haddock	1%	Camembert	23%	Dairy ice cream	7%
...lamb (shoulder)	26%			Edam	23%	Milk (full cream)	5%
...pork sausages	25%			Cheese spread	23%	Milk (homogenised)	4%
Roast leg of pork	20%			Cottage cheese	4%	Yoghurt	1%
Fried beefburgers	17%					Skimmed milk	Less than 1%
Grilled rump steak	12%						
Casseroled pigs liver	8%						
Stewed steak	7%						
Casseroled chicken	7%						
Fried lamb kidneys	6%						
Tinned ham	5%						

CONTROLLING CHOLESTEROL LEVELS — WHICH FOODS TO EAT

Food group	Advisable	In moderation	Not advised
CEREAL FOOD	Wholemeal flour, oatmeal, wholemeal bread, wholegrain cereals, porridge oats, crispbreads, wholegrain rice and pasta, sweet corn	White flour, white bread, sugar-coated breakfast cereals, white rice, pasta	Fancy breads e.g. croissants, savoury cheese biscuits, cream crackers
FRUIT AND VEGETABLES	All fresh and frozen vegetables, dried beans and lentils, fresh fruit, dried fruit	Chips if cooked in suitable oil or fat, avocados, olives	Potato crisps, chips cooked in unsuitable oil or fat
NUTS	Walnuts	Almonds, brazil nuts, chestnuts, hazelnuts, peanuts	Coconut
FISH	All white fish, oily fish e.g. herrings, tuna	Shellfish occasionally	Fish roe
MEAT—LEAN	Chicken, turkey, veal, rabbit, game	Ham, beef, pork, lamb, bacon, lean mince, liver and kidney occasionally	Visible fat on meat (including crackling), sausages, pate, duck, goose, streaky bacon, meat pies, meat pasties
EGGS AND DAIRY FOODS	Skimmed milk, skimmed milk cheese e.g. cottage and curd cheese, egg whites (3 yolks per week only)	Edam cheese, Camembert, Parmesan	Whole milk, cream, hard cheese, Stilton, cream cheese, excess egg yolks
FATS	All fats should be limited	Margarine labelled 'high in polyunsaturates', corn oil, sunflower oil, soya oil, safflower oil	Butter, dripping, suet, lard, margarine not 'high in polyunsaturates', cooking/vegetable oil of unknown origin
MADE-UP DISHES	Skimmed milk puddings, skimmed milk sauces, pastry puddings, cakes and biscuits made with suitable margarine or oil and wholemeal flour	Pastry puddings, cakes and biscuits made with suitable margarine or oil and white flour, ice cream	Tinned or whole milk puddings, dairy ice cream, pastry puddings, cakes, biscuits and sauces made with whole milk, eggs or unsuitable fat or oil, all proprietary puddings and sauces, mayonnaise
SWEETS, PRESERVES AND SPREADS	Bovril, Oxo, Marmite	Meat and fish pastes, boiled sweets, fruit pastilles, peppermints, etc., jam, marmalade, honey, sugar	Peanut butter, chocolate, toffees, fudge, butterscotch, lemon curd, mincemeat
DRINKS	Tea, coffee, mineral water, unsweetened fruit juices, clear soups, homemade soups e.g. vegetable, lentil	Packet soups, alcohol	Cream soup

CHOLINE

One of the B-group vitamins, choline is

lecithin, liver, green leafy vegetables, nuts, fruit and wholemeal cereals. Symptoms of deficiency include fatty infiltration of the liver, kidney damage, atherosclerosis and muscle weakness.

Choline has been used in the treatment of liver disease in combination with a high protein diet, and serves the important preventive health function of maintaining healthy arteries. Unofficial RDA : 1000 mg.

CHOROID

The middle coating of the eye. This membrane is located between the sclera and the retina.

CHROMIUM

A mineral needed by the body only in very small amounts, but essential for the metabolism of sugars and fats. Some diabetics are helped by taking chromium which acts togeter with insulin to metabolise sugars. Chromium is also thought to help reduce cholesterol levels. People in Asia generally have much higher levels of chromium in their bodies, and the incidence of diabetes and hardening of the arteries is much lower. Sources of chromium include brewer's yeast, unrefined wholegrain cereals, clams, mushrooms, black pepper, liver and beer.

CHROMOSOME

A rod-shaped body which appears in the nucleus of a cell during cell division. Chromosomes contain genes — or hereditary factors — and are of a constant number for any given species.

CHRONIC

A term used to describe a health disorder

An enzyme derived from the sap of the green pawpaw (papaya) fruit. Chymopapain appears to be a valuable treatment for people suffering from lower back herniated discs — commonly referred to as 'slipped discs'. When chymopapain is injected into the vertebral disc it causes the jelly-like substance in the centre to dissolve, shrinking the disc and relieving pressure on root-nerves. Chymopapain treatment was first used in 1964 and has now been tested internationally in medical centres in Canada, the United States, Europe and Australia. It appears to be a useful adjunct to chiropractic and osteopathy, and a far more appropriate treatment than surgery. Only one injection of the substance is required and most patients are able to walk satisfactorily within 6 hours of treatment. Recurrence of disc pain is rare and the treatment is usually free of complications.

CILIA

The eyelashes. *See also Cillosis*.

CILLOSIS

A continuous trembling of the upper eyelid.

CIRCADIAN RHYTHMS

Biological and physiological functions which occur approximately once a day (Latin: *circa*, 'about', *dies*, 'day'). These include sleep patterns and fluctuations in urine and blood pressure. The existence of these rhythms lends some credibility to the concept of biorhythms. *See also Biorhythms* (Part 2).

CLAVICLE

The collar bone, which articulates with the shoulder blade to form the pectoral arch.

CO-CARCINOGEN

A substance which is not in itself a carcinogen but which stimulates or acts as a catalyst for substances which are. For example, the controversial artificial sweetener cyclamate is considered by the American Food and Drugs Administration (FDA) to be a possible co-carcinogen.

COCCYX

The triangular bone located at the base of the spinal cord.

COCHLEA

The spiral passage in the inner ear through which sounds are received and then transformed into nervous impulses.

COD-LIVER OIL

An oil extracted from the livers of the codfish *(Gadus morrhua)*, and traditionally used to treat rickets, which is caused by vitamin D deficiency. In addition to vitamin D the oil also contains vitamin A, bromine, iodine and a fatty acid EPA *(Eicosapentaenoic acid)* that helps prevent the formation of blood clots which can cause thrombosis. A further fatty acid contained in the oil is DHA *(Docosahexaenoic acid)*, which is thought by scientists to be necessary for the early phases of brain development. The 2 fatty acids convert into prostaglandins — biological substances which control blood pressure, blood clotting and digestion.

Two teaspoons of cod-liver oil taken daily is sufficient to reduce high blood cholesterol levels. The oil is also recom-

mended for pregnant up to the age of n

COITUS

Sexual intercourse

COLD PRESS

A category of oi safflower, soya bean, kernel oils. Cold-pressed good source of unsaturated fatty

COLIC

A sharp, intermittent pain in the abdomen. The term originally referred to pain in the colon or large intestine, but is now used to refer to periodic pain in several organs. Colic is common in infants around 3 months old.

COLITIS

Inflammation of the colon, or large intestine.

COLLAGEN

The inter-cellular 'cement' which bonds tissues together in the body. Collagen is a vital protein ingredient in blood vessels, fibrous tissue in scars, and the matrix of hard tissue like bone and cartilage. It represents approximately 35 per cent of the body's protein, and provides the fibre in the connective tissue which supports the body. Vitamin C is required for the synthesis of collagen, and without this substance the slightest wound in the body would prove fatal.

Collagen is used in skin-care treatment to replace damaged or disfigured tissue. Therapeutic collagen is taken from cattle and is highly purified. It is then injected into the skin at the specific location where scarring or wrinkling have occurred. Collagen implanting may be used in cases of severe facial disfigurement which cannot be easily removed with surgery. It is commonly used as a treatment for wrinkles, frown lines on the forehead and between the eyes, and for creases from the nose to the corner of the mouth. It is not used, however, as a treatment for the receding hairline. Collagen is injected into the skin's while scar particularly run from the surface of the skin straight through to a deeper level underneath. Collagen treatment is effective for about a year.

COLOSTRUM

The thin, yellowish, milky fluid secreted by the breasts prior to the birth of a baby, and also immediately following the birth. Colostrum contains vitamins, minerals and antibodies, and flows until real breast milk is produced.

COMPLEMENTARY PROTEIN FOODS

Protein foods which combine together to produce a balanced intake of amino acids. Proteins may be found in grains, seeds, legumes and dairy products. Good combinations include bread and cheese; cereal grains and milk; rice-bean casserole and wheat-soy bread; humus and lentils-rice; tahini sesame seed paste and bean salad; sunflower seeds and legumes. *See also Protein.*

COMPLETE PROTEIN FOOD

A protein food containing the 8 essential amino acids in the correct amounts for dietary absorption. Examples include meat and eggs. *See also Protein.*

CONGESTION

An excessive quantity of fluid in any given part of the body.

CONJUNCTIVA

The mucous membrane which lines the eyelid. Inflammation of this membrane is known as conjunctivitis.

CONNECTIVE TISSUE

The structural tissue in the body which has a binding role and provides the foundation for nerves, organs and blood vessels.

CONSTIPATING FOODS

Foods which may induce constipation, or a clogging effect in the bowels. These foods include cheese, eggs, white bread and pastries, salted and pickled meats, and rice.

CONSTIPATION

The clogging of food wastes in the bowel, often associated with a diet including refined flour, decreased fibre intake and excessive amounts of red meat. (Dietary fibre helps to exercise the intestinal and bowel muscles.)

When the bowels become sluggish the wastes tend to accumulate and harden. Chronic constipation can exacerbate varicose veins and hernias, and also lead to the possibility that toxic wastes could be reabsorbed into the system (a possible contributing cause of cancer of the colon).

CONTAGIOUS DISEASE

A disease which is spread as a result of direct body contact; for example, venereal disease.

COPPER

A mineral needed by the body in only very small quantities for the formation of haemoglobin in red blood cells, and for healthy bones, skin and hair. It is abundant in many foods including nuts, legumes, whole rice, mushrooms and seafoods. It is possible to have too much copper in the diet, and this can lead to irritability, insomnia and depression.

CORNEA

The transparent membrane which forms part of the outer surface of the eyeball.

CORONARY HEART DISEASE

Known as coronary atherosclerosis, the impairment of heart function due to a reduction of blood flow to the heart — *see Atherosclerosis.*

CORTEX

The outer layer of any given organ.

CRAMP

A painful spasm in a muscle, often associated with exposure to cold, or with poor circulation.

CRANIUM

The bones of the skull.

CRESS, watercress, scurvy grass, stime, tall nasturtium *(Nasturtium officinale)*

A peppery-flavoured plant which commonly grows in ditches and streams, but can be cultivated in very wet, shady soil. It is widely used in salads and as a garnish. It is a particularly nutritious food, being exceptionally rich in vitamins C and E, and in minerals. Cress contains significant amounts of iron, manganese, sulphur, iodine and phosphorus, and if eaten regularly, either raw or made into a tea, it will keep the complexion healthy, clear up pimples and sores, and stop hair falling out. It stimulates digestion and purifies the blood, and acts as a general illness preventive. It is sometimes recommended for respiratory complaints such as catarrh and for kidney stones, but should not be eaten excessively as it can cause throat and stomach inflammations and kidney problems. Cress was mentioned by the early Anglo-Saxons as one of the 9 sacred herbs used to repel evil.

Land cress *(Lepidium sativum)*, also known as dittander, karse or curled cress, has similar properties to water cress; it is grown in gardens or on sprouting trays.

CROUP

A health disorder, common in children, in which the larynx becomes infected and the small air passage blocked. This results in hoarseness, coughing and breathing difficulty.

CUTANEOUS

That which relates to the skin.

CYANOCOBALAMIN —
see Vitamin B12

CYST

A collection of fluid in an area of the body, sometimes as a result of a blocked oil-producing gland.

CYSTINE

A non-essential amino acid of the neutral class. It is important for healthy development of red corpuscles, mammary glands and hair, and helps the tissues to resist infections. Food sources include carrot, cauliflower, onion, garlic, apples, pineapples, and brazil and hazel nuts.

CYSTITIS

Infection of the bladder, associated with a burning sensation during urination. It is usually caused by bacterial infection.

D

DANDRUFF

A scalp disorder characterised by a dry, flaky scalp or the blockage of overactive sebaceous glands. Dandruff symptoms can be caused by stress and trauma, but may also be nutritionally related. Dandruff sufferers often consume more starch and sugar than those without dandruff, and the preventive measure is therefore to eliminate processed carbohydrates (cakes, pastries, white bread and sugar) from the diet as far as possible. Naturopaths use vitamin B-complex, vitamin B12 and vitamin C as dietary supplements to treat dandruff.

DEGENERATIVE DISEASE

A disease in which the body tissue deteriorates, loses its functional purpose, and is either converted to or replaced by some other type of tissue. For the most part, degenerative diseases are non-contagious. Heart disease and cancer are examples.

DEHYDRATION

Loss of water in the body.

DEPRESSION

A common emotional illness which can be caused by a variety of factors. Very often it is related to stresses in one's daily lifestyle, deriving from the perception that there are seemingly insurmountable obstacles impeding one's happiness, fulfilment or self-esteem. Alternatively, one's existence may seem to be increasingly meaningless following a breakdown in relationships, or some other form of emotional crisis.

Depression may, however, also have tangible nutritional causes. It can be caused by hypoglycaemia (low blood sugar), food allergies, a lack of B vitamins, mineral imbalances in the body, inadequate vitamin C, or lack of the amino acid L. tryptophan.

Naturopaths have noted that depression before a menstrual period or menopause is often related to vitamin B6 deficiency, and that post-natal depression following pregnancy may result from a deficiency of vitamin B12 and the B-group vitamin folic acid. Nutritional supplements, allergy tests and glucose tolerance tests are thus possible ways of highlighting and remedying depression caused by specific nutritional factors.

DERMATITIS

Inflammation of the deeper layers of the skin.

DERMIS

The so-called 'true skin' or deeper levels of the skin beneath the epidermis.

DEXTROSE — *see Glucose*

DIABETES

A health disorder caused by the body's inability to utilise carbohydrates or sugary foods. Carbohydrates provide energy for the body and the assimilation process involves the production of insulin in the pancreas. In diabetics the pancreas is not able to make sufficient insulin and the sugar accumulates instead of being used as energy. The kidneys endeavour to excrete the excess sugar with the result that diabetics also pass more urine than is normal. Diabetics are treated with insulin and must monitor their dietary intake very carefully.

DIARRHOEA

Abnormally fluid stools, or a condition in which the bowels are more open than usual and liquid faecal matter is passed. Diarrhoea can result from infection or over-consumption of fat.

DIASTOLIC PRESSURE
— *see Sphygmomanometry*

DIETARY FIBRE — *see Fibre, dietary*

DIET, BALANCED

Adequate nutrition based on a varied choice of foods which provide nutrients, energy, dietary fibre and fluids in proportions appropriate for health. Food is often divided by nutritionists into 5 basic groups:

Bread and cereals — which supply energy, fibre, vitamins and minerals
Fruit and vegetables — which supply fibre, vitamins and minerals, especially vitamin C from citrus fruits
Meat or meat substitute — which supply body-building protein, energy, vitamins and minerals
Milk and dairy products — which supply bone and teeth-building calcium, body-building protein, energy, vitamins and minerals
Butter and margarine — which supply energy, vitamins A and D, and essential fatty acids

Most nutritionists recommend that for a balanced diet one should select from the 5 basic groups and eat moderately. Wholegrain cereals are preferred and care should be taken to reduce salt and fat intake, decrease consumption of sugars, and restrict alcohol consumption to a moderate level.

Vegetarians can also make use of the 5 food-group categories while substituting plant foods like fruit, nuts, cereals and vegetables for flesh foods like meat, fish and poultry. It is generally acknowledged that some intake of eggs and dairy products makes the vegetarian diet easier to balance because these foods are a good source of calcium, riboflavin, quality proteins and vitamins A, D and B12.

DIETETICS

The science of regulating the diet for a therapeutic and hygienic purpose. According to naturopathic practice, the intake of natural foods enhances the natural functions of the body and is therefore an ideal approach in maintaining health. The basic food categories under consideration are proteins, carbohydrates, fats, vitamins, minerals and cellulose (fibre) — *see separate listings*.

DIGESTION

The process of breaking down foods so that they can be absorbed into the body. *See also Digestive tract.*

DIGESTIVE TRACT

The body system involved with the digestion of food. It includes the mouth, pharynx, oesophagus, stomach, small and large intestines, liver, gall bladder and pancreas.

DIGLYCERIDE

One of a group of edible fats and oils, a diglyceride is a fatty acid ester of the alcohol glycerol in which 2 of the 3 hydroxyl groups are joined to a fatty acid.

DISEASE

A sickness, illness or disorder affecting the body or some specific organ or limb. Naturopaths regard disease as a manifestation of imbalance and a sign that the body is endeavouring to rid itself of elements which are intrinsically unnatural; for example, the presence of toxins in the system. 'Vitalist' concepts of health, like acupuncture, acupressure and polarity balancing, which regard health in terms of the flow of energy through the body, are more inclined to regard disease in terms of 'blockages' to the life-force in the body (for example, the *chi* energy which is said to travel through the meridians of the body). It is common in the alternative health modalities to talk of the dis-ease of the body, thereby emphasising that, in this state, the body is out of harmony with itself.

DISLOCATION

A situation in which a bone slips out of place at a joint; for example, a shoulder dislocation in which the head of the humerus slips out of the hollow in the shoulder. Dislocations are a common form of sports injury and can be extremely painful.

DNA

Deoxyribonucleic acid — a double helix molecule, contained in chromosomes, which relays through its structure the patterns of hereditary traits.

DRIED FRUITS

A healthful alternative to sweets, and an excellent source of minerals, vitamins, fructose, plant cellulose and fibre, dried fruits are a valuable source of nutrients.

They include the following:

Apricot: rich in carotene (which the body converts into vitamin A), copper and iron
Nectarine: A good source of plant cellulose and vitamin B-complex
Peach: includes the mineral salts potassium, phosphorus, copper, calcium and iron, as well as vitamin B-complex
Pear: includes vitamin B1 and B2, calcium and phosphorus
Prune: rich in vitamin A, the B vitamins and iron, and also well known for its regulatory bowel function
Seeded raisin: an excellent source of carbohydrate, iron, potassium, phosphorus, calcium, magnesium and several of the B vitamins.

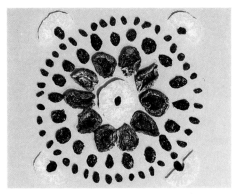

Dried fruits are an excellent source of minerals, vitamins and fibre

DUCT

An enclosed channel in the body, the function of which is to conduct liquid; an example is the bile duct.

DUODENUM

The first section of the small intestine, located next to the stomach. It is so-called because in man it is approximately 12 finger-breadths long (Latin: *duodecim*, 'twelve').

DYSMENORRHOEA — *see*
Menstruation

On balance, eggs may be regarded as an excellent source of nutrients. Recommended intake: 2–3 per week.

ELEMENTS, MACROBIOTIC THEORY OF

The concept of macrobiotics draws not only on the Chinese idea of *yin* and *yang*, but also on the fivefold classification of the elements. The traditional Chinese elements are wood, fire, earth, metal and water, and each of these is associated with a colour, various body organs, a season of the year, and different types of food. According to macrobiotic theory we should harmonise with the food offerings of a given season and rectify deficiencies that might be present by choosing foods from the appropriate seasonal phase or colour group.

The following tables include several macrobiotic correlations:

ELEMENT	COLOUR	SEASON	ORGAN
Wood	green	spring	liver, gall bladder, eyes
Fire	red	summer	heart, small intestines
Earth	yellow/orange	late summer	spleen, pancreas, stomach
Metal	white	autumn	lungs, large intestines
Water	black/blue/grey	winter	kidneys

EMBOLUS

A clot, piece of fat, group of cells or air-pocket which is blocking a blood vessel in the body.

EMETIC

Any substance which causes vomiting.

EMOLLIENT

Any substance which softens, relaxes and soothes the skin. Emollients may be applied in poultices, fomentations and liniments to any inflamed part of the skin in order to soften the tissues and remove

ECOSYSTEM

The total range of relationships of living and non-living things in an environment.

ECTOPIC PREGNANCY

A pregnancy which occurs outside the womb. This can take place when a fertilised ovum lodges in a fallopian tube and begins to grow, causing pain in the lower abdomen. Ectopic pregnancies require surgery but do not affect fertility.

ECZEMA

An itchy and inflammatory, but non-contagious, skin condition. Eczema can result from an irritant (clothes, detergent, jewellery), or from allergens and dietary deficiencies. Naturopaths may use supplements of vitamin C, vitamin A, and vitamins B2 and B6, zinc and oil of evening primrose to treat the symptoms, but eczema has also been successfully treated with acupuncture and hypnotherapy (since it is sometimes also a psychosomatic condition).

EGGS

A fine source of complete protein, vitamin A and vitamin B12, as well as lecithin, potassium, magnesium, calcium, zinc and selenium. Eggs also contain vitamins B2, D, E and niacin. Egg yolks have a comparatively high cholesterol content, which has made them unpopular with many nutritionists — including the late Nathan Pritikin — but there is no scientific evidence that eating eggs increases the risk of the average person having a heart attack. On the positive side, the amino acid content of eggs helps remove metal pollutants from the body.

any irritation. Examples include olive oil and vaseline.

EMPTY CALORIE FOODS

Foods and beverages which are high in calories but virtually devoid of nutrients; for example, white sugar and soft drinks. This is a nutritional term for 'junk food'.

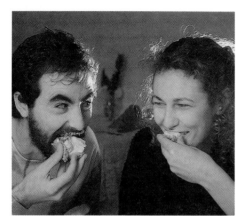

Empty calorie foods — the polite term for 'junk foods'

EMULSIFIERS

Modifying agents used in food and drink to produce a specific constancy. Emulsifiers are used for a number of effects — to maintain texture, to bond ingredients which might otherwise separate, and — in the case of margarine — to reduce splattering when used for cooking. Some emulsifiers are produced synthetically — for example, by chemically modifying the glycerides of fatty acids — but others are natural. One of these is lecithin, found in eggs and soya beans.

ENDOCRINE GLANDS

Ductless glands which manufacture secretions or hormones that pass directly into the blood or lymphatic systems, closely affecting physical growth and sexual development. Included among the endocrine glands are the pancreas, pituitary, thyroid, thymus, adrenals, ovaries and testes.

ENDOMETRIOSIS

A condition in which endometrium tissue from the uterus transfers to the fallopian tubes or pelvic cavity. The tissue cells become embedded on the outer walls of the uterus, fallopian tubes, or on the pelvic organs, and begin to grow, causing considerable pain. High doses of oestrogen and progesterone are generally successful as a treatment, and becoming pregnant usually cures it, as well. Supplements of vitamin E have also been effective in some cases.

ENDORPHINS

Naturally occurring opiates in the brain which produce a state of pain relief and even euphoria. Endorphins are triggered by intense sports like jogging and long-distance running, and produce a type of 'high' as a result; some sportspeople experience corresponding withdrawal symptoms if they are not able to regularly engage in these activities.

Endorphins are also released by acupuncture stimulation and are responsible for the analgesic, or pain-killing effect which results when the needles are placed in position along specific acupuncture meridians.

ENDOSPERM

Starch granules found in cereal grains. Grains produce a one-seeded fruit which includes the germ, or embryo, together with the endosperm; these are enclosed by the seed coat. The endosperm provides food for the germ. In the case of wheat it is the source of refined white flour.

ENKEPHALINS

Pain-killing peptides (small chains of amino acids) which inhibit the passage of pain impulses up the spinal cord to the brain. Enkephalins form part of the protein betalipotropin.

ENTERITIS

Inflammation of the intestines.

ENZYME FOOD ADDITIVES

Enzymes are sometimes used in the preparation of specific foods where they do not occur naturally. For example, the plant enzymes bromelain, papain and ficin are present in some types of beer, and papain is sometimes used to tenderise meat. Health authorities usually require food labels to indicate the presence of enzyme additives. *See also Enzymes.*

ENZYMES

Protein molecules, made up of amino acids, which act as catalysts in the body. In solution, enzymes produce fermentation and chemical changes in other substances without apparently undergoing changes themselves. Enzymes are responsible for breaking down or building up cellular raw material within specific body tissues or organs.

There are over 5500 different enzymes in the body and their construction in the cell is directed by the genetic message coded in the genes.

EPIDERMIS

The outer, protective layer of the skin which covers the dermis, or 'true skin' underneath.

EPITHELIAL TISSUE

Cellular tissue found in the skin, digestive system, nose, throat and lungs, and which has the function of protecting and secreting.

EPSOM SALTS

The popular name for magnesium sulphate heptahydrate, a saline purgative. It is also used as an anticonvulsant, and in ointments for its water-drawing and anaesthetic effect.

ERYTHEMA

Non-infectious and non-contagious dark red rash on the skin.

ERYTHROCYTE

A red blood corpuscle.

ESSENTIAL AMINO ACIDS

Amino acids which cannot be produced by the body and must therefore be obtained through the diet. Eight amino acids fall into this category: isoleucine, leucine, lysine, methionine, phenylalanine, threonine, tryptophan and valine. Two other amino acids, histidine and arginine, are required for the healthy growth of children. *See Amino acids.*

ESSENTIAL FATTY ACIDS

Unsaturated liquid oils, usually vegetable in origin, which enable oxygen to be more easily transported by the bloodstream to cells, tissues and organs. They help lubricate the cells and combine with protein and cholesterol to produce living membranes which bind the body cells together. Essential fatty acids also provide the body with the means for producing potent prostaglandins — fatty acid hormone-like substances which help to regulate blood clotting and blood viscosity. The fatty acids also work with vitamin D to make calcium available to the body tissues, help facilitate the assimilation of phosphorus, and aid the conversion of carotene to vitamin A. Unsaturated fatty acids are more readily metabolised by the body than saturated fatty acids.

Essential fatty acids cannot be synthesised by the body, and must therefore be obtained from the daily diet. Essential fatty acids fall into two classes: N6 and N3.

The first of these classes contains linoleic acid, which is found mainly in seed oils like sunflower and safflower, and especially in evening primrose oil, which also contains gamma-linolenic acid.

The second class of essential fatty acids occurs in linseed oil and contains alpha-linolenic acid.

ESTROGEN — *see Oestrogen*

EUSTACHIAN TUBE

The connecting passage between the middle ear and pharynx. It admits air which equalises pressure on either side of the ear drum and allows it to vibrate.

EXCRETION

The passing of waste materials, or toxins, from the body.

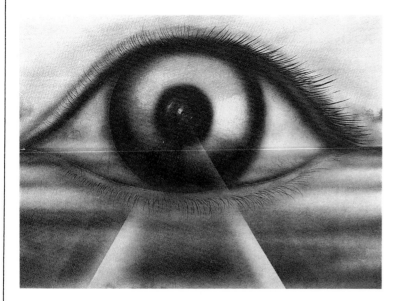

EXCRETORY ORGANS

Organs with the function of eliminating waste materials from the body. These organs include the intestine, kidneys, lungs and skin.

EXPECTORANT

A substance which facilitates the ejection of mucus or phlegm from the throat or lungs.

EXTREMITIES

A popular term for the hands and feet, or arms and legs.

EYE PROBLEMS

Deteriorating vision may be attributed to a variety of causes, including a dietary deficiency of vitamin A or vitamin B2 (riboflavin), or a high intake of sugars and refined carbohydrates. The American ophthalmologist William H. Bates found that many eye problems could be solved by exercising the muscles surrounding the eyeball, through techniques such as palming and cupping. Chiropractors and osteopaths may also treat eye problems by correcting spinal faults impinging on nerves which service the eyes. Some naturopaths have found vitamin C helpful in preventing glaucoma and cataracts. *See also Bates Method, Palming, Cupping* (Part 2).

F

FAECES

Solid waste matter consisting of by-products from the digestive process and secretions of the body, excreted through the rectum. Chemical substances and undigested matter may also be present. *See also Stool.*

FALLOPIAN TUBES

The 2 tubes or canals through which ova pass from the ovary to the uterus. They are named after the Italian anatomist Gabriel Falloppio (1523–62).

FASCIA

The layer of fibrous connective tissue between two muscles, or between the skin and deeper levels of tissue.

FATS

Fats are generally divided into saturates and unsaturates. Saturated fatty acids are characterised by straight molecules with no 'double bonds' — which tends to make the fat firm. Examples of fats rich in saturates include butter, beef dripping, lard and coconut oil, and with the exception of the last of these, they are sold at room temperature.

Unsaturated fatty acids contain double bonds and are characterised by 'bent' molecules which make the fat softer. For this reason they are liquid at room temperature. This category of fatty acids may in turn be differentiated as *mono-unsaturates* containing only 1 double bond (a type found in olive oil and some fish oils) and *polyunsaturates* containing 2 or more double bonds (a type found in fruits, nuts and vegetable oils).

The most significant dietary poly-unsaturated fatty acid is linoleic acid, which is 18 carbons long and contains 2 double bonds. An essential fatty acid, it cannot be produced in the body and must be consumed in the diet. People whose diet is high in polyunsaturates usually have low serum cholesterol levels and are less at risk from heart disease. Ideally consumption of fats should not exceed 30 per cent of kilojoule intake. *See also Essential fatty acids.*

FATTY ACID

A constituent of fats consisting of a long chain of carbon atoms with an acid group (carboxyl group) at one end. Fatty acids come in various categories. Examples include palmitic and stearic acid (saturated); oleic acid (unsaturated) and linoleic, linolenic and arachidonic acids (polyunsaturated). *See also Essential fatty acids.*

FDA

The American Food and Drugs Administration.

FEVER

A condition in which the body temperature exceeds 100°F (38°C) in an adult, or 102°F (39°C) in a child. The normal temperature of the human body is 98°F (37°C).

When the body is invaded by harmful bacteria the immune system causes an increase in temperature to destroy the disease micro-organisms and improve body efficiency.

In general, naturopaths resist using treatments designed to curtail a state of fever, maintaining that fever is a natural response by the body to rid itself of disease.

AMOUNT OF FIBRE IN SELECTED FOODS

Source of dietary fibre	Average serve	Fibre per average serve (g)	Fat (g)
High source (over 6.5 g per serve)			
Lentils, cooked	1 cup	9.2	0.6
Baked beans	½ cup	9.1	0.6
Dried figs	3	7.4	0.5
Dried apricots	4–5 halves	7.2	0.1
Kidney beans, cooked	⅓ cup	7.0	1.0
Good source (5.0–6.5 g per serve)			
Corn, tinned	110 g	6.3	0.7
Loganberries, stewed	100 g	5.2	—
Raspberries, canned	100 g	5.0	—
Spinach	Average serve	5.0	0.2
Moderate source (2.5–5.0 g per serve)			
Broad beans	½ cup	4.6	0.4
Corn, on the cob	1 medium	4.5	1.2
Almonds	⅓ cup	4.3	16.1 ✦
Broccoli	Average serve	4.2	0.3
Coconut, fresh, 30 g	1 piece	4.1	10.6 ✦
Wholemeal bread	2 slices	4.0	1.4
Bananas	1 medium	3.4	0.3
Prunes	3 large	3.4	0.2
Desiccated coconut	1 tablespoon	3.3	8.8
Peas	⅓ cup	3.1	0.2
Carrots	1 medium	3.1	0.2
Potato with skin	1 medium	3.0	0.1
Brussels sprouts	4 medium	2.9	0.3
Avocado	½ medium	2.8	19.0 ✦
Strawberries	½ punnet	2.8	0.6
French beans	⅓ cup	2.6	0.2
Mushrooms	100 g	2.5	0.3
Cabbage	Average serve	2.5	0.2
Small amounts (less than 2.5 g per serve)			
Cauliflower	Average serve	2.5	0.2
Brown rice, cooked	1 cup	2.4	1.2
Peanuts, 30 g	1 tablespoon	2.4	14.6 ✦
Pear	1 medium	2.4	0.4
Apple	1 medium	2.3	0.4
Oatmeal, cooked	½ cup	2.1	2.3
Sultanas	30 g	2.1	—
Orange	1 medium	2.0	0.3
Wholemeal flour	1 tablespoon	1.9	0.5
Tomato	1 medium	1.8	0.2
Macaroni, white cooked	1 cup	1.7	0.8
White bread	2 slices	1.6	0.9
Peanut butter	Average on sandwich	1.5	9.7 ✦
Melon	½ large rockmelon	1.5	0.6
Fruit cake, boiled	1 slice	1.4	7.5 ✦
White rice, cooked	1 cup	1.4	0.1
Olives	6	1.3	3.9
Grapefruit	½ medium	0.9	0.3
Pumpkin	Average serve	0.6	0.2
Plain sponge, 40 g	1 slice	0.4	3.7
Lettuce	2 large leaves	0.4	0.1
White flour	1 tablespoon	0.3	0.3

FIBRE, DIETARY

That part of food which is not digested in the small intestine. There are two types of fibre — insoluble and soluble. Insoluble fibre is material which has the ability to speed the transit-time of waste through the digestive tract and therefore promote bowel health. Soluble fibre has little effect on 'regularity', but lowers serum cholesterol levels in human beings and animals, whereas insoluble fibre does not.

Wheatbran and beans are both high in soluble fibre and have been shown experimentally to be effective in reducing blood cholesterol.

Fibre includes a number of different components: pectin (in fruit), cellulose (in all vegetables), hemi-cellulose (found especially in cereal husks), lignin (in cereals and vegetables) gums, saponins and waxes.

Dietary fibre is not broken down substantially by the digestive enzymes, but once it reaches the large intestine it undergoes a bacterial fermentation process. This produces short-chain fatty acids which nourish the bowel cells, influence the way in which the body uses cholesterol, and also affect the manner in which blood sugars are utilised. Dietary fibre also slows the digestive process in the upper section of the intestinal tract, thereby producing a slow release of nutrients into the bloodstream.

A daily intake of 20–30 g of dietary fibre is recommended. The following table gives the amount of fibre in some commonly eaten foods.

FIBRIN

A protein which provides the structural cause of a blood-clot. It is present in newly shed blood.

FIBROSITIS

A rheumatic condition caused by the inflammation of fibrous tissues. It is characterised by pain and stiffness in the muscle sheaths and fascia.

FIBROUS

Consisting of fibres, or bundles of thread-like tissues.

FIBULA

The slender outer bone located between the knee and ankle in the leg. *See also Tibia.*

FLATULENCE

Distension of the stomach or intestines associated with excessive accumulation of wind or gas. Flatulence causes belching.

FLORA

A term used medically to describe micro-organisms present in the intestines.

FLUID RETENTION

A condition commonly found in women as a result of hormonal imbalance, extended periods on the Pill, or prior to the onset of menstruation. It can be related to food or chemical allergies and may also be caused by excessive salt intake or inadequate consumption of protein. Many herbs — including juniper, nettle and dandelion — serve as diuretics when taken as teas, and these may alleviate the symptoms. Vitamins B6, C and E also have diuretic actions.

FLUORIDE

A chemical which has been shown to prevent or reduce dental decay. It is used in toothpaste and by dentists, and is added to the drinking water in many areas. Although it has significantly improved the state of children's teeth in those areas, many natural health practitioners disapprove of its use, partly because it has been claimed to cause cancer and to inhibit the body's absorption of vitamin C. Some people choose to purify their water and remove the fluoride by adding fresh wheat grass.

FLUORINE

A non-metallic element present in small amounts in bones and teeth. Very little is needed by the body and this can be obtained from vegetables, particularly garlic and watercress.

FOETUS (or FETUS)

The unborn offspring which develops in the womb. The term also refers to the young of all vertebrate animals between the embryonic and independent states.

FOLIC ACID

One of the B-group vitamins, folic acid is a co-enzyme to vitamin B12 and is essential for red blood cell formation and for the formation of new cells. It is also essential for efficient brain functioning, and is important in the production of antibodies.

Folic acid is water soluble and occurs naturally in green leafy vegetables, yeast, mushrooms, nuts, milk, liver and wheatgerm. Symptoms of deficiency include megaloblastic anaemia, diarrhoea, mental sluggishness, menstrual and skin problems, and inflammation of the tongue. Folic acid is used to treat anaemia and intestinal disturbances, especially during pregnancy. It is also useful in treating alcoholism, atherosclerosis, coeliac disease and Hodgkin's disease (malignant inflammation of the lymph nodes).
RDA: 400 mcg.

FOLLICLE

From the Latin *folliculus*, 'a little bag', a secretory sac or gland; for example, hair follicles which are found at the base of hairs on the body.

FOOD ADDITIVE NUMBERS

Numbers approved by government authorities in Europe and Australia for the identification of food ingredients. Under agreed guidelines, food labels must now list, in descending order by mass, all the ingredients which have gone into the food in the package.

Additives are not specified by name in the new system but by a number code. For those who are allergic to certain additives, or who are following a restricted diet, a knowledge of constituents is vital. The code numbers for food additives are as follows (in Europe these numbers are preceded by a capital E):

FOOD ADDITIVE NUMBERS
Numbers approved by the National Health and Medical Research Council for approved food additives

No.	Food additive
100	Curcumin
101	Riboflavin
102	Tartrazine
107	Yellow 2G
110	Sunset yellow FCF
120	Cochineal, carminic acid
122	Carmoisine
123	Amaranth
124	Brilliant scarlet 4R
127	Erythrosine
132	Indigo carmine
133	Brilliant blue FCF
140	Chlorophylls
142	Green S
150	Caramel
151	Brilliant black BN
153	Carbo medicinalis vegetalis (charcoal)
155	Chocolate brown HT
160	Carotenoids
160(a)	Carotene, alpha-, beta-, gamma-
160(b)	Annatto (bixin, norbixin)
160(e)	Beta-apo-8' carotenal

No.	Food additive
160(f)	Ethyl ester of beta-apo-8' carotenoic acid
161	Xanthophylls
161(g)	Canthaxanthine
162	Beetroot red, betanin
163	Anthocyanins
170	Calcium carbonate
171	Titanium dioxide
172	Iron oxides and hydroxides
200	Sorbic acid
201	Sodium sorbate
202	Potassium sorbate
203	Calcium sorbate
210	Benzoic acid
211	Sodium benzoate
212	Potassium benzoate
213	Calcium benzoate
220	Sulphur dioxide
221	Sodium sulphite
222	Sodium bisulphite
223	Sodium metabisulphite
224	Potassium metabisulphite
234	Nisin
249	Potassium nitrite
250	Sodium nitrite
251	Sodium nitrate
252	Potassium nitrate
260	Acetic acid
261	Potassium acetate
262	Sodium acetates
263	Calcium acetate
270	Lactic acid
280	Propionic acid
281	Sodium propionate
282	Calcium propionate
283	Potassium propionate
290	Carbon dioxide
296	Malic acid
297	Fumaric acid
300	Ascorbic acid
301	Sodium ascorbate
306	Tocopherol-rich extracts of natural origin
307	Synthetic alpha-tocopherol
308	Synthetic gamma-tocopherol
309	Synthetic delta-tocopherol
310	Propyl gallate
311	Octyl gallate
312	Dodecyl gallate
320	Butylated hydroxyanisole (BHA)
321	Butylated hydroxytoluene (BHT)

No.	Food additive
322	Lecithins
325	Sodium lactate
326	Potassium lactate
327	Calcium lactate
330	Citric acid
331	Sodium citrates
332	Potassium citrates
333	Calcium citrates
334	Tartaric acid
335	Sodium tartrates
336	Potassium tartrates
337	Sodium potassium tartrate
339	Sodium orthophosphates
340	Potassium orthophosphates
341	Calcium orthophosphates
350	Sodium malates
351	Potassium malates
352	Calcium malates
353	Metatartaric acid
354	Calcium tartrate
355	Adipic acid
363	Succinic acid
380	Tri-ammonium citrate
400	Alginic acid
401	Sodium alginate
402	Potassium alginate
403	Ammonium alginate
404	Calcium alginate
405	Propylene glycol alginate
406	Agar
407	Carrageenan
410	Locust bean gum
412	Guar gum
413	Tragacanth
414	Acacia
415	Xanthan gum
416	Karaya gum
420	Sorbitol
421	Mannitol
422	Glycerol
433	Polyoxyethylene (20) sorbitan mono-oleate
435	Polyoxyethylene (20) sorbitan monostearate
436	Polyoxyethylene (20) sorbitan tristearate
440(a)	Pectin
442	Ammonium phosphatides
450	Sodium and potassium polyphosphates
460	Microcrystalline cellulose, powdered cellulose

No.	Food additive
461	Methylcellulose
464	Hydroxypropyl-methylcellulose
465	Ethylmethylcellulose
466	Carboxymethyl-cellulose
471	Mono- and diglycerides of fatty acids
472(e)	Mono- and diacetyltartaric acid esters of mono- and diglycerides of fatty acids
473	Sucrose esters of fatty acids
475	Polyglycerol esters of fatty acids
476	Polyglycerol polyricinoleate
481	Sodium stearoyl-2-lactylate
482	Calcium stearoyl-2-lactylate
491	Sorbitan monostearate
500	Sodium carbonates
501	Potassium carbonates
503	Ammonium carbonates
504	Magnesium carbonate
508	Potassium chloride
509	Calcium chloride
529	Calcium oxide
536	Potassium ferrocyanide
541	Sodium aluminium phosphate
551	Silicon dioxide
553(b)	Talc
554	Sodium aluminium silicate
558	Bentonite
559	Kaolins
570	Stearic acid
572	Magnesium stearate
575	Glucono deltalactone
621	Monosodium glutamate
627	Sodium guanylate
631	Sodium inosinate
637	Ethyl maltol
900	Dimethylpolysiloxane
901	Beeswaxes
903	Carnauba wax
904	Shellac
905	Paraffins
909	Stearic acid
920	L-Cysteine and its hydrochlorides
924	Potassium bromate
925	Chlorine
926	Chlorine dioxide

SOME ADDITIVES THAT MAY CAUSE PROBLEMS

Additive	Foods in which the additive may be found*	Possible problems
Allura red AC (red colouring)	Any food to which colour may be added.	Has been reported as causing tumours in rats.
Amaranth (red colouring)	Any food to which colour may be added.	Banned in US in 1976. Linked to hyperactivity in children. Large doses cause cancer in female rats. Prevents pregnancy and causes stillbirths in rats. Can cause allergic and respiratory reactions
Anethole (flavouring)	Beverages, confectionery, ice cream.	Occurs naturally in anise, fennel and star anise. May cause irritation of skin or mouth.
Aspartame (artificial sweetener)	Approved for use in diet food and soft drinks.	Toxic to people suffering from phenylketonuria as it breaks down to release phenylalanine.
Benzoic acid, benzoates (preservative)	Condiments, cordials, fruit juices, jams, maraschino cherries.	Occurs naturally in berry fruits and tea. Can cause allergic reactions.
Benzoyl peroxide (bleaching agent)	Flour.	Can cause allergic reactions.
Brilliant blue FCF (blue colouring)	Any food to which colour may be added; toothpaste.	Can cause allergic reactions. Suggested link with hyperactivity in children.
Butylated hydroxyanisole-BHA (antioxidant)	Chewing gum, ice cream, instant potatoes, margarine, vegetable oils, shortenings.	Can cause allergic reactions and affect liver and kidney function.
Butylated hydroxytoluene-BHT (antioxidant)	Pecan nut and walnut kernels.	Can cause allergic reactions, affect kidney function and large doses given to pregnant mice affected the brain functioning of offspring. Prohibited in UK.
Calcium silicate (anti-caking agent)	Dried milk powder, salt.	On FDA list of additives that need further study.
Cyclamates (artificial sweetener)	Diet food and soft drinks.	Large doses cause cancer of the bladder in rats.
Erythrosine (red colouring)	Any food to which colour may be added.	Can cause allergic and respiratory reactions. Suggested link with hyperactivity in children.
Licorice (flavouring)	Beverages, confectionery, ice cream, medicines.	Eating licorice regularly can raise blood pressure, cause headaches and muscle weakness.
Monosodium glutamate (flavouring)	Condiments, pickles, snack foods, tinned soups.	Occurs naturally in tomatoes, mushrooms, parmesan cheese and sweet corn. Can cause allergic reactions, asthma, and discomfort in sensitive individuals. On FDA list of additives that need further study.
Nitrites	Canned fish and meat, cured fish and meat, salami.	May cause cancer, if converted to nitrosamines.
Saccharin (artificial sweetener)	Diet food and soft drinks.	Large doses cause cancer of the bladder in several species.
Sorbitol (humectant)	Almond paste, confectionery, desiccated coconut, dietary foods, modified starches used to thicken many canned goods.	May alter the absorption of drugs; may cause diarrhoea.
Sulphur dioxide, sulphites, metabisulphites (preservative)	Biscuits, cakes, cheese pastes, fruit juices, gelatin, mince, preserved fruit and vegetables, sausages and sausage mince.	Can cause allergic and respiratory reactions.
Sunset yellow FCF (yellow colouring)	Any food to which colour may be added.	May cause allergic reactions. Suggested link with hyperactivity in children.
Tartrazine (yellow colouring)	Any food to which colour may be added.	Can cause allergic reactions, particularly in people allergic to aspirin and benzoic acid. Suggested link with hyperactivity in children. US requires items containing tartrazine to list it on the label.

*The additives may be present in foods other than those listed

FOOD ALLERGY MUSCLE TEST

Based on a technique utilised in applied kinesiology, the food allergy muscle test is performed as follows: the tester stands facing the subject and pulls down reasonably quickly on the extended arm to test the strength of the deltoid muscle, while asking the subject at the same time to resist.

To test for food allergy, a small portion of the food is placed on the subject's tongue and the muscle test is repeated. If the subject is allergic to the food it will be impossible to resist the downward thrust applied by the tester on the arm.

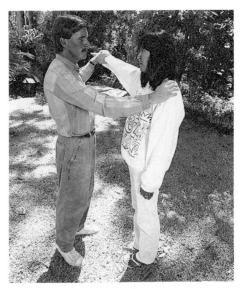

Muscle-testing for food allergies

FOOD CHALLENGE

A food allergy test in which the subject resists eating 'suspect' foods for a period of time, preferably during a 5-day fast. A portion of 1 of these foods is then eaten and reactions to it are noted in a diary. The food challenge is most effective if common allergens are avoided for 2 weeks prior to the test. These include wheat products, eggs, tomatoes, milk and dairy products, and foods containing yeast.

FOOD INTOLERANCE

Allergies related to the intake of specific foods. Some foods are allergens because they are inadequately digested as a result of a missing enzyme (as in lactose intolerance), while other diseases like Crohn's disease or colitis are associated with food sensitivities. Sometimes proteins from wheat or milk are only partially digested and then act on the brain in a manner resembling hormones. These peptides are known as exorphins and have been linked to some mental disorders. Other food peptides lead to inflammation and degeneration in the bones, joints or soft body tissues.

The major offenders among food allergens are cow's milk, wheat and yeast-containing foods like brewer's yeast, bread, beer and wine. Food intolerance is normally treated through an elimination diet which seeks, over a period of time, to isolate the specific offending foods. The Food Allergy Muscle Test may also be useful. *See Allergy, Food allergy muscle test.*

FOOD IRRADIATION

A technique of preserving foods for a longer period by subjecting them to gamma-ionising or radionuclide radiation. This form of radiation is similar to the type produced by such radioactive substances as cobalt 60 and uranium, although current techniques of irradiation do not make food radioactive.

Foods which are at present subject to irradiation include wheat, flour, garlic, onions, white potatoes, and some herbs and spices. In the United States pork may also be irradiated.

Food irradiation has been widely criticised by natural health practitioners throughout the world, for the following reasons:

• Gamma or ionising radiation produces deleterious or uncharacterised effects on nutrients; fat and water-soluble vitamins, essential amino acids, nucleic acids and enzymes are depleted or destroyed.

- Irradiation produces radiolytic chemical by-products in foods. These free-radical medicated chemical by-products have not been tested for long-term latent toxicity.
- Irradiation may convert a wide variety of herbicides, insecticides, pesticides, fungicides, colourants, antibiotics, steroids, preservatives and stabilisers to chemical by-products which pose substantial toxic risk to consumers.

Food irradiation — a potential health risk?

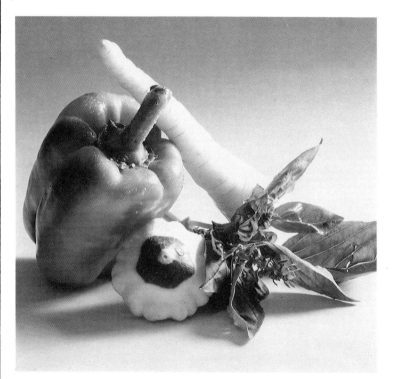

FOOD PRESERVATIVES

Substances used to control the presence of undesirable moulds, odours and tastes in foods. Usually the processes of decomposition and decay in food are unacceptable, although bacteria are required for the production of cheese and yoghurt, and the fermentation process is utilised in manufacturing breads and wines.

Many methods of food preservation have been used traditionally, including drying, smoking, pickling, salting and sugaring, and in recent times pasteuris-ation, canning and refrigeration have evolved as additional methods. Most canned foods do not include preservatives because the canning process eliminates harmful micro-organisms, but preservatives are often used commercially in such foods as bread, cakes, pastries, soft drink, dried fruits, fruit juices and various meat products. Common food preservatives include nisin, sorbic acid, benzoic acid, natamycin and sulphur dioxide.

FOOD SUGARS

The main sugars in food are the carbohydrates sucrose ('sugar'), glucose (dextrose), fructose (fruit sugar), lactose (milk sugar) and maltose (malt sugar). With the exception of lactose, these have varying degrees of sweetness.

These sugars each contribute about the same amount of energy (approximately 16 kilojoules per gram). Artificial sweeteners like saccharin, cyclamate and aspartame, however, do not provide substantial amounts of energy and some sweeteners of this type have an unpleasant after-taste.

FREE FATTY ACID

A fatty acid which is in a 'free' state, not combined with glycerol. Fatty acids occur in this state in trace amounts in most cells and tissues.

FRUCTOSE

Fruit sugar; a carbohydrate sweetener which serves as an energy source in the diet. Fructose supplies 1660 kilojoules (395 calories) of energy per 100 grams. *See also Food sugars.*

G

GALL BLADDER

A small hollow organ attached to the liver. The gall bladder receives bile from the liver and transfers it into the duodenum, where it aids digestion. In some cases gallstones — consisting largely of cholesterol — may be formed in the gall bladder. *See Gallstones.*

GALLSTONES

Deposits which form in the gall bladder, especially when the flow of bile from the liver becomes thick and sluggish. In traditional allopathic medicine gallstones are removed by surgery, but many naturopaths employ nutritional supplements to treat or prevent their formation. Preventive measures include reducing intake of both polyunsaturated and saturated fats, and taking supplements of vitamin E, since a deficiency of this vitamin is thought, in some cases, to produce gallstones. A high-fibre diet including fresh fruits, vegetables and grains is both beneficial and highly recommended as a general measure. Daily lecithin supplements break down cholesterol deposits, and bile salts may be taken to break down the gallstones themselves, although with the latter treatment medical or naturopathic supervision is recommended because prolonged use can result in gallbladder irritation.

GAMETE

A protoplasmic body, such as an ovum or sperm, which unites with another of the opposite sex, for conception.

GASTROINTESTINAL TRACT — *see Alimentary canal*

GENE

The hereditary factory transmitted by each parent to its offspring, thereby determining hereditary characteristics.

GENITALS

The external sexual organs: the penis and testicles in the male, and the vulva in the female.

GERMS

A popular term for bacteria, viruses or micro-organisms which invade the body and cause disease. Examples include staphylococcus, which produces boils; streptococcus, which causes tonsillitis; and the viruses which cause influenza.

GERSON THERAPY

A cancer therapy developed by German physician Dr Max Gerson (1881–1959) over a period of 30 years of clinical experimentation. The therapy is based on the concept that cancer patients have reduced immune defences and generalised tissue damage, especially in the liver.

Gerson therapy focuses on a high potassium, low sodium, low fat diet, and keeps animal protein to a minimum. The juices from raw fruits, vegetables and raw liver are used to provide active oxidising enzymes to help restore the liver and repair damaged body tissue elsewhere in the body. Iodine and niacin supplementation is used, and coffee enemas are frequently employed to facilitate excretion of toxic cancer breakdown products from the body.

Gerson therapy regards cancer as one of several degenerative diseases and is effective in treating other conditions of this type, such as osteoarthritis, multiple sclerosis and heart disease. Gerson actually developed the method to cure his own debilitating migraines, and he subsequently found his treatment to be effective against tuberculosis, asthma and diabetes, as well as all types of cancer.

Gerson's idea that there was an important link between nutrition and cancer has now been taken up in earnest by the American Cancer Society, the National Cancer Institute and the National Academy of Sciences, among other institutions. (The Gerson Institute: PO Box 430, Bonita, California 92002, USA)

GESTATION

The act of carrying the young in the womb during pregnancy. The term is also used to describe the length of time from conception to birth, which in humans is approximately 266 days.

GINGIVITIS

Inflammation of the gums.

GLANDS

The lymphatic glands are approximately the size of a pea and are distributed over the body, filtering out toxins which are produced when bacteria invade the body. Glands with a duct, known as exocrine glands, produce substances used in the healthy functioning of the body. The sweat glands in the skin and the salivary glands in the mouth are examples.

GLOSSITIS

Inflammation of the tongue.

GLUCOMANNAN — *see Konjac*

GLUCOSE

A simple carbohydrate which is the form of sugar carried in the bloodstream to all cells of the body. As a sweetener it is also known as dextrose, and occurs naturally in grapes and various other fruits. It serves as an energy source in the diet, supplying 1660 kilojoules (395 calories) of energy per 100 grams. However, it is not as sweet as sucrose. *See also Food sugars.*

GLUTAMIC ACID

A non-essential amino acid of the acidic group. It is important for digestion, for manufacturing insulin, for disinfecting and for preventing anaemia. Food sources include carrots, string beans, celery, parsley, lettuce and pawpaw.

GLUTEN

The rubbery substance which remains when wheat flour (or the flour of other cereal grains) is washed to remove the starch. Gluten contains approximately 80 per cent of the protein in wheat flour and has the same chemical structure as albumin.

GLYCERIN

An antiseptic, syrupy substance derived from various fats like palm oil. Glycerin is sweet, odourless and colourless, and is used extensively in medicine (as well as in the manufacture of explosives). It serves as a laxative when taken internally and is used as a preservative in certain herbal mixtures.

GLYCINE

A non-essential amino acid of the neutral group. It is important for building cartilage and muscle fibre, and for controlling the hormones. Food sources include carrots, celery, parsley, garlic, oranges, watermelon and almonds.

GLYCOGEN

Animal starch; it is in this form that the body stores carbohydrates, especially in the liver which converts it into glucose. Glycogen is also found in the muscles and is converted into energy as required.

GOITRE

An enlarged thyroid gland, caused by either excess or insufficient thyroxine. Deficiency causes tiredness and may lead to an overweight condition (myxoedema), which excess thyroxine speeds the body up, causes the heart to beat faster and leads to weight loss (thyrotoxicosis). Goitre can also be caused by iodine deficiency in the diet.

GONAD

The germ gland in the testis of the male or the ovary of the female.

GOUT

A disease condition which occurs when uric acid salts accumulate around the joints, especially in the big toe. The crystalline deposits produce pain and inflammation, and also affect lubrication of the joints.

Uric acid is normally metabolised in urea and excreted through the kidneys, but if there is an enzyme deficiency in the body this process may not occur so effectively. Some naturopaths have found daily supplements of vitamin B6 and B-complex to be a useful antidote. As a preventive measure, intake of meat, eggs, dairy products, sugar and refined carbohydrates should be reduced, since they produce uric acid in the body. Foods high in potassium—for example, bananas and green leafy vegetables—are also helpful in minimising the onset of gout.

GRAINS

A general term for a wide variety of carbohydrate nutrients, including wheat, rice, millet, oats, barley, buckwheat, corn and rye. Whole grains provide energy and fibre in the diet, and also a certain amount of primary protein. They are a healthful constituent of a wide range of breads and cereals. *See separate listings.*

GRAPE DIET

A mono diet recommended by some health practitioners as a treatment for cancer, on the basis of its detoxifying effects. It is also suitable for cases of constipation.

A kilogram (2 lb) of red grapes are eaten on the first day, followed by an additional ½ kg (1 lb) each day until a 6 kg (12 lb) maximum is reached. No other foods are consumed.

The grapes should be washed so they are completely free of chemical contaminants. *See also Mono diet.*

GRAS

Abbreviation used by the American Food and Drug Administration with reference to food additives which are 'generally regarded as safe'. *See also Food additive numbers.*

GREYING, PREMATURE

A hair condition often related to extended or intense stress, but also thought to respond to nutritional therapy. Naturopaths have used a variety of supplements to prevent premature greying, including vitamin B5 (pantothenic acid), folic acid and zinc. Beneficial food sources include brewer's yeast, sunflower seeds, kelp and royal jelly. *See also Mineral trace elements.*

GUELPHE FAST

A fasting practice in which solid or semi-solid food is replaced by liquids and juices. Juices extracted from fruits and vegetables are acceptable, and in certain cases only one type is consumed—for example, lettuce juice. Herbal teas are also permitted during a Guelphe fast. Normally this type of fast extends for only one day.

GUM DISEASE — *see Pyorrhoea*

H

HAEMOGLOBIN

The red-coloured substance in human blood cells which carries oxygen to the tissues. Haemoglobin is a protein and contains an iron atom in its molecular structure.

HAEMORRHAGE

A discharge of blood from the blood vessels; bleeding can be either external or internal.

HAEMORRHOIDS

Dilated or varicose veins occurring in the anal canal. Haemorrhoids can be prevented by increasing the amount of fibre in the diet, either through fresh fruit and vegetables or bran. Naturopaths treat haemorrhoids with supplements of vitamin E to improve the blood circulation, and vitamin C and the bioflavonoids rutin and hesperidin to enhance the elasticity and strength of the

vessel walls. Aloe vera cream may be applied externally.

HALITOSIS

Bad breath, a condition caused by a variety of factors including poor mouth hygiene, pyorrhoea and gum disorders, dental decay, mouth and throat infections, and digestive disorders. If teeth and gum disorders are not the cause, poor stomach functioning may be to blame and to this extent effective treatment consists of preventive and curative dietary measures. These include reduced intake of animal protein, and increased use of raw foods and herbs like gentian (to boost the liver), goldenseal, rosemary and meadowsweet to stimulate effective digestion. Parsley juice is also a specific against halitosis, and a tablespoon may be taken in the morning in combination with carrot or apple juice to neutralise stomach acids and cleanse the system.

HAY FEVER

An irritation of the mucous membranes in the nose, often caused by dust, pollen from hay grasses, or other allergens. It is characterised by headache, sneezing and catarrh.

HDL CHOLESTEROL

High density lipoprotein, a form of cholesterol in the bloodstream which is sent to the liver to be processed out of the body through the gall bladder and intestines. *See LDL and HDL cholesterol.*

HEALTH

From the Greek *holos*, 'whole', a state of personal balance and well-being: soundness of body, mind and spirit. Although practitioners of orthodox medicine sometimes define health as the absence of disease, practitioners of natural health prefer to emphasise the positive aspect of health as a state in which the physical and mental processes of one's life are functioning in harmony.

HEART

A specially adapted muscle beneath the chest wall, which pumps blood continuously in order to nourish the tissues and distribute oxygen to the body. Air is taken into the body through the lungs, where there is a network of tiny blood capillaries. These in turn absorb the oxygen, and the oxygenated blood is passed to the heart and then distributed, via the arteries, to the body.

The heart consists of 4 chambers: the right and left atria receive blood, and the right and left ventricles pump it out. The heart normally beats at 70–80 times per minute.

HEART ATTACK

A sudden impairment of heart function, often due to a reduction of blood supply caused by a blockage in a coronary artery. *See Atherosclerosis.*

HEARTBURN

A burning sensation, sometimes experienced in the oesophagus after eating a large meal. It is caused by acidic fluids rising up from the stomach some 15 minutes after the food has been consumed.

HEMIPLEGIA

A condition in which half the body is paralysed, often after a stroke. This involves paralysis of the same side of the face as the side of the brain affected, and the opposite side of the body. There are several cases of hemiplegic patients who have been successfully treated with acupuncture, although the usual treatment is remedial physiotherapy. *See also Paraplegia.*

HEMOGLOBIN — *see* *Haemoglobin*

HERNIA

The external protrusion of any internal organ through the enclosing membrane. The term often refers to the protrusion of the bowel through the muscular wall of the abdomen. Hernias are generally caused by strain or injury (rupture).

HIATUS HERNIA

A protrusion of part of the stomach into the thoracic cavity. *See also Hernia.*

HISTIDINE

An essential amino acid of the heterocyclic class. It is important for the formation of glycogen in the liver, for controlling mucus, and as a component of haemoglobin and semen. Food sources include carrot, celery, garlic, onion, alfalfa, apples and pawpaw.

HIVES

Red, itchy patches of skin which are raised up in a temporary swelling, usually as a result of an irritation or allergy.

HOLLOW BACK — *see* *Lordosis*

HOMEOSTASIS

The internal stability maintained in the physiological system. One example is internal body temperature, which is maintained within specific limits by a homeostatic mechanism.

HONEY

The viscous fluid made by bees for use as their own food, but collected by humans since ancient times and traditionally highly valued both as a food and for its healing qualities. Honey is a particularly good instant energy boost as it is assimilated very quickly. Many people use it to replace sugar as a food and drink sweetener as honey, especially if it is dark, contains several important minerals (iron, magnesium, potassium and silica) as well as vitamin B and sometimes vitamin C, depending on its source. Honey also has antiseptic and antibiotic qualities and was used by the ancient Egyptians to dress burns. This practice is still followed in some English hospitals. It is an important ingredient in many cough medicines and throat lozenges and, especially with hot lemon juice, is a popular folk remedy for a head cold or sore throat. Honey is also a natural laxative and is easier for small children to digest than is sugar, though it could be argued that they do not need either. Many people claim that chewing honeycomb will relieve hay fever and sinusitis.

The main constituents of honey are moisture (17%), levulose (40.6%), dextrose (34.3%), sucrose (1.9%), maltose (4.35%), dextrins and gums (1.6%) and trace minerals (0.25%).

Honey is a source of minerals and natural sugars

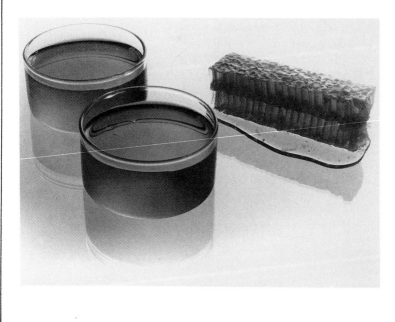

HORMONE

A chemical substance which is secreted by a gland and affects the metabolism of other cells and organs in the body. Hormones usually circulate by means of the bloodstream and affect only specific organs or tissues.

HUMECTANT

Any substance which attracts and holds water to the skin. Humectants are used in hand-creams and skin-care products. Examples include glycerin and rosewater.

HYDROXYGLUTAMIC ACID

An amino acid similar to glutamic acid.

HYDROXYPROLINE

A non-essential amino acid important for the emulsification of fats, for the liver and gall bladder, and for the red blood corpuscles. Food sources include carrots, lettuce, cucumber, apricots, grapes, oranges and almonds.

HYPER-

An increase in level of any given health condition; for example, hypersensitivity, hypertension.

HYPERCHOLES-TERAEMIA

Excessively high level of cholesterol in the blood.

HYPERLIPO-PROTEINAEMIA

Excessively high level of lipoproteins in the blood.

HYPERTENSION

High blood-pressure, a stress-related disease associated with the risk of stroke or heart attack. Contributing factors include obesity, excessive quantities of salt in the diet, lack of cardiovascular fitness, and extreme response to stressors. Hypertension is treated through a combination of dietary controls and relaxation techniques which utilise the progressive relaxation of different muscle groups in the body.

HYPERTONIC

A state of excessive tone or tension in a blood vessel or muscle. In Reichian therapy this state is associated with body armour and holding patterns. *See Reichian therapy, Body armour* (Part 2).

HYPERVITAMINOSIS

Excessive intake of fat-soluble vitamins, producing severe symptoms. Excess vitamin A, for example, can lead to peeling skin, hair loss, an enlarged liver and nausea (a situation which can occur if one drinks too much carrot juice). *See Megadose, toxic.*

HYPO-

A decrease in level of any given health condition; for example, hypoglycaemia, hypothyroidism.

HYPOGLYCAEMIA

A condition characterised by low blood glucose and often accompanied by severe or prolonged stress. Physical symptoms include fatigue, dizziness, sweating, shakiness, blackout, palpitations and blurred vision. Mental symptoms include emotional instability, anxiety, depression and, occasionally, anger or irritability.

Some doctors regard hypoglycaemia as a 'mimic disease' similar in nature to the manic depressive syndrome, but it seems unwarranted to dismiss hypoglycaemia simply as an emotional state. Physical symptoms are relieved by eating or drinking some form of carbohydrate, including sugar or sucrose. Some naturopaths also treat patients with high potency B vitamins in the initial stages of treatment and carefully monitor the diet thereafter.

HYPOTENSION

Low blood pressure.

HYPOTHALAMUS

A region of the brain with the function of regulating the metabolism of carbohydrates and fats. It also helps regulate water balance, body temperature, sexual functions and such basic functions as thirst, sleep and hunger.

HYPOTHERMIA

Abnormally low body temperature, especially in elderly people or children. The normal temperature of the human body is 98°F (37°C).

HYPOTHYROIDISM

A condition in which the thyroid gland is functioning below optimal level. Hypothyroidism is characterised by fatigue, dry or coarse skin, lethargy, obesity and migraines, and may also be associated with premature ageing. The most common cause of hypothyroidism is iodine deficiency. Naturopathic treatment includes iodine supplementation or increased intake of various forms of sea-vegetable which are rich in iodine. *See also Goitre.*

I

ICHTHYOSIS

Dry scaly skin.

ILEUM

The lower part of the small intestine.

IMMUNE RESPONSE

The response of the body to the intrusion of foreign cells, such as invading bacteria. *See Immune system.*

IMMUNE SYSTEM

When disease or infection invades the body in the form of viruses or bacteria, immune system cells in the body fight to hold them at bay. Alzheimer's disease, AIDS and systemic lupus are examples of diseases related to a poorly functioning immune system.

In 1979 *The Journal of the American Medical Association* suggested that certain nutrients were involved in the maintenance of a healthy immune system and these included vitamin A, • vitamin C, • the B group vitamins, vitamin E and zinc.

Vitamin A defends the body against pollutants and the presence of zinc helps this vitamin to perform more effectively. Vitamin C is utilised by the lungs to guard against respiratory infection, and it also acts as a natural antihistamine for asthmatics by reducing the swelling in sinuses and nasal passages. The B vitamins, especially pantothenic acid, vitamin B6, folic acid and vitamin B12 are all vital for the health of the immune system, and vitamin E helps produce more defender cells. Zinc nourishes the lymphocyte cells that battle infection and aid the body in the production of antibody cells.

Other nutritional sources of reduced immune function include protein deficiency (which is uncommon in most developed Western nations), and continued intake of denatured, refined foods.

Emotions also play an important role in personal resistance to disease. Stress factors can be measured by checking the thymus gland; this gland produces T-cells, or T-lymphocytes, and these are the main mechanism for cellular immunity. They help protect the body from viruses, bacteria, foreign cells, allergens and fungi, and a decline in the production of T-cells causes ageing.

Scientific studies indicate that many diseases, including colitis, multiple sclerosis, rheumatoid arthritis, diabetes and even cancer, result from defective T-cell function. It is also apparent that among ageing couples, severe stress factors (caused, for example, by a partner's major illness or death) can lead to a reduction of thymus gland activity, making the body vulnerable to attack from different organisms. This may be why the second partner often dies soon after the death of the first.

The late Dr Ainslie Meares, an internationally recognised clinical hypnotherapist, believed that specific forms of meditation could reduce the stress factors in disease and physiologically bolster the immune system by lowering cortisone levels in the body (a correlate of stress). This is the basis of the meditative approach to cancer — *see Cancer. See also T-lymphocytes.*

IMPOTENCE

The inability of a male to perform sexual intercourse. This can be caused by psychological factors or physical causes like excess alcohol consumption or internal damage to the urethra.

INCOMPLETE PROTEIN FOOD

A protein food which does not contain all of the 8 essential amino acids required for a balanced dietary intake. Vegetable proteins are generally considered to be 'incomplete'. However the soya bean provides a very valuable source of vegetable protein because its amino acid composition comes closer to the composition of human protein than that of other grains. Soya beans consist of about 40% protein in combination with 20% oil and 30% carbohydrate. *See also Protein.*

INCONTINENCE

The inability to control the emptying of waste matter from the rectum or bladder.

INCUBATION PERIOD

The time-span between exposure to an infectious disease and the manifestation of symptoms.

INDIGESTION

Discomfort or pain following an upset in the normal digestion process. Indigestion may refer to a number of conditions including acidosis, dyspepsia, flatulence, or the presence of duodenal or gastric ulcers.

INFECTION

The invasion of the body by disease micro-organisms. A disease is considered infectious when germs can be spread indirectly from one person to another, as with the common cold.

INFERTILITY

The inability to conceive, usually as a result of poor quality or insufficient sperm, blockages in the fallopian tubes, erratic ovulation, ulcers on the neck of the womb, or inadequate diet.

INFLAMMATION

From the Latin *inflammare*, 'to set on fire', a disease condition in any part of the body, either internal or external, characterised by heat, redness, swelling and pain. Inflammations are red because the small blood vessels are opened and are painful because the nerve-endings are irritated.

INFLUENZA

A viral infection associated with a variety of symptoms, including fever, aches and pains in the limbs, a hot and shivery sensation, watery eyes, sore throat and coughing. Influenza is self-limiting and usually passes within a few days. Antibiotics are not especially effective against influenza, and the best treatment is for the patient to rest in bed.

INOSITOL

A B-complex vitamin which facilitates ribonucleic acid (RNA) and biotin synthesis, assists zinc absorption, and helps lower blood cholesterol levels. It is important for healthy heart muscles and brain cell nutrition. Inositol is water soluble and occurs naturally in brewer's yeast, corn, citrus fruit, liver, milk, nuts, lecithin and wholegrain cereals.

Inositol deficiencies manifest in eye problems, hair loss, and eczema. Naturopaths use supplements of inositol to treat atherosclerosis, constipation and high blood cholesterol levels, and also to maintain healthy hair. RDA: not established but similar to choline: 1000 mg.

INSOMNIA

The inability to fall asleep. Insomnia affects approximately 1 in 5, and many people resort to sleeping pills to remedy this problem. There are, however, several natural approaches to overcoming insomnia. These include avoiding tea, coffee or cola because of their caffeine content, and replacing them instead with a herbal beverage like chamomile or catnip; gentle music as an environment accompanied by soothing massage from a partner, or a long soak in a herbal bath scented with rosemary or lavender oil. It may also help to adopt a special breathing rhythm in which the in-breath takes twice as long as the out-breath.

INSULIN

A hormone secreted by the pancreas. Insulin enters the bloodstream, facilitating the combustion of the dextrose content of the blood.

INTERFERON

A protein produced in the body cells as a natural response to viral infection. High blood levels of vitamin C also stimulate the production of interferon.

IN UTERO

In the womb.

IODINE

A non-metallic element with a purplish metallic lustre. Although toxic in its pure form, iodine can be made into a tincture and used as an antiseptic for cuts and wounds. Iodine is essential for the formation of the hormone thyroxine by the thyroid gland, and deficiencies, which are common in some areas, cause enlarged thyroid gland or goitre. Other symptoms of iodine deficiency are cold hands and feet, irritability, dry hair and hardening of the arteries. Good sources of iodine are seafood, kelp, iodised salt, spinach and milk (in countries like Australia and New Zealand chemicals containing iodine are used to clean dairy equipment). Eggs, mushrooms, potatoes and many other vegetables contain iodine, unless they have been grown in areas where the water contains little iodine. If chlorine has been added to an area's drinking water, this speeds up the loss of iodine from the bodies of residents in the area. Iodine may be taken internally in solution with potassium and iodide as Lygol's solution, which has been used to treat polio, TB, syphilis, ovarian cysts and thyroid disorders. Most people excrete any excess amount of iodine as it is highly soluble, but some people may develop some dysfunction of the thyroid gland if they take in large amounts of iodine.

IODOGORGOIC ACID

A non-essential amino acid which is important for the functioning of all glands. It is found in kelp, carrot, celery, spinach, tomato, lettuce and pineapple.

IRON

An essential mineral for the formation of haemoglobin in the red blood cells which carry oxygen around the body. Although the body contains only about 4 mg of iron, the recommended daily intake is at least 10 mg for men and children, and up to 20 mg for pregnant or menstruating women and teenagers. Much of the iron consumed in food is not absorbed by the body, so it is very important to regularly eat foods which are rich in iron. The most common symptom of iron deficiency is anaemia, which occurs in quite a large number of people, particularly women, children and infants over 6 months old who are fed bottled milk only. People with insufficient iron in their diet are often pale, listless, short of breath, and depressed or irritable. Their nails and hair are brittle and lustreless, and they may have swollen ankles. Good sources of iron are meat (red or white, but particularly liver and kidneys), eggs, dark green leafy vegetables and cooked pulses, dried fruits, wheat germ, wholegrain unrefined cereals and molasses. Vitamin C helps the absorption of iron. Too much iron in the diet can cause liver damage, diabetes and even scurvy, as the iron drains the body's supply of vitamin C, so it is best to take iron supplements only when really necessary.

ISOCALORIC

Containing an equal number of calories.

ISOLEUCINE

An essential amino acid important for the functioning of the thymus, spleen and pituitary, for the production of haemoglobin and the regulation of the metabolism. Food sources include pawpaw (papaya), avocado, coconut, and most nuts except peanuts and cashews.

J

JAUNDICE

A yellow discolouration of the skin and eyes caused by bile pigments in the blood. Jaundice is associated with disorders of the liver or bile duct, and is also a symptom of hepatitis.

JEJUNUM

The section of the small intestine adjoining the duodenum.

JOINTS

Articulation points for 2 or more bones in the body. To facilitate easy movement the joints require lubrication, and the body produces synovial fluid for this purpose. The cells which produce the fluid may, however, be damaged by the presence of chemical pollutants or other toxins — resulting in poor joint lubrication.

Degenerative joint conditions are common and include rheumatoid arthritis and osteoarthritis. Rheumatoid arthritis is characterised by swelling and pain in the joints, while osteoarthritis involves the hardening and thickening of tendons and ligaments — especially as a result of calcium deposits. The limbs become stiff and sore, and occasionally 'nodules' appear around the joints.

Naturopaths treat rheumatoid arthritis with a variety of approaches. These may involve eliminating from the diet allergens which are capable of causing inflammation in the joints (for example, dairy products, potatoes, tomatoes or aubergines); the use of antioxidant dietary supplements (for example, vitamin E, vitamin C); or the use of nutrients (for example, evening primrose oil) to stimulate an anti-inflammatory prostaglandin response.

Osteoarthritis may be treated naturopathically with supplements of vitamin B3 (niacinamide) to improve joint mobility; vitamin B5 to stimulate bone growth; vitamin B6 and C to assist the formation and quality of synovial fluid, and vitamin E as an antioxidant. Dietary supplements of calcium, zinc, magnesium and manganese may also be useful.

JUGULAR VEINS

The veins in the neck.

K

KAOLIN

An absorbent substance used to remove toxins from the alimentary canal. For this reason it can be used to treat diarrhoea. It may also be used externally as a poultice to absorb moisture. *See also Poultice* (Part 2).

KELP

A controversial seaweed extract recently subjected to close scrutiny by several health authorities. Much of the controversy surrounds the undoubted presence of minute traces of arsenic in kelp, and whether kelp should properly be classified as a food or as a therapeutic medicine. The World Health Organisation specifies a safe maximum intake of arsenic as 3000 millionths of a gram, and to reach this level one would need to consume 300–400 kelp tablets per day; the normal nutritional intake is 2–6 tablets.

On the positive side, kelp is a rich source of nutrients, including vitamin C, vitamin B12 and iodine. It is useful as a treatment for goitre (caused by iodine deficiency), thyroid regulation and excessive menstrual bleeding.

KERATIN

A protein found in the hair, nails and epidermis.

KIDNEYS

Glandular organs located in the lumbar region of the abdominal cavity. The kidneys excrete urine and also control the electrolyte balance in the body.

KIDNEY STONES

Deposits formed in the kidneys or bladder, often consisting of calcium oxalate. Naturopathic treatments for the prevention of kidney-stone formation include supplements of vitamin B6 (to lower the oxalate levels in the urine), and magnesium (to balance body calcium levels and decrease the possibility of calcium deposits). Herbalists use a variety of herbs to remove or reduce kidney stones; these include catnip, chamomile, knotgrass and cranberry juice.

KILOCALORIE

A unit of energy in food. A kilocalorie is 1000 times the amount of energy required to raise 1 cubic centimetre of water by 1°C. In food technology a kilocalorie is simply referred to as a calorie for practical purposes.

KONJAC

A vegetable root, traditionally used in Japan to prevent weight gain. The root extract is known as glucomannan — a natural fibre which is said to assist reduction of blood cholesterol levels when taken as a dietary supplement. Konjac is generally taken in tablet form, in a glass of water prior to meals. It results in the sensation of 'feeling full', thereby reducing the appetite.
Note: Glucomannan tablets have attracted medical and legal controversy because they may expand in the throat, causing possible blockages. Readers are advised to check with their doctor or naturopath.

KYOLIC

The brand name for a form of garlic grown in specially composted soils which are monitored for their germanium and selenium minerals — garlic attracts these from the soil. Kyolic garlic oil is cold-pressed and aged by a fermentation process. The concentrated oil is odourless, has its enzymes intact, and acts as a blood purifier. It is a natural chelating agent, helping to eliminate toxic heavy metals from the body. Kyolic is available in liquid and tablet form. *See also Garlic* (Part 1), *Chelation therapy* (Part 2).

KYPHOSIS

A postural condition in which the head

drops, the back is rounded, and the chin drags down, sagging the chest. This condition is commonly referred to as 'round back'.

L

LACTASE

An enzyme required in the body for the breakdown of lactose (milk sugar) to glucose and galactose. Failure of the body to perform this function, a comparatively common occurrence among Asians and some other racial groups, is known as lactose intolerance. *See Lactose intolerance.*

LACTIC ACID

A carbon compound produced in the muscle cells following anaerobic respiration. It is also the substance produced by the fermentation of lactose (milk sugar) and is contained in yoghurt.

LACTOSE

A sugar found in milk. A disaccharide, it yields 2 simple sugars, D-galactose and D-glucose, and does not have a sweet taste. *See also Food sugars, Lactase.*

LACTOSE INTOLERANCE

A form of food intolerance characterised by the inability to digest lactose as a result of lactase deficiency. This can lead to allergy attacks associated with aching muscles, stomach cramps and flatulence. The highest rates of lactose intolerance are among Filipinos, Japanese, Taiwanese and other Asians. Black Americans and Arabs also appear to be vulnerable. The problem is less prevalent among white Americans and northern Europeans. *See also Lactase.*

LAETRILE

Sometimes referred to as vitamin B17, a compound with the chemical name of laevo-mandelonitrilebeta glucuronoside. Laetrile occurs in the bitter almond, apricot kernels, millet seeds and raw buckwheat, and has been advocated as a cancer treatment by American health practitioner Dr Ernst Krebs Sen. and his son Dr Ernst Krebs Jun. Laetrile liberates hydrocyanic acid in tumours but not in healthy cells, because the rhodanase enzyme neutralises its effect. This process helps to kill tumour respiration.

Laetrile is a controversial cancer treatment and is not recognised by the American Food and Drugs Administration (FDA).

LARYNGITIS

Inflammation of the larynx, or voice box, characterised by a 'tickling' sensation low in the throat as well as coughing and a hoarse voice. Laryngitis usually clears within a week.

LARYNX

The upper part of the trachea, or windpipe, containing the vocal cords.

LAXATIVE

From the Latin *laxus*, 'loose', any substance which lessens constipation and assists regular bowel movements. Most healthy people have at least 2 bowel movements per day.

Natural laxatives are high in fibre content, and include apples, bran, raw cabbage, carrots, celery, grapes, lettuce, oatmeal, prunes, raisins, spinach and wholegrain wheat.

LDL AND HDL CHOLESTEROL

There are two forms of cholesterol: LDL or low-density lipoprotein, and HDL or high-density lipoprotein — the preferred form. A higher ratio of LDL cholesterol in the bloodstream brings with it a high risk of heart and/or artery disease. During normal body functioning, cholesterol is produced in the liver as LDL and this cholesterol is required by the body to manufacture hormones and form cell membranes. Cells excrete excess cholesterol which is then, normally, processed out of the system. However, the LDL:HDL ratio may be upset if not enough cholesterol is eliminated. In this case plaque forms on the artery walls, they harden, and this leads to the possibility of blood clots. If the artery becomes narrower and blocks the blood supply, heart attack or stroke may result. *See also Cholesterol.*

Legumes, a rich source of vegetable protein

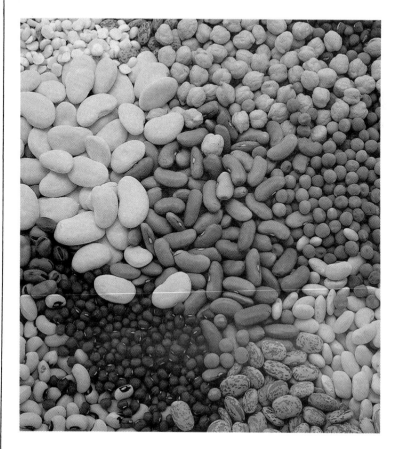

LECITHIN

A naturally occurring emulsifier and antioxidant which is important for the transport of fats in the body. Chemically it is a mix of phospholipids — derivatives from phosphatidic acid. It consists of saturated and unsaturated fatty acids (depending on whether its source is animal or vegetable), choline, inositol and phosphorus. It also contains small amounts of calcium, magnesium, iron, vitamin B6, vitamin K and folic acid.

In the blood, lecithin helps to dissolve cholesterol and reduce the size of lipid particles in the bloodstream. Some lecithin is produced in the body itself (it is found in some tissues, semen, bile and the blood), but it is also found in vegetable oils, nuts, egg yolks, whole wheat cereal and wheat germ.

Commercially available grades of lecithin vary considerably, and its use extends beyond its function in relation to cholesterol. The best quality commercial lecithin has a level of over 30 per cent phosphatidyl choline, used to manufacture the neurotransmitter acetyl choline (ACH), a substance involved in learning capacity, REM sleep and motor activity. Good quality lecithin is often used to treat those suffering from memory loss or Alzheimer's disease. RDA: 1–2 tablespoons.

LEGUMES

Members of the pea family, (Leguminosae), including alfalfa, peas, lentils, beans and peanuts. They are a rich source of incomplete protein with thiamine, riboflavin, niacin and iron. Sprouted legumes are also rich in vitamin C.

LENTIL *(Lens esculenta)*

Cultivated especially in the Middle East and Mediterranean countries, the lentil is a member of the bean family. It grows on a bushy plant and produces flat, oblong pods containing 2 seeds approximately the size of small peas. These seeds are harvested when mature and are rich in nutrients — including calcium, iron, vitamin B-complex, protein and carbohydrates.

Lentils are considered an important vegetarian health food because they contain a higher percentage of protein than lean meat. They are usually soaked in water overnight prior to use, and are a popular ingredient in soups and stews.

LESION

Any injury to, or adverse change in, the structure and function of the living tissues of the body; for example, boils and wounds. (From the Latin *laedere*, 'to hurt'.)

LEUCINE

An essential amino acid which acts as a counterbalance to isoleucine and is found in the same food sources.

LEUCOCYTES

The white corpuscles in the blood which are capable of destroying bacteria and other micro-organisms. An abnormal increase in leucocytes is referred to as leucocythaemia, and is often accompanied by glandular swelling.

LEUKAEMIA

A disease in which the white blood corpuscles multiply indiscriminately instead of performing their normal role of defending the body against invading micro-organisms. As a result, the production of red blood cells and other blood constituents is suppressed, leading to anaemia and swelling of the spleen and liver, among other symptoms. Leukaemia is sometimes referred to as cancer of the blood.

LEUKOCYTES — *see Leucocytes*

LEVULOSE

Also known as grape sugar, or fructose. Levulose is white and crystalline. *See Fructose.*

LIGAMENTS

The strong, fibrous bands of tissue which connect the bones of the body and hold the joints together.

LINOLEIC ACID

An essential fatty acid found in several fats and oils including soya bean, peanut, corn, sunflower seed and poppyseed. It is also found in linseed oil in the form of a glyceride. *See also Essential fatty acids.*

LIPIDS

A general term for a group of fats, fatty acids and waxes which are insoluble in water, but which dissolve in alcohol, ether and other solvents. Lipids, together with carbohydrates and proteins, provide the intrinsic components of all living cells. *See Fats, Essential fatty acids.*

LIPOMA

A soft painless lump which forms under the skin as a result of the uneven distribution of fat. Lipomas are harmless but are sometimes removed surgically for cosmetic reasons.

LIPOPROTEIN

A combination of a lipid and a protein but including general properties of proteins. High-density lipoproteins (HDL) carry cholesterol from the cells for re-utilisation, while the presence of low-density lipoproteins (LDL) serves as a measure for the risk of atherosclerosis. A high HDL/LDL ratio is the ideal pattern for good health. *See also LDL and HDL cholesterol.*

LIPOXIDASE

An enzyme that catalyses a chemical reaction between various polyunsaturated fats and molecular oxygen. Lipoxidase is active in the bleaching of carotene and in the oxygen uptake of fatty acids present in flour.

LIVER

An organ which facilitates the breakdown of protein, the storage of sugar and fat, the maintenance of blood composition, and detoxification. The liver also secretes bile, which is stored in the gall bladder, and aids the digestion of fatty substances.

Liver overload can be avoided by eliminating or reducing intake of fatty and sweet foods, and those with artificial additives. Good foods for the liver include fresh fruits, wholegrains, green vegetables and garlic.

Dandelion coffee is a liver booster and acts as a tonic. Dietary supplements which help prevent liver problems include vitamin C (as a detoxifying agent), vitamin B6, zinc and magnesium.

LORDOSIS

A postural condition in which the back is pulled in and the buttocks pushed out. This condition is commonly referred to as 'hollow back'.

LUBRICANT

A substance which facilitates the smooth interaction between moving parts or organs which brush against each other as they move. Lubricants are usually oils. In massage, for example, safflower oil is used as a lubricant and may be scented with additional aromatic essences.

LUMBAGO

Rheumatic pain in the lumbar muscles of the lower back, resulting from inflammation of the fibrous tissues.

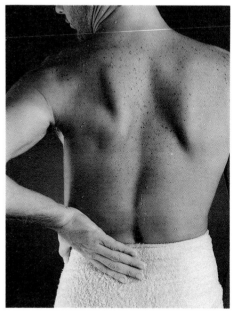

Lumbago is pain in the lower back

LUMBAR

That which relates to the lower back.

LUNGS

The organs of respiration. Breathing is an automatic body function and approximately 1800 litres (400 gallons) of air are taken in daily. The fine hairs, or cilia, which line the lungs, serve as a defence against air pollutants like cadmium, ozone and nitrous oxide, which are common in the urban environment.

LYMPH

A watery, alkaline fluid contained in the tissues and organs of the body. Lymph resembles blood plasma and helps transport leucocytes and various nutrients around the body. It also spreads infection and disease in the body because of its role as a transport system.

LYMPHATICS

Small vessels in the body containing lymph.

LYMPHOCYTE

A small cell in a lymphatic gland which becomes a white blood corpuscle.

LYMPH SYSTEM

The circulatory system in the body which transports lymph towards the heart — *see Lymph.*

LYSINE

An essential amino acid of the basic class. It is important in the liver and gall bladder, in the regulation of the pineal and mammary glands and the ovaries, and in the prevention of cell degeneration. Food sources include carrot, cucumber, parsley, alfalfa, apples, apricots and pears.

M

MACROBIOTICS

A concept developed by Japanese philospher George Ohsawa in relation to healthy diet. The term derives from the Greek *macro* ('large') and *bio* ('life'), and was first mentioned in Ohsawa's book *Zen Macrobiotics* (1962).

According to Ohsawa, the preparation and selection of foods is critically import-ant for health and longevity. So too is an appropriate balance of *yin* and *yang* energy, for imbalance leads to disease. Ohsawa classified foods as predominantly *yin* or *yang*.

YIN	YANG
Grown in a hot climate	Grown in a cold climate
Generally acidic	Generally alkaline
Grown high above the ground	Grown below the ground
Fruits, leaves	Roots, seeds
Sweet and hot foods	Salty and bitter foods
Foods that are purple, blue or green in colour	Foods that are red, yellow or orange in colour
Foods that contain more water and perish quickly	Foods that are dry and store well

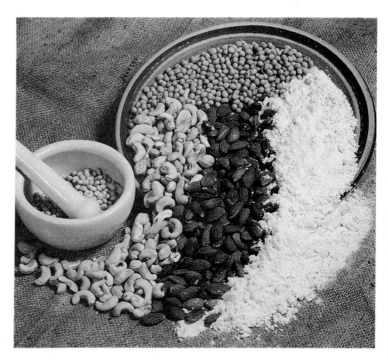

According to macrobiotic theory the diet should be carefully balanced and should draw on foods available in season. Cereal grains are favoured because they combine seed and fruit (*yang* and *yin*), and span the complete vegetal cycle. They comprise 50–60 per cent of the recommended macrobiotic diet and include whole wheat, barley, oats, brown rice, maize

In macrobiotics, foods are divided into yin *and* yang

and rye. Fresh fruits and vegetables comprise 20 per cent of the diet. Nuts and sea vegetables (seaweed) are also consumed, and if animal protein is required fish is preferred to meat. Milk, cheese, butter and eggs are usually avoided or kept to a minimum in the macrobiotic diet, as are sugar, refined flour and other processed products. The extremely *yin* foods like potatoes, tomatoes and aubergines do not feature strongly in macrobiotic diet either.

MACRO-NUTRIENTS

The major nutrients required by the body for growth, repair, maintenance and energy. They include proteins, carbohydrates and fats *(see separate listings)*. *See also Micro-nutrients.*

MACROPHAGES

Large white blood cells that act as scavengers in the body. Macrophages are vital for the immune defence system and circulate in the blood, destroying invading viruses, bacteria, fungi and parasites. They also help organise and repair body tissue. Some macrophages which infiltrate solid tissue have the capability of attacking cancer cells, and medical scientists anticipate that in the near future specific forms of protein will be developed which can stimulate this type of protective function in the body.

MACULA (or MACULE)

A coloured spot or blemish on the skin which is not raised above the skin surface. *Compare with Hives.*

MAGNESIUM

A mineral found in all vegetable and animal tissue; in humans it is found mainly in the bones and teeth. In the proper balance with calcium, magnesium helps regulate the heart, muscles and nerve transmission, and acts as a catalyst in the metabolism of carbohydrates. Deficiency is generally considered rare, but may cause nervous disturbances, extreme sensitivity to heat, cold or noise, sleeplessness, severe constipation, overweight, and gallstones. Magnesium has been used to treat stress and heart disease. Some mineral therapists claim magnesium deficiency is much more common than is generally supposed, and research has shown that alcoholics need increased amounts of magnesium. Good sources are green vegetables like spinach and parsley, egg yolk, honey, kelp and seafood.

MALTOSE

Malt sugar, a carbohydrate sweetener produced by the action of malt on starch. Maltose serves as an energy source in the diet, supplying 1660 kilojoules (395 calories) of energy per 100 grams. However, it is not as sweet as the sugars fructose and sucrose. *See also Food sugars.*

MAMILLA

The nipple of the female breast.

MAMMARY GLANDS (or MAMMAE)

The breasts, or milk-secreting organs in the female, used for nourishing the young. Mammary glands are a characteristic of all mammals.

MANDIBLE

The lower jaw bone of the skull.

MANGANESE

A mineral found mainly in the bones; it is important for transmitting nerve impulses to the muscles, and for metabolism, tissue growth, production of sex hormones, and the synthesis of ribo-nucleic acid (RNA) and deoxyribonucleic acid (DNA). Deficiences are not con-sidered common but may cause dizziness, lack of muscle coordination, nervous tremors, asthma and allergies. Diabetics have been successfully treated with manganese, as have people suffering from shaking tremors caused by long-term use of tranquillisers. Good sources are green leafy vegetables, legumes, unprocessed whole grains, coffee, tea, nuts, liver, bananas and pineapples. Miners or chemical workers who deal with manga-nese may absorb excessive amounts and suffer weakness, sleeplessness, apathy and nervous disturbances.

MANNITOL

A form of sugar with a diuretic action (i.e. it increases the volume of urine excreted from the body).

MARROW

Soft vascular tissue present in the central cavities of bones, and composed primar-ily of fat and white corpuscles. It is also known as the medulla.

MASTURBATION

Sexual self-gratification, involving stimu-lation of the sexual organs in order to achieve an orgasm.

MAXEPA

The trade name for a substance found in the fatty tissues of several cold-water fish, and thought to substantially reduce blood-fat levels, thereby lessening the risk of heart disease.

Greenland Eskimos have a fat intake sometimes exceeding 600 g per day and a very high intake of flesh protein, and yet they are not prone to heart disease. The relevant factor is the type of fat con-sumed. Fish and marine mammals are generally higher in unsaturated fatty acids relative to saturated fats than land-based animals, and it is the latter which predominate in the Western diet.

Cod-liver oil is an excellent source of maxEPA and recent tests at the Baker Medical Research Institute in the United States show that a daily dose of maxEPA can reduce cholesterol and blood-fat levels by 90 per cent over a period of only a few weeks. *See also Omega-3 fish oils.*

MAXILLA

The upper jaw bone of the skull which helps define the face on either side of the nose.

MEAT

In recent years the subject of meat con-sumption has been vigorously debated by devotees of natural health. Vegans and vegetarians prefer not to eat meat for a range of reasons, the most common objections being the cruelty inflicted on animals in the testing and slaughtering processes, and the toxic chemicals (ferti-lisers, etc.) consumed by animals while grazing. However, it is also true that many vegetarians are prone to iron deficiency and red meats are an excellent source of iron.

Meat is easily digested and is a 'com-plete protein' food containing the full range of essential amino acids. About 20% of the iron present in meat is absorbed, while the absorption rate from other foods is substantially lower (spinach 1.4%, wheat 5%, soya beans 7%). Red meat is a good source of zinc, which is required for healthy skin, eyes and physi-cal growth. Meat is also a good source for B vitamins; vitamin B12 is usually avail-able only from animal sources (sea vege-tables appear to be an exception).

Vegetarians emphasise that cholesterol is only found in foods of animal origin and there is no doubt that the intake of saturated fats and cholesterol needs to be carefully monitored by those who eat meat. However lean meat contains a rela-tively moderate amount of cholesterol (90–130 mg per serve), and chicken contains approximately 100 mg per serving. This is considerably lower than seafood (250 mg), eggs (250 mg) and offal (500 + mg).

As a result of these findings, many nutritionists now recommend a modest intake of lean meat to complement the increased consumption of fresh fruit and vegetables.

MEDULLA

Bone marrow, especially that of the spinal vertebrae. The term is also used to refer to the central parts of some organs, such as the kidneys, and to the cellular inner part of animal hair. *See also Marrow.*

MEGADOSE, TOXIC

An often unintended side effect of megadose vitamin therapy, toxic megadosing can arise when vitamin supplements are taken in such large quantities that the vitamins become drugs rather than nutrients. Megadose quantities are those 10 times or more in excess of the recommended daily intake, and toxic effects have now been established for several of the vitamins available to consumers.

It used to be thought that the water-soluble B vitamins were non-toxic in any

Vitamin supplements should be used as nutrients, not as drugs

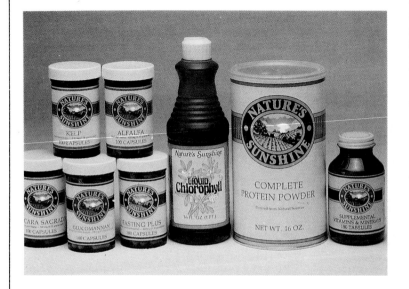

quantity because they were rapidly cleared from the body. However toxic megadosing is possible with both water-soluble and fat-soluble vitamins.

Niacin (niacinamide B-complex) is water-soluble, but megadoses are associated with a variety of symptoms, including abnormal heart rhythms, cramps, nausea, abnormally low blood pressure and elevated blood sugar.

Vitamin B6 (pyridoxine) is used in megadose quantities in body-building regimens, to relieve pre-menstrual tension, and for autistic or hyperactive children (sometimes in quantities 1000 times in excess of the recommended dose). B6 megadosing can result in neurological problems including numbness, sharp pains and loss of normal reflexes. Vitamin C megadosing can also result in problem symptoms, despite Dr Linus Pauling's advocacy of this form of therapy for the common cold. Untoward effects include diarrhoea, abdominal cramps and, in some cases, kidney stones. If the body is allowed to become dependent on vitamin C megadoses and these are then withdrawn suddenly it is also possible for scurvy to result.

Among the fat-soluble vitamins, toxic megadosing is most commonly reported for vitamins A and D. Vitamin A poisoning is characterised by a variety of symptoms, including dehydration, hyper-irritability, headaches, nausea and vomiting, loss of skin and hair, fatigue or sleeplessness, haemorrhages, enlargement of the liver, and double-vision. If megadose quantities are consumed during pregnancy, vitamin A can also cause birth defects.

Vitamin D at megadose levels can produce abdominal pain, nausea and vomiting, dangerously high levels of blood calcium, bone pain, cataracts and kidney failure.

MELAENA

Excessively dark faeces, resulting from blood in the faeces. This can be a warning sign for bowel cancer.

MELANIN

A brown-black pigment found in the eye, hair and skin. Deposits of melanin appear as freckles on suntanned skin, and as brown deposits on the skin of the elderly.

MELANOMA

A skin tumour, usually black, or brown in colour. Melanomas are so-called because they occur in the melanin-forming cells. They may become malignant, spreading rapidly and leading to secondary growths in the liver.

MENADIONE — *see Vitamin K*

MENARCHE

The onset of menstruation in females following puberty.

MENOPAUSE

Also known as the 'change of life' in women: the cessation of function in the female reproductive organs. Menopause usually begins around the age of 45, but can vary considerably. At this time menstruation becomes irregular and eventually ceases, but the transition can be marked by flushing, excessive bleeding and nervous disorders.

Menopause is characterised by a diminishing oestrogen supply in the body; this is the cause of flushing, especially in states of stress which place pressure on the adrenal glands where oestrogen is made. Adrenal functioning can be boosted by supplements of royal jelly, vitamin B5, vitamin C, vitamin E and zinc.

MENORRHAGIA — *see Menstruation*

MENSTRUATION

The female 'period' — the monthly discharge from the womb of blood and tissue debris from the lining of the uterus when the latter has not been implanted by a fertilised ovum. Menstruation begins at puberty, around the age of 14, and ceases at menopause. Failure to menstruate (amenorrhoea) may be caused by anaemia, depression, or some glandular disorders, while painful menstruation (dysmenorrhoea) may result from womb spasm. Excessive discharge (menorrhagia) can occur as a result of inflammation within the womb.

MENTAL DISORDER

A general term for mental ill-health encompassing 4 main categories. These are *mental illness*, in which normally intelligent people become disordered; *severe abnormality*, in which the mental disorder becomes so extreme that the person is incapable of leading a normal life; *subnormality*, in which specialist health care and training can help overcome incomplete mental development, and *psychopathic disorder*, in which a person may or may not be of normal intelligence but acts in either an irresponsible or overly aggressive way when not under medical treatment. *See also Psychopathic disorder.*

METABOLIC

That which relates to the metabolism — *see Metabolism.*

METABOLISM

The molecular processes of building up and breaking down, which are vital in living organisms to sustain life and growth, assisting, for example, in the building of body tissues and facilitating their ongoing functioning. Metabolism in the human body refers to a variety of processes including ingestion and digestion of food, absorption of nutrients, transportation through the circulatory system, respiration and excretion of waste matter.

METHIONINE

An essential amino acid which is a constituent of haemoglobin and serum, and is important for the functioning of the spleen, pancreas and lymph. Food sources are cabbage, cauliflower, chives, garlic, apples, pineapples and brazil nuts.

MICROBE

A micro-organism, especially the type of bacteria associated with disease symptoms or the process of fermentation.

MICRO-NUTRIENTS

A category of nutrients which do not supply energy to the body but which are essential for other reasons. They include:
Vitamins which facilitate chemical reactions in the body known collectively as metabolism. These reactions include the conversion of fats and carbohydrates into energy and the utilisation of proteins to repair damaged tissue.
Minerals which, like vitamins, are also involved in chemical reactions essential for human nutrition but which may also act as components of important body structures like bones, teeth and soft body tissue, as well as the blood.
Fibre which is not strictly a nutrient at all but which assists the digestive process by softening bile waste and speeding the elimination of undigested food.
See also Macro-nutrients.

MIGRAINE

A severe recurrent headache caused by the constriction and dilation of blood vessels in the brain. During the period of constriction the sufferer often experiences flashing colours and this is followed, during the dilation, by severe headache. Migraines are sometimes accompanied by vomiting.

MILK

As a general term 'milk' can refer to cow's milk, human breast milk, goat's milk and soy milk. These have different vitamin and mineral constituents and varying degrees of water, fat and carbohydrate.

Whole cow's milk is widely consumed in modern Western society, where estimated average consumption is approximately 2 litres per week, per person. Fresh cow's milk consists of around 88% water, and the balance divides into 37% lactose, 31% fat, 27% protein and a variety of vitamins and minerals, including vitamins A, B1, B6, B2, B5 and B12, C, D and E, folic acid, calcium, potassium, phosphorus and sodium.

Pasteurisation removes approximately 25% of the vitamin C and 10% of vitamin B1, but these elements are usually supplied by other foods in the diet.

Many nutritionists recommend consumption of dried skim milk since it provides good value and has a substantially lower fat content.

Another milk consumed as a beverage is goat's milk, which has a lower nutrient score than cow's milk (particularly in its folic acid content) but is more easily digested than cow's milk and is a useful

Skimmed milk is substantially lower in fat content

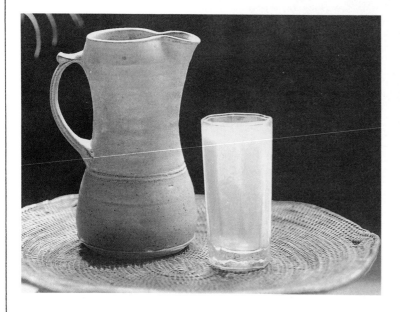

alternative for those who are allergic to cow's milk. Soy milk is also popular, especially with vegetarians and vegans who consume no dairy products. Soy milk, extracted from soya beans, contains no cholesterol and is not mucus-forming. It, too, is easily digestible and it is high in sodium, potassium and magnesium. Some commercial soy milks contain barley and the sea-vegetable *kombu*.

MINERAL THERAPY —
see separate listings under individual minerals and Blackmore's celloids

MINERAL TRACE ELEMENTS

Minerals required in very small amounts by the body. These are essential nutrients in the diet but the RDA is not universally agreed upon by dietitians. For example, zinc is sometimes classified as a trace element and around 10–15 mg are required each day in the diet.

The essential mineral elements include calcium, chromium, cobalt, copper, fluorine, iodine, iron, magnesium, manganese, molybdenum, nickel, phosphorus, potassium, selenium, silicon, sodium, vanadium and zinc.

MINERAL WATERS

Waters occurring naturally in mineral springs and which are utilised for drinking or bathing. Consumption of mineral waters assists bowel and kidney function, while bathing in mineral springs helps keep the skin pores open and healthy.

MIOSIS

Reduction in the size of the pupil of the eye.

MIRACULIN

A glycoprotein which, although it is taste-less on its own, makes other foods taste sweet — often several hours after the miraculin is consumed. Miraculin was first isolated from a West African berry.

MISO

Highly regarded in the Orient, miso is generally derived from a mix of soya beans and grains like rice and barley. (*Hatcho* miso is the main exception: this form of miso is made from soya beans only.) *Koji* mould is employed to produce enzymes which then convert the oils, starches and proteins to more fermentable compounds. Sea salt and well water are added, and the mixture is then aged in cedarwood kegs for up to 2 years. The liquid which rises to the surface is known as *shoyu* or *tamari* (soy sauce), but the solid mixture which remains is miso, and this is used extensively in macrobiotic cooking.

The varieties of miso range from rich and salty to light and sweet. Miso can be used as a spread or as an ingredient in soups and sauces. It is comparatively high in salt, but contains vitamin B12, an essential nutrient rarely found in vegetable foods.

MOLASSES, BLACKSTRAP

The residue which remains after the extraction of sugar from cane or beet. A stronger tasting sweetener than honey, molasses contains calcium, iron, potassium, vitamin E, several B vitamins, copper, magnesium and phosphorus. It is used medicinally to treat constipation, varicose veins, colitis, psoriasis, eczema, arthritis, ulcers and various nervous problems. RDA: 1 tablespoon dissolved in warm milk or water.

MONILIASIS

Infection by the yeast-like organism monilia.

MONO DIET

A diet in which, for a given time, only 1 item of food is consumed. Different dietary authorities have proposed a variety of foods for mono diets — for example, grapes, grapefruit, rice, prunes and wheatgrass — although most nutritionists recommend a carefully balanced diet as being preferable. A variant on the mono diet is the alternating diet of Dutch nutritionist Dr C. M. De Vos, in which only wholemeal or wholegrain bread is eaten on alternating days, and a normal diet maintained on the others.

MONOGLYCERIDE

One of a group of edible fats and oils, a monoglyceride is a fatty acid ester of the alcohol glycerol in which only 1 of the 3 hydroxyl groups is joined to a fatty acid.

MONO-UNSATURATES
— *see Fats*

MORBIDITY

A state of disease. The term also relates to the prevalence of disease in a given social district: i.e. the ratio of sick to well persons in the community.

MUCIN

A white glutinous fluid which is the main constituent of mucus and saliva — *see Mucus.*

MUCOUS MEMBRANE

Thin skin containing cells which secrete the lubricant mucus. Mucous membranes occur on the internal surfaces of the body, such as the lining of the mouth, the eyelids, the breathing and digestive passages, and the genital tract.

MUCUS

A sticky secretion consisting mainly of water, mucin and salts, which forms a protective covering for mucous membranes. *See also Mucous membrane.*

MULTIPLE SCLEROSIS

A chronic disease of the central nervous system characterised by progressive destruction of the nervous tissue. In this process the white fatty material contained in the sheaths of nerve fibres becomes hard scar-tissue. The result is increasing loss of muscle function accompanied by tremors, paralysis and defective speech and sight. Multiple sclerosis is thought to be viral in origin.

MUSCULAR DYSTROPHY

An inherited disorder in which the muscles gradually become weaker and waste away as a result of a fault in metabolism. There are various forms of muscular dystrophy and the condition is difficult to treat. Physiotherapy is often beneficial.

MUTAGENIC

That which induces genetic mutation — a permanent transmissible change in an offspring caused by a genetic change in the parent.

MYALGIA

Pain felt in the muscles.

MYOCARDIAL INFARCTION

Death of part of the heart muscle as a result of cessation of blood flow to the area; for example, coronary thrombosis.

MYOCARDIAL INSUFFICIENCY

Insufficient blood flow to parts of the heart muscle.

MYOCARDIUM

The muscular area of the heart.

MYOPIA

Short-sightedness, resulting from the lens of the eye being more convex than usual, or the axis of the eyeball being elongated. In this situation incoming light is focused before it reaches the retina. In optometry the error is corrected by concave lenses, but treatments such as the Bates Method, which stimulate the muscles around the eye, may also be effective. *See Bates Method* (Part 2).

N

NASAL CATARRH

Inflammation of the mucous membrane of the nostrils, associated with the discharge of rheum from the mucous glands. The condition is also known as rhinitis.

NECROSIS

The death of body tissue. This may occur in individual cells, in groups of cells, or in small localised areas of the body.

NEONATAL

Pertaining to the newborn child in the first month of life.

NEPHRITIS

Inflammation of the body of the kidney, characterised by an accumulation of fluid under the skin all over the body, back pain, and fever. Nephritis is treated with rest, purgatives and vapour baths.

NERVES

Specialised cells in the body through which its activities are initiated and controlled. Nerves are present in large numbers in the grey matter of the brain and in the central nervous system. Long fibres branch out to all parts of the body, transmitting brain commands to the muscles, the organs of sensation, the digestive system, etc. Much nerve functioning is automatic and is not called to consciousness except through specific modalities like biofeedback, which in some cases enables autonomic functions like heart-rate to be affected by the conscious will.

NEURALGIA

Severe pain felt along the track of a nerve but not caused by nerve inflammation. Neuralgia can arise as a result of exhaustion or illness, or because of displacement of the discs between the vertebrae, leading to conditions like sciatica.

NEURITIS

Inflammation of a nerve or group of nerves following infection, injury or poisoning by toxins.

NEURON

A nerve cell and its appendages. The neuron is the basic structural unit of the nervous system.

NEURO-TOXINS

Toxic substances which poison the brain or nervous system, leading to behavioural abnormalities, depression, memory loss or hallucinations. These toxins include ethoxyethanol, an ingredient in various commercial lacquers and dyes, and carbon disulphide, a substance formerly used as an anaesthetic and now used in the manufacture of rubber. Ethoxyethanol has no immediate effects on adult subjects but may have damaging neurological effects on one's offspring, while carbon disulphide affects work capacity, psycho-motor function, neuromuscular speed and the intelligence itself. Other neuro-toxins include methyl-n-butyl ketone, which affects psycho-motor function and memory; lead, which can cause learning difficulties, mental retardation, hyperactivity or poor concentration; mercury, which can cause neuromuscular incoordination, and selenium which, in high doses, causes neurological impairment and a rare heart condition called Keshan disease. Several pesticides, including DDT, can also have a toxic effect on the nervous system.

NEUROTRANSMITTER

A chemical in the brain which is released from one neuron into the synaptic junction or space between it and another neuron: for example, serotonin.

NIACIN — *see Vitamin B3*

N-NITROSO COMPOUNDS

Chemical compounds, some of which can induce cancers in animals and possibly in man. The compounds are formed when nitrates (nitrogen-containing compounds) combine with amides, urea or amines. This chemical reaction, called nitrosation, can occur either in the environment or within the body.

It has been discovered, however, that the process of nitrosation can be blocked by vitamin C and that, provided no N-nitroso compounds have already been formed, vitamin C exerts a protective effect against the development of cancer. This is particularly relevant in the case of stomach cancer: subjects whose diet is rich in vitamin C are less prone to this form of the disease.

NODULE

A small, rounded mass or lump; for example, a small, knotty tumour or ganglion (swelling under the skin).

NON-ESSENTIAL AMINO ACIDS

Amino acids which can be produced by the body as long as there are sufficient nitrogen-containing foods in the diet. The non-essential amino acids include alanine, aspartic acid, arginine, citrulline, cystine, glutamic acid, glycine, hydroxyglutamic acid, hydroxyproline, norleucine, proline, serine and tyrosine. *See Amino acids.*

NUTRIENT

A food substance taken into a living organism to sustain its existence, promoting growth and providing energy.

NUTRITION

The relationship between food and the requirements of the human body for health. The essential nutrients are proteins, carbohydrates, lipids, vitamins, minerals and water, and these provide the basis for healthy growth and development, efficient body functioning, energy, and resistance to infection.

Proteins are responsible for the growth and development of body tissue. Carbohydrates provide energy and assist in the assimilation of other foods. Lipids also provide energy, aid digestion, insulate the body and assist in the absorption of the vitamins A, D and E. Vitamins and minerals serve as activators in the absorption of proteins, carbohydrates and lipids, while water is required for absorption, digestion and elimination. *See separate listings.*

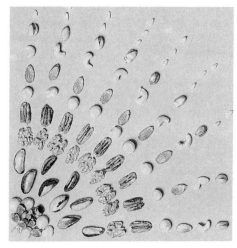

Nuts provide ideal vegetable protein

NUTS

A food source high in unsaturated fatty acids, protein and fibre. They contain calcium, iron, copper and phosphorus, and varying degrees of vitamin E and the B vitamins. Nuts can be combined with grains and legumes as an excellent protein alternative to meat, and some nuts — especially almonds and cashews — may be blended to make a milk. Brazil nuts are an excellent source of the amino acid methionine. Pine nuts have the highest protein content, and pistachios the highest iron content. Almonds contain the highest proportion of fibre — around 14 per cent.

NYSTAGMUS

Rapid involuntary movements of the eyeball. This sometimes occurs in people who work in cramped quarters and poor light.

O

OATS

One of the most popular grains in the Western diet, and grown since Roman times, oats are available as whole grain cereal, rolled oats or in gritted, hulled or 'quick-cook' forms. Whole oats are a rich source of inositol, vitamin B1, silicon, iron and calcium, and contain around 14 per cent primary protein. An ingredient in authentic forms of muesli, oats aid the development of strong bones and teeth, help reduce blood cholesterol levels, and are a good food source for treating arthritis.

OBESITY

Excessive fatness. Obesity may derive from a variety of factors including genetic variables, glandular problems associated with thyroid malfunction, and nutritional patterns. A hypoactive thyroid is indicated by body temperatures consistently below 97.8°F (36.5°C), and may be remedied by foods like sea-vegetables and shellfish which contain iodine. However, the most common cause of obesity is lack of exercise combined with a diet high in refined, low-fibre foods. In this case obesity can be countered by increased intake of fresh fruits and vegetables, whole grains, legumes and brown rice. *See also Overweight, Weight-for-height ratio.*

OCULAR

Pertaining to the eye.

OEDEMA

An accumulation of fluid, either in tissue spaces or body cavities, resulting in swelling.

OESOPHAGUS

The tube which connects the pharynx and the stomach. The oesophagus is part of the intestinal tract, or alimentary canal.

OESTROGENS

Hormones produced in the ovaries and placenta in the female and, to a much smaller extent, in the testes of the male. Oestrogens are involved in the development of the female sex organs and influence such factors as body hair, the growth of breasts and the shape of the figure. They are also responsible for the changes in the body during ovulation.

Synthetic oestrogens are used to treat menstrual disorders, delayed puberty and various fertility problems, as well as to treat acne and the 'hot flushes' experienced during menopause.

OILS

Liquid fats which may have value as nutrients, fuels, lubricants or medicines. Oils are an integral part of such seeds as soya beans, jojoba and corn, and also leaves such as those of the eucalyptus and tea-tree. The extraction of oils is performed either mechanically — by crushing, adding water, and then heating and cooking the seeds — or by using a variety of chemical solvents to extract the oil from the shattered seeds. In the latter case the solvent is boiled off but trace elements invariably remain.

Most vegetable oils become rancid after a time but jojoba oil, a natural skin moisturiser, is an exception. *See also Lipids, Fats.*

OLEATES

Solutions of medicines in oleic acid. These are alkaloids or mineral salts.

OLFACTORY NERVE

The nerve responsible for the sense of smell.

OMEGA-3 FISH OILS

Fish oils rich in polyunsaturated fatty acids which are believed to lower levels of cholesterol and triglycerides — the blood fats associated with heart disease. Omega-3 oils are thought to assist in preventing blood clots and in retarding the development of atherosclerosis. They may also lower blood pressure, help relieve arthritis, and have a positive effect on skin disorders like eczema and psoriasis.

Found in certain species of cold-water fish, Omega-3 oil was isolated as a result of scientific investigation of the Eskimo diet. Eskimos have a high-fat diet but a low incidence of heart disease, and it appears that the Omega-3 oils protect the body from the accumulation of blood clots. Omega-3 oils produce prostacyclin, a substance which prevents platelets from sticking together. Dietary tests have shown that the oil may reduce blood cholesterol levels by up to 20 per cent.

OMEGA-3 RATINGS FOR SELECTED FISH SPECIES

Common name	Omega-3 fatty acids (g per 100 g)	Total fat (g per 100 g)
Salmon, Chinook, canned	3.04	16.0
Mackerel, Atlantic	2.18	9.8
Salmon, pink	1.87	5.2
Tuna, albacore, canned, light	1.69	6.8
Sablefish	1.39	13.1
Herring, Atlantic	1.09	6.2
Trout, rainbow (US)	1.08	4.5
Oyster, Pacific	0.84	2.3
Bass, striped	0.64	2.1
Catfish, channel	0.61	3.6
Crab, Alaska King	0.57	1.6
Ocean perch	0.51	2.5
Crab, blue, cooked, canned	0.46	1.6
Halibut, Pacific	0.45	2.0
Shrimp, different species	0.39	1.2
Flounder, yellowtail	0.30	1.2
Haddock	0.16	0.66

Omega-3 oil also substantially reduces blood triglyceride levels. The oil is now available as a health supplement. The following table shows Omega-3 ratings for different fish species.

OPTIC NERVE

The nerve responsible for the sense of sight.

ORAL

Relating to the mouth. Oral medicines and treatments are those which are taken through the mouth.

ORANGE

A fruit rich in vitamins A and C, and several of the B vitamins. Oranges also contain calcium, potassium and the bioflavonoids, as well as having an astringent effect, which helps loosen mucus and tighten the membrane linings. Oranges are recommended as a food to help ward off colds and aid sinusitis and respiratory infections. They are not recommended, however, for people suffering from arthritis, eczema or hives.

ORGAN

A distinct part of the body which has a particular, specialised function; for example, the liver, heart and stomach.

ORGANIC FOOD

Food which is grown without the use of pesticides, fungicides, weedicides and other chemical substances. Organic fruits and vegetables are grown only with natural fertilisers.

ORGASM

An emotional peak, or climax, following sexual arousal. In men it is accompanied by the ejaculation of semen, while in women clitoral and vaginal stimulation builds to a plateau of intense excitement. Orgasm is followed by physical and mental relaxation. For Wilheim Reich the orgasm was of profound importance for the relief of accumulated tension and the basis for deep and extended personal relationships — *see Reichian therapy* (Part 2).

ORIFICE

A natural opening in the body; for example, the mouth, anus and vulva.

OROTATES

The mineral salts of orotic acid (vitamin B13), produced as nutritional supplements which allow for the intake of minerals in combination with organic molecules. They include magnesium, potassium and calcium orotate, and also formulae containing amino acids like tryptophan.

OROTIC ACID

Also known as vitamin B13, orotic acid is thought to assist liver function and prevent the premature ageing of the body cells. It is found in whey.

Organic food is grown without chemical fertilisers

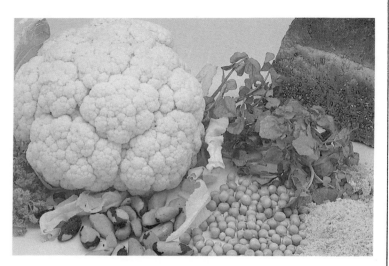

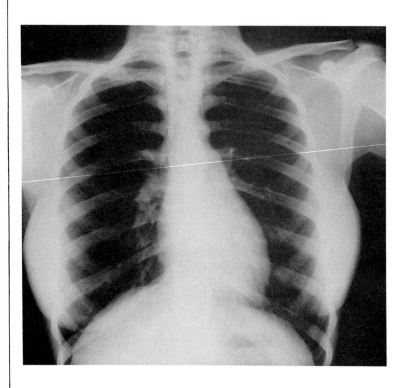

In osteoporosis the bones become weak and brittle

weight for a given height, age and sex. *See Obesity, Weight-for-height ratio.*

OVUM

The egg-cell produced from the ovaries in the female. The term also refers to the embryo after fertilisation by the male sperm. (Plural: *ova*).

P

PABA *(Para-aminobenzoic acid)*

A water-soluble sub-vitamin essential for all aspects of metabolism and associated with a variety of specific functions in the body. PABA is a constituent of folic acid, aids blood cell formation, and helps maintain healthy skin and hair. PABA occurs naturally in green vegetables, brewer's yeast, dairy products, liver and wholegrain cereals. Deficiency symptoms include eczema and other skin disorders, fatigue, anaemia, greying hair, growth retardation and reproduction failure. Naturopaths use PABA to treat burns and vitiligo (white patches on the skin), and also to restore hair colour. RDA (non-official): 10 mg.

OSTEOPOROSIS

Demineralisation of the bones, leaving them weak and brittle. Osteoporosis is thought to be due to a high intake of animal protein, especially from beef, and this protein intake releases calcium from the bones which is then excreted in the urine. A diet rich in calcium, as well as protein, lessens the severity of the complaint, but a diet low in calcium and high in protein can lead, in later life, to bone breakages and lower back problems.

OVARIES

The reproductive organs in the female in which the ova, or female egg-cells, are formed and developed. The ovaries are located inside the abdominal cavity, on each side above the womb. They also help to control menstruation.

OVERWEIGHT

A situation in which an individual weighs 20 per cent or more above the average

PAIN

A warning signal in which the body is alerted by nerves which carry messages to the brain. When these are irritated or injured, the result is pain. *See also Reflex.*

PALSY

A defect in nervous function characterised by loss of the power of movement or feeling.

PANCREAS

A gland located near the stomach which supplies digestive juice to the duodenum and also secretes insulin — a hormone which induces the combustion of dextrose in the blood.

PANGAMIC ACID

Also known as vitamin B15, pangamic acid benefits the nervous and glandular systems, and helps maintain and increase the supply of oxygen to the cells and tissues. Natural sources include brewer's yeast, seeds, nuts and brown rice.

PAPULE (or PAPULA)

A pimple, or raised area, on the skin.

PARALYSIS

The complete or partial loss of the power of movement or sensation in the body — for example, following a stroke or injury. Some forms of paralysis have been effectively treated by acupuncture; in these instances a meridian is stimulated which feeds into the paralysed area. Paralysis can also be treated through special forms of remedial exercise.

PARAPLEGIA

A specific form of paralysis in which all parts of the body below an injury or lesion to the spinal cord are paralysed. *See also Hemiplegia.*

PARATHYROIDS

Four small glands arranged in pairs and located near the outer lobes of the thyroid gland in the neck. They produce a hormone called parathormone which controls calcium metabolism and thus regulates the healthy growth of bones.

PAROTID GLANDS

The largest salivary glands in the body. There are two parotid glands and they are located just in front of, and below, the ear near the jaw.

PATELLA

The kneecap. (*Adjective*, patellar: relating to the kneecap).

PATHOGEN

Any micro-organism or substance capable of producing disease.

PATHOLOGY

An abnormal health condition.

PEACH MEAT

An extract from the centre of the peach stone, used for a medicinal purpose. Peach meat can be dissolved in a cordial and taken as a tonic after illness. It aids the stomach and is useful after bouts of dysentery.

PECTIN

A carbohydrate found in ripe fruit, especially apples. It has an intrinsic congealing function, and can be used in the treatment of diarrhoea.

PECTORAL

Relating to the external surface of the breast or chest.

PELLAGRA

A disease characterised by the onset of diarrhoea, cracked skin and — in

251

extreme cases — mental disorders. Pellagra is caused by a deficiency of niacin, a form of vitamin B3.

PELVIS

The large basin-shaped bone on which the spine rests, and onto which the thigh bones move.

PENIS

The male sex organ. The penis contains a canal called the urethra through which urine is passed from the bladder. The penis is usually relaxed but when sexually excited it becomes stiff and erect. During the climax of sexual intercourse the penis discharges semen through the urethra.

PEPSIN (or PEPSINE)

An enzyme formed in the gastric juice as an aid to digestion, specifically to break down proteins.

PEPTONE

A soluble compound arising as a result of the action of pepsin on proteins — *see Pepsin, Protein.*

PEPTONISATION

The conversion of food into peptones as a result of the enzyme pepsin, thus making the food more easily digested. *See also Pepsin.*

PERISTALSIS

Rhythmic constrictions and relaxations of different parts of the gastrointestinal tract, allowing material to move through it. Practitioners of bioenergetics utilising the technique of 'psychoperistalsis' maintain that the peristaltic rhythm is subject to considerable modification by influences from the central nervous system, including emotional factors. Bodywork techniques applied to the viscera can therefore result in abreaction. *See also Psychoperistalsis, Abreaction* (Part 2).

PERITONEUM

The membrane which lines the abdominal cavity and the viscera.

PERNICIOUS ANAEMIA

Anaemia caused by deficiency of vitamin B12, a vitamin not normally present in plant foods (spirulina, fermented soya beans and certain sea-vegetables being an exception). Vegetarians and vegans are prone to pernicious anaemia, which causes damage to nerve cells, tiredness, shortness of breath and weakness in the arms and legs. *See also Vitamin B12.*

PHARYNX

The cavity at the back of the mouth which connects the mouth and nasal passages with the oesophagus.

PHENYLALANINE

An essential amino which is important in controlling kidney and bladder function, and the elimination of waste products from the body. Food sources include carrot, spinach, parsley, tomato, apple and pineapple.

PHLEBITIS

The inflammation of a vein so that it becomes hard and can be felt like a cord under the skin. Phlebitis can arise from disease or injury, or as a development of varicose veins.

PHOBIA

A fear without any basis in fact.

PHOSPHOLIPID

A lipid which contains phosphorus. An example is lecithin, which is found in plant and animal cells, and also in egg yolk.

PHOSPHORUS

A mineral which, when combined with an equal amount of calcium, helps build strong bones and teeth, regulates heart, nerve and muscle activity, and helps to maintain the acid–alkali balance in the blood and other tissues. Plentiful supplies of phosphorus are found in eggs, fish, milk, meat, wholegrain cereals (especially oats), yeast, nuts and many other foods — so deficiencies are quite rare. However, if increased calcium is taken then it should be supplemented by extra phosphorus, and if one takes large amounts of yeast, liver or wheat germ, it may be necessary to add calcium to the diet to balance the extra phosphorus. Phosphorus absorption is controlled by the parathyroid, and if this is not functioning properly it may cause phosphorus deficiency; this can lead to nervous disorders, fatigue, tooth, gum and bone weakness, appetite loss and weight problems.

PILES — *see Haemorrhoids*

PITUITARY GLAND

A ductless gland located at the base of the brain. The gland secretes hormones which regulate growth: oxytocin, which stimulates muscular contractions of the uterus, and vasopressin, which affects the re-absorption of water into the kidneys and stimulates the muscular walls of blood vessels to contract.

PLATELETS

Substances which assist the clotting mechanism of the blood.

PLETHORA

An over-abundance of red corpuscles in the blood.

PLEURA

The membrane lining the chest and covering the thoracic cavity. Inflammation of this membrane results in pleurisy.

POLYP

A small, pear-shaped growth on the internal surfaces of the body. Polyps are usually benign and are found typically in the colon (where they sometimes become malignant), the nose (where they restrict breathing), and in the womb (where they can cause bleeding). Polyps are generally cause by chronic infection.

POLYPEPTIDE

A compound which consists of 2 or more amino acids, and is formed by the breaking down of proteins.

POLYUNSATURATES —
see Fats

POTASSIUM

A mineral which is found in quite large quantities (about 120 grams) in the human body, and is important for regulating the heart, blood flow, kidneys, muscles and nervous system. In the correct balance with sodium, it keeps the blood pressure low. Potassium is plentiful in fresh fruits (particularly oranges and bananas) and vegetables, whole grains, and dried fruits. However, potassium deficiency does occur, especially in people who are on special diets with very little raw fruit or vegetables, or who are being treated with diuretics or cortisone. People suffering from some diseases such as leukaemia, diabetes, epilepsy and some kidney and heart conditions often have low levels of potassium and may be helped by supplements. Potassium levels can also be lowered by too much salt, sugar, coffee or alcohol in the diet, and by stress. Symptoms of potassium deficiency include fatigue, muscle weakness, high blood pressure, poor circulation, cramps, irritability and digestive problems.

PRECURSOR

A nutrient required for the manufacture of a given substance in the body. For example, carotene is a precursor of vitamin A and tryptophan is a precursor of niacin, a form of vitamin B3.

PREGNANCY

Pregnancy — 40 weeks on average

The fertilisation of the female ovum by the sperm, and its development in the lining of the womb. The normal duration of pregnancy is 40 weeks, and during this time the monthly period ceases, the breasts become larger and the abdomen becomes progressively more protrusive. *See also Natural childbirth* (Part 2).

PREMATURE BIRTH

Any birth occurring before the 37th week and after the 28th week of a pregnancy — *see Pregnancy*.

PRE-MENSTRUAL TENSION (PMT)

A female disorder which occurs up to 2 weeks preceding menstruation and which is thought to affect up to 70 per cent of women. PMT is characterised by states of depression and other severe mood changes, like outbursts of rage or anxiety, as well as feelings of considerable physical discomfort. Other symptoms include fatigue, headaches, tender breasts, acne, and bloating of the legs or abdomen.

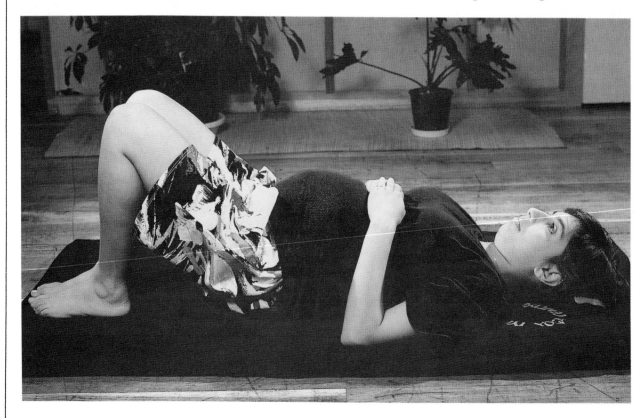

Some women also experience cravings for sugar.

PMT is now thought to be related to an imbalance in the ratio of the 2 hormones produced by the ovarian gland — oestrogen and progesterone. In the 2 weeks prior to menstruation these hormones are produced in greater quantities and this has a metabolic effect on nearly all organs in the body. The ratio of these hormones in the blood also affects neurotransmitters in the brain, thereby influencing the emotions.

Naturopathic treatment for PMT includes vitamin and mineral supplementation (especially vitamin B complex, zinc, magnesium and manganese), accompanied by fresh fruits to ensure sufficient nutrients to manufacture the female hormones, and vitamins C and E, as well as regular exercise to ensure the ovarian glands have adequate circulation and oxygen supply.

Some aspects of PMT may also be stress-induced and some doctors are now asking PMT sufferers to record their symptoms over a number of cycles, paying close examination to day-to-day feelings. Counselling for stress factors and negative emotional associations can therefore also be effective as an adjunct to nutritional and hormonal treatments for PMT.

PRENATAL

Occurring prior to birth.

PRITIKIN DIET

A diet developed by American nutritionist Nathan Pritikin (1916–85) to highlight the importance of reducing fat and cholesterol levels in the body. As a young researcher, Pritikin rejected the then prevalent notion that heart disease was stress-related: he found that the incidence of heart attacks in England and Wales in 1944 was 50 per cent lower than before the war. Later he discovered that only those countries which had greatly reduced rations of high fat and cholesterol foods

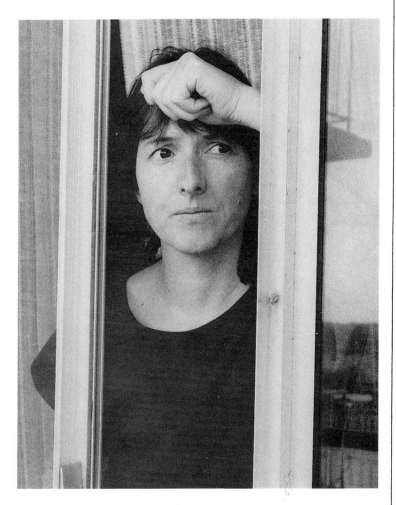

PMT, thought to be related to hormonal imbalance

had a drop in heart disease and diabetic deaths. Pritikin also found that the typical American diet followed a high-fat, high-cholesterol pattern. His own level in the early 1950s was close to 300 mg per 100 ml, when it should have been no higher than 160. Pritikin later came to regard 220 as the danger threshold.

The Pritikin Diet is almost 80 per cent carbohydrate and emphasises wholegrains, fresh fruit and vegetables. Only 8–12 per cent of the total calories are fat, and red meat is avoided. Pritikin himself was not averse to non-fat milk, or to white meats (fish, chicken and turkey, the latter with the skin removed), but most Pritikin Diet adherents are substantially vegetarian. Pritikin's ideas are contained in his books *The Pritikin Programme for Diet and Exercise* (1979) and *The Pritikin Promise* (1983).

PROGESTERONE

A hormone associated with the female sex cycle and the maintenance of pregnancy. One of its main roles is to prepare the womb lining for the fertile egg. It is also active in preparing the breasts for lactation and helps prevent the release of an egg during pregnancy.

Progesterone-type substances are used medically as contraceptives and to treat some menstrual problems. They are often used in combination with oestrogen hormones.

PROLAPSE

The falling down of a part of the body, such as the womb or rectum, from the position it normally occupies.

PROLINE

A non-essential amino acid which forms part of the white blood corpuscles and is involved in the emulsifying of fats. Food sources include carrot, lettuce, cucumber, apricot, grapes, oranges, coconut and almond.

PROPOLIS

A sticky, antibacterial, antiviral substance gathered by bees from buds and bark, and used to disinfect the hive. Propolis contains a number of vitamins, minerals, resins, balsams, waxes and aromatic essential oils, and is used naturopathically to treat infections, colds and influenza. Propolis lozenges are available in health food shops.

PROSTAGLANDINS

Hormone-like substances found in minute quantities in most body tissues. They help to regulate cell behaviour and stimulate or relax smooth muscle tissue. It is thought that they may prove useful as contraceptive agents, in inducing labour or delayed menstruation, and in restricting high blood pressure. They are also used in treating conditions like asthma, alcoholism and gastric ulcers.

PROSTATE

A gland which is located near the urethra and lower part of the bladder, and secretes a fluid that is part of semen. Disease of the prostate may interfere with the flow of urine or cause its retention. It is sometimes the site of benign or cancerous tumours.

PROTEIN

The world 'protein' means 'of the first importance' and was coined by Gerardos Johannes Mulder, who recognised the significance of these constituents in biochemistry.

Proteins are primarily responsible for the growth and development of body tissue. They consist of amino acids and occur in a variety of forms: for example, as albumins in blood plasma, as globulins in muscle tissue, as protamines and histones in nucleic acids, and as scleroproteins in skeletal and connective tissue. They combine with lipids to form lipoproteins (found especially in the blood) and with carbohydrates to form glycoproteins.

Our bodies consist of 18–20 per cent protein by weight. Our skin, muscles, organs, bones, hair and nails, for example, are mostly fibrous protein. While protein is the main body-building substance, it also helps the body to fight infection and repair damaged tissue. Protein can also supply fuel to the body when energy is not supplied by carbohydrates and lipids, but this is not its principal function.

As nutrients, proteins are usually divided into animal and vegetable. Animal protein derives from meat, eggs, dairy products and fish, and vegetable protein from grains, nuts, legumes, etc. Meat is regarded as a 'complete' protein since all of the 8 essential amino acids are present

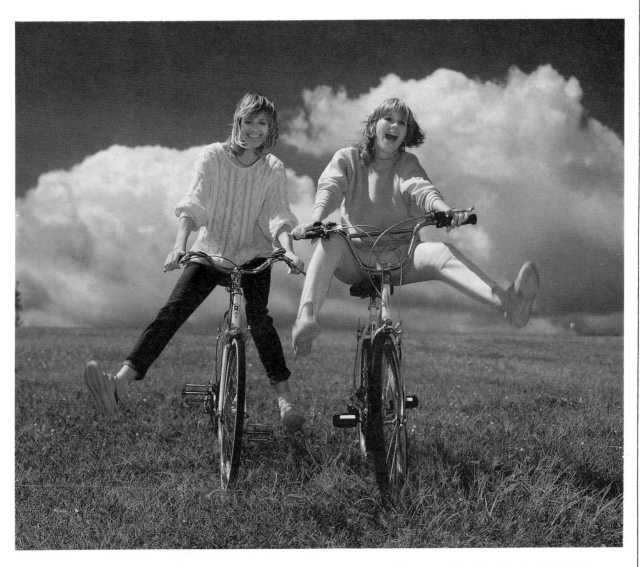

Proteins build body tissue

in their correct amounts. Red meats, however, are prone to toxic by-products and bacteria, so many people on a natural health diet avoid red meats entirely, or limit their intake substantially. People who rely solely on vegetable protein are, however, vulnerable to protein deficiency and may require additional foods to balance their amino acid intake. *See also Complete protein food, Incomplete protein food, Complementary protein foods.*

If a food contains 'complete protein', all the essential amino acids are present in amounts appropriate for growth and the maintenance of life. 'Incomplete proteins' are not able to support growth or life.

Animal protein is high quality, complete protein, while plant protein usually lacks the essential amino acids lysine, methionine, threonine and tryptophan. *See also Complete protein food, Incomplete protein food, Amino acids.*

PROTEIN QUALITY

An assessment of protein in terms of the amount of amino acids which are present.

PROTEOLYTIC

Relating to the breakdown of protein.

PSORIASIS

A skin disease characterised by thick red patches of skin covered by white, heavy scales. Psoriasis rashes usually occur in the joints: for example, the elbows, and the back of knees, behind the ears, under the arms. The scales shed in flakes, leaving a red itchy rash.

Psoriasis is often due to lecithin deficiency — either because of poor nutrition or because the body is unable to absorb it adequately. Lecithin supplements may be taken, or a lecithin cream applied directly to the rash.

PSYCHODIETETICS

A term coined by Doctors Emanuel Cheraskin and W. M. Ringsdorf to describe the relationship between diet and emotional well-being. According to Cheraskin and Ringsdorf, many emotional disorders have their origin in improper diet and nutrition. According to principles of psychodietetics, food intake can be modified to have a positive and preventive effect for good health in the future: 'The shortage of a single essential vitamin, mineral element, amino or fatty acid' they claim in their book on this topic, 'will create a shock wave that spreads to affect the utilisation and/or function of every other essential nutrient'.

The pulse may be taken at the wrist

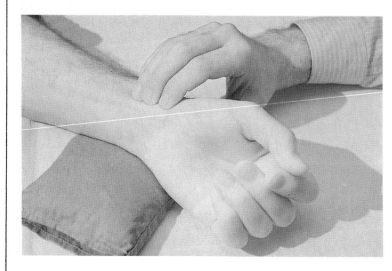

PSYCHOPATHIC DISORDER

A state of mental ill-health in which a person acts in either an irresponsible or overly aggressive way when not under medical treatment. Examples include schizophrenia, paranoia and manic depressive insanity.

PSYCHOSIS — *see Mental disorders*

PSYCHOSOMATIC DISEASE

From the Greek *psyche* ('the mind') and *soma* ('the body'), any illness which has a mental or emotional cause. Psychosomatic illness often arises from stress, and this may manifest as general irritability, depression, impulsive and aggressive behaviour, inability to concentrate, accident-proneness, emotional tension, or sexual problems. Insomnia, migraines, eczema, obesity and high-blood pressure may also be brought about by psychosomatic factors, and in these cases can be treated by such therapies as clinical hypnosis, guided imagery and meditation.

PULMONARY

That which relates to the lungs.

CHECK YOUR PULSE RATE

Fitness level	18–26 years		33–57 years	
	Men	Women	Men	Women
Excellent	69–75	76–84	63–76	73–86
Good	76–83	85–94	77–90	87–100
Average	84–92	95–105	91–106	101–117
Fair	93–99	106–116	107–120	119–130
Poor	100–106	117–127	121–134	131–144

PULSE

The throbbing of the heart and blood vessels, which can be felt as a rhythmical beat in peripheral arteries, especially at the wrist.

PULSES

The edible seeds found in various legumes; for example, peas, beans and lentils.

PUPIL

The small circular opening in the centre of the iris of the eye, through which light rays pass to the retina.

PURGATIVE

Any substance which is used to relieve constipation — *see Constipation*.

PUS

A fluid consisting of dead body tissue and white blood cells.

PYORRHOEA

A dental disease involving the destruction of the supportive tissue of the teeth. It is characterised by the discharge of pus from the gums around the roots of the teeth.

R

RAW FOOD

Food consumed without any form of preparation. This includes vegetables, fruits, cereals, nuts, herbs and certain seeds such as sunflower and pumpkin seeds.

Raw food generally contains more fibre than prepared food, and has not lost vitamins as a result of processing or cooking. Most fruits and vegetables are alkaline-forming foods (with the exception of sweet potatoes), and counteract the acid-forming tendency of egg yolks, beef, poultry, fish and milk. Among the main alkaline fruits and vegetables are apples, apricots, avocados, bean sprouts, broccoli, cabbage, carrots, celery, corn, leeks, melons, oranges, spinach and tomatoes. Dates, prunes and raisins are especially alkaline-forming.

The vitamins are retained in raw food

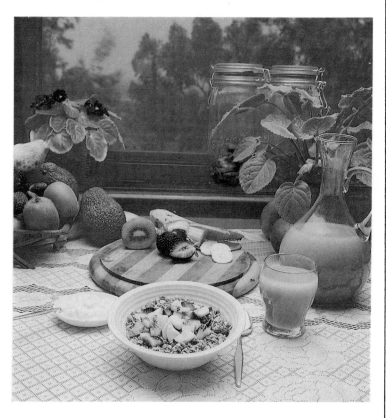

Advocates of a raw-food diet emphasise that many of the body's illnesses are caused by excessive acidity, so a diet of 80 per cent raw fruit and vegetables is recommended for preventive health care. Nevertheless, the diet needs to be balanced, encompassing protein-rich nuts, cheese and cereals, as well as a natural sweetener like honey which, together with fruit sugars, supplies carbohydrate content. Fruit and vegetables alone do not supply sufficient protein for daily requirements.

The rebounder is ideal for aerobic exercise

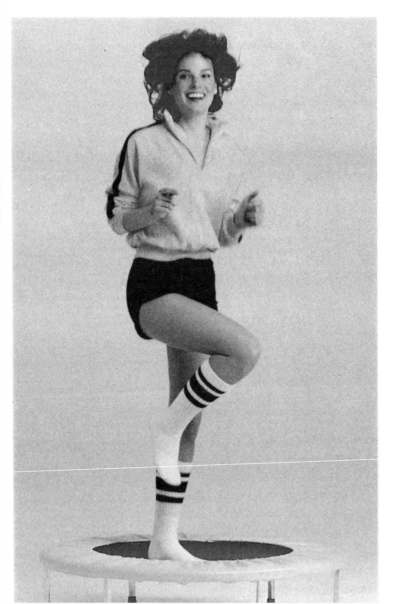

REBOUNDER

A small circular trampoline which can be used for aerobic exercise. During a session of 5 minutes bouncing on a rebounder, the body cells are forced to adjust to increased gravitational force and thus become stronger. Rebounding is less stressful on the body joints than jogging, enhances the cardiovascular system, and stimulates lymphatic activity. Rebounders are reportedly useful for treating arthritis, bad backs, asthma, diabetes and other degenerative complaints. Some practitioners recommend rebounding to music. *See also Aerobics.*

RECEPTOR

A nerve-ending or sense-cell which is sensitive to a stimulus.

RECOMMENDED DIETARY ALLOWANCE (RDA)

Levels of nutrients considered essential, on a daily basis, for the maintenance of good health. Established in the United States in the 1940s, the system of RDAs is only a guide, for the genetic makeup and physical condition of each person are unique. Nevertheless, the RDA provides a useful indicator of minimum levels required to prevent a state of nutrient deficiency disease in most people. The RDA is also known as the RDI (Recommended Daily Intake).

The following tables provide RDAs, for both adults and children, for major nutrients:

RECOMMENDED DAILY DIETARY ALLOWANCES FOR ADULTS WITH GUIDE TO DEFICIENCY SYMPTOMS*

Vitamin or mineral	RDA for adults	Possible deficiency symptoms*
A	5000 IU, men 4000 IU, women	Night blindness; abnormal dryness of the eyeballs; dry, rough, itchy skin; susceptibility to respiratory infection
B_1 (thiamine)	1.4 mg, men 1.0 mg, women	Confusion; weakness of eye muscles; loss of appetite; uncoordinated walk; poor memory; inability to concentrate
B_2 (riboflavin)	1.6 mg, men 1.2 mg, women	Discoloured tongue; anaemia; cracks at corners of mouth; scaly skin; burning, itchy eyes
Niacin	18 mg, men 13 mg, women	Dermatitis; insomnia; headache; diarrhoea; dementia
B_6 (pyridoxine)	2.2 mg, men 2.0 mg, women	Depression; skin lesions; extreme nervousness; water retention; lethargy
B_{12}	3.0 μg	Anaemia, accompanied by symptoms such as heart palpitations, sore tongue, general weakness; weight loss
Folacin	400 μg	Anaemia; dizziness; fatigue; intestinal disorders; diarrhoea; shortness of breath
C	600 mg	Easy bruising; spongy, bleeding gums; dental problems; slow wound healing; fatigue; listlessness; rough skin
D	200 IU	Softening of bones (osteomalacia); bone pain; susceptibility to bone fracture (osteoporosis); excessive tooth decay
E	15 IU, men 12 IU, women	Muscle degeneration; anaemia; nerve dysfunction
Calcium	800 mg	Susceptibility to bone fractures (osteoporosis); softening of bones (osteomalacia); periodontal disease
Iron	10 mg, men 18 mg, women	Anaemia, accompanied by symptoms such as weakness, fatigue, headache, heart palpitations, mouth soreness
Magnesium	350 mg, men 300 mg, women	Foot and leg cramps; muscle weakness; irregular pulse; nervousness
Zinc	15 mg	Slow wound healing; skin and hair problems; poor resistance to infection

These symptoms can, of course, suggest medical conditions other than nutrient deficiencies. For a proper diagnosis of symptoms, see your doctor.

RECOMMENDED DAILY DIETARY ALLOWANCES FOR CHILDREN

	Age (years)	Protein (g)	Vitamin A (IU)	Vitamin D (IU)	Vitamin E (IU)	Ascorbic Acid (mg)	Folacin (μg)	Niacin (mg)	Riboflavin (mg)	Thiamin (mg)	Vitamin B_6 (mg)	Vitamin B_{12} (μg)	Calcium (mg)	Phosphorus (mg)	Iron (mg)	Magnesium (mg)	Zinc (mg)
Infants	0.0–0.5	kg × 2.2	1400	400	4	35	50	5	0.4	0.3	0.3	0.3	360	240	10	60	3
	0.5–1.0	kg × 2.0	2000	400	5	35	50	8	0.6	0.5	0.4	0.3	540	400	15	70	5
Children	1–3	23	2000	400	7	40	100	9	0.8	0.7	0.6	1.0	800	800	15	150	10
	4–6	30	2500	400	9	40	200	12	1.1	0.9	0.9	1.5	800	800	10	200	10
	7–10	36	3300	400	10	40	300	16	1.2	1.2	1.2	2.0	800	800	10	250	10
Boys	11–14	44	5000	400	12	45	400	18	1.5	1.4	1.6	3.0	1200	1200	18	350	15
	15–18	54	5000	400	15	45	400	20	1.8	1.5	2.0	3.0	1200	1200	18	400	15
Girls	11–14	44	4000	400	12	45	400	16	1.3	1.2	1.6	3.0	1200	1200	18	300	15
	15–18	48	4000	400	12	45	400	14	1.4	1.1	2.0	3.0	1200	1200	18	300	15

Extracted from Recommended Daily Dietary Allowances, Food and Nutrition Board, National Academy of Sciences, National Research Council, Revised 1974.

RECTUM

The lower end of the large intestine from the sigmoid flexure to the anus. It is this section of the bowel which stores faeces.

RECUPERATION

Slow recovery from an illness. This may involve progressively strengthening the body with mild forms of exercise and a healthy diet, and gradually returning to optimal physical and mental condition.

REFINED CARBOHYDRATE

A carbohydrate, such as starch or sugar, which has been artificially separated from other substances with which it is usually associated in the natural state. Refined white flour, for example, consists substantially of endosperm separated from bran and wheat germ.

REFLEX

An involuntary response by an organ, gland or muscle to a given stimulus. This stimulus is picked up by sensory receptors and the impulse is relayed through the body's nervous system via the spinal cord. Further impulses are then sent back to that organ, gland or muscle to produce a response to the original stimulus. Withdrawing one's hand from a source of pain is an example of this process.

REFLUX

The flowing back of gastric material into the oesophagus — *see Heartburn*.

REMISSION

A cessation of the anticipated progression of the disease process. Spontaneous remission occurs without any obvious cause and may be associated with symptoms of psychosomatic origin once a stressor is removed or overcome.

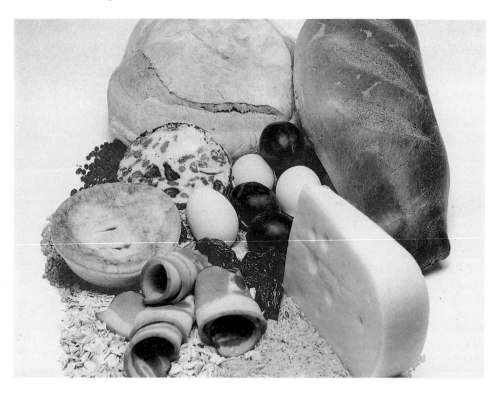

In a restricted diet, acid-forming foods such as these could be contra-indicated

RENAL

That which relates to the kidneys.

RENNIN

A casein-digesting enzyme in gastric juice which curdles milk. It is present in the stomachs of infants and aids the coagulation of milk products. *See also Casein.*

REPETITIVE STRAIN INJURY (RSI) — *see*

Tenosynovitis

RESPIRATION

The process of breathing with the lungs in which there is an exchange of oxygen and carbon dioxide. This exchange of gases between the inhaled air and the blood capillaries occurs in the alveoli — *see Alveoli.*

RESPIRATORY SYSTEM

The body system responsible for taking air into the lungs and facilitating the exchange of oxygen, which is inhaled, and carbon dioxide, which is exhaled. The respiratory tract includes the nose, mouth, larynx, pharynx, trachea, bronchi, bronchioles and the alveoli in the lungs.

RESTRICTED DIET

A diet in which the intake of certain foods is restricted. This may be for any number of reasons, including food allergies, religious or economic factors, metabolic disorders or because of specific health requirements (for example, reducing salt intake to help lower blood pressure). Food intake is also restricted during times of fasting. On these occasions it is usually limited to water or diluted fruit juice.

RETINA

The inner layer of the eye from which sensory impressions are relayed to the brain. Light rays pass to the retina through the pupil. *See also Pupil.*

RETROVERSION

The backward displacement of an organ in the body, such as the uterus.

RHEUM

Fluid secreted by the mucous glands and discharged from the eyes or nostrils when the mucous membranes are inflamed.

RHINITIS

Inflammation of the mucous membrane of the nostrils, more commonly known as hay fever, or nasal catarrh.

RIBOFLAVIN — *see Vitamin B2*

Rhinitis — more commonly known as hay fever

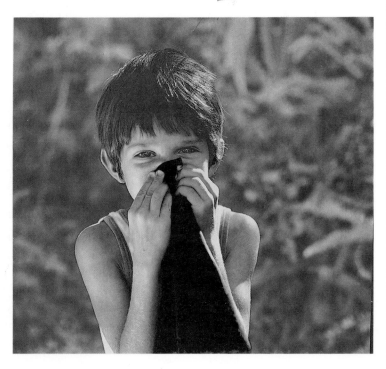

RICE

Rice has been consumed as a food in China for at least 7000 years, and in India for about 5000 years. It is an energy food rich in complex carbohydrates, protein, B vitamins (especially thiamine, and riboflavin) and minerals like calcium and iron. Complex carbohydrates act as a special fuel for working muscles and are stored in the body as glycogen. They are also absorbed slowly into the bloodstream — a vital aspect for diabetics and those suffering from hypoglycaemia.

Rice is an ideal food for people in this category because it is low in fat and salt, as well as providing fibre and carbohydrate. Regular rice consumption may also assist in reducing high blood pressure and preventing such diseases as bowel cancer and coronary heart disease — making it an ideal component in modern Western diet. It is also suitable for people who are slimming, for it provides an ideal accompaniment to many vegetable and lean meat dishes. Half a cup of cooked rice supplies 350 kilojoules, or 85 calories — the equivalent of one thick slice of bread, one large potato, a medium-size apple or pear, or a small glass of milk.

Rice is low in fat and salt

RICKETS

An infantile disease of the bones, characterised by bow-legs and knock-knees. Rickets is due to defective development of the bones and results from a deficiency of vitamin D in the diet.

RNA

Ribonucleic acid, a substance found in the nuclei of living cells. RNA relays instructions from DNA in the cell nucleus to cell polyribosomes, and this leads to the formation of new proteins. RNA is involved in the synthesis of hormones and glandular secretions, which are in turn active in metabolic processes. *See also DNA.*

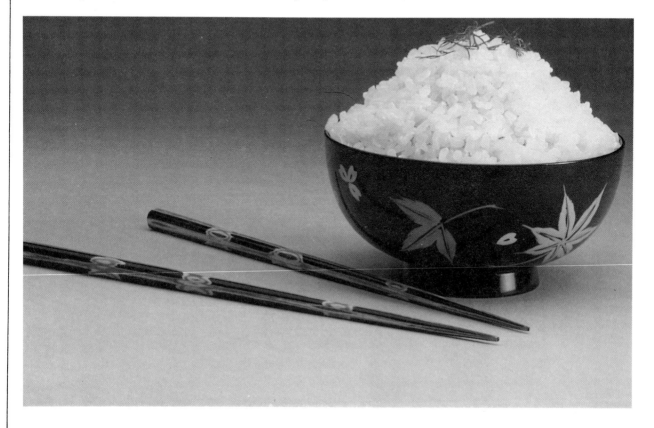

ROUNDBACK — *see Kyphosis*

ROYAL JELLY

A milky susbstance generated by the salivary glands of worker bees specifically for the development of the queen bee. The selected larvae which are fed royal jelly become twice as large and live 30 times longer than the other larvae which do not receive this special nutrient. This has led to interest in the substance as a dietary supplement for humans.

Royal jelly is a rich source of vitamin B5 (pantothenic acid) and contains other vitamins, minerals, amino acids and hormones. It rejuvenates the body, helps regulate blood pressure and also enhances the healthy functioning of the adrenal glands. Royal jelly may be taken as is, or mixed with honey. Normal dose: ½ teaspoon, 1–2 times per day, for 1–5 months.

RUPTURE

A breaking or bursting apart of a body organ, often as a result of increased pressure; examples include ruptured blood vessels or spleen.

RUTIN

One of the bioflavonoids, formerly known collectively as vitamin P. Bioflavonoids occur naturally with vitamin C in citrus fruits, plums, blackcurrants, cherries and grapes, and are also found in buckwheat and the herb, rue. Bioflavonoids, have antioxidant properties and protect the function of vitamin C in the body. Rutin works specifically to strengthen the walls of small blood vessels, and assists in reducing toxic levels of copper in the body. *See also Bioflavonoids*.

S

SAC

A bag, pouch or cavity which serves as a receptacle, usually for fluid.

SACCHARIDES

A category of carbohydrates of varying sweetness. They include glucose, sucrose and ribose.

SACRUM

A triangular composite bone consisting of 5 vertebrae fused together. It forms part of the hip-girdle at the base of the vertebral column.

SALICYLIC ACID

The substance from which aspirin is derived. When applied to the skin it has an antibacterial and antifungal action.

SALT, COMMON

Sodium chloride is a major ingredient in many popular and processed foods, and is frequently associated with high blood pressure in those who consume excess quantities. The average intake of salt in modern Western countries averages around 8–12 g per day — a dietary pattern reinforced by increasing dependence on 'fast foods', many of which have a high salt content. Sodium is also taken into the diet through sodium nitrites and nitrates — used in curing meats — and through mono-sodium glutamate, a flavour-enhancing agent found in many commercially prepared foods, especially Chinese cuisine.

Fresh meats, eggs and dairy products have higher sodium levels than grains, fruits or vegetables. A 100 g serving of steak contains around 93 mg of sodium; a similar quantity of chicken 79 mg; 100 g of milk contains 58 mg of sodium and an egg 69 mg. However, ½ cup red kidney beans contains only 8 mg, the same quantity of shredded raw cabbage 9 mg, and a medium-size apple, banana or orange, around 2 mg of sodium.

The US National Research Council recommends the following daily sodium levels as safe and adequate:

Infant aged up to 6 months: 115–350 mg

Baby aged from 6–12 months: 250–750 mg

Child aged from 4–6 years: 450–1350 mg

Child aged from 7–10 years: 600–1800 mg

Adults: 1100–3300 mg

See also Sodium.

METABOLIC FUNCTIONS OF TISSUE SALTS

Remedy	Function	Indications
Calcium fluoride	Maintains tissue elasticity	Relaxed conditions, muscular weakness, poor circulation, dental decays.
Calcium phosphate	Tissue-cell builder	Constituent of bones, teeth, connective tissue, blood corpuscles and gastric juices. Aids vitality and endurance, chief remedy for teething disorders.
Calcium sulphate	Blood cleanser	Skin problems, helpful in clearing pimples during adolescence, wounds that are too slow to heal. Purifies and tones the system.
Iron phosphate	Oxygen carrier	Assists with the oxygenation of the blood stream, supplies energy and vitality, aids feverish colds and chills, sore throats and all inflammatory conditions particularly in alternation with potassium chloride.
Potassium chloride	Blood conditioner	Congested conditions, respiratory disorders, coughs and colds particularly in alternation with iron phosphate. Sometimes referred to as the 'liver' salt.
Potassium phosphate	Nerve nutrient	Nourishes the nerves and brain, strengthens mental powers, depression, nervous headaches. For fatigue and all nerve complaints.
Potassium sulphate	Oxygen exchanger	Maintains the skin and indicated in treatment of minor skin ailments, disorders of the scalp, hair, nails and mucous membranes. For relief of brittle nails alternate with silicon oxide.
Magnesium phosphate	Nerve stabiliser	Relaxes and steadies the nerves. For the relief of spasmodic, darting pains, cramps, neuralgia. Will usually act more rapidly taken with little hot water.
Sodium chloride	Water distributor	Assists in the control of dryness or excessive moisture and important for relief of runny nose, loss of smell or taste.
Sodium phosphate	Acid neutraliser	Aids digestion, particularly in the relief of acidity and heartburn. Used in the treatment of rheumatic ailments.
Sodium sulphate	Excess water eliminator	Assists with the body water balance. Indicated in the treatment of biliousness, liver upsets, water retention and influenza.
Silicon	Cleanser and conditioner	Assists in the treatment of pimples and spots. For brittle nails in alternation with potassium sulphate.

Source: Richard B. Judge

SATURATED FATTY ACIDS — *see Fats*

SATURATES — *see Fats*

SCABIES

A contagious skin disease resulting from female itch-mites burrowing under the skin and causing infection.

SCAPULA

The shoulder blade, a flat triangular bone which articulates with the clavicle, or collar bone, to form the pectoral arch.

SCHUESSLER TISSUE SALTS

The so-called 'biochemic' system of medicine developed by Dr Wilhelm H. Schuessler, a German medical practitioner sympathetic to the homeopathic approach of Samuel Hahnemann.

Dr Hahnemann had himself researched the therapeutic value of minerals — specifically sodium, potassium, calcium and silica — and included mineral dilutions among his remedies. Then in March 1873 Schuessler published an article titled 'An Abridged Homeopathic Therapeutics' in a German homeopathic journal, and identified 12 'tissue salts' which he had analysed in human blood, and in the ash of human remains. These salts seemed to be essential for healthy body function and Schuessler believed that they could be given in homeopathic potencies. (He used what is known in homeopathy as the 6x potency, that is 1:1 000 000.) The following list includes both the English and German names of these tissue salts, and their common abbreviation:

ENGLISH NAME	GERMAN NAME	ABBREVIATION
Calcium fluoride	*Calcarea fluorica*	Calc. Fluor.
Calcium phosphate	*Calcarea phosphorica*	Calc. Phos.
Calcium sulphate	*Calcarea sulphurica*	Calc. Sulph.
Iron phosphate	*Ferrum phosphoricum*	Ferr. Phos.
Potassium chloride	*Kalium muriaticum*	Kali. Mur.
Potassium phosphate	*Kalium phosphoricum*	Kali. Phos.
Potassium sulphate	*Kalium sulphuricum*	Kali. Sulph.
Magnesium phosphate	*Magnesia phosphorica*	Mag. Phos.
Sodium chloride	*Natrum muriaticum*	Nat. Mur.
Sodium phosphate	*Natrum phosphoricum*	Nat. Phos.
Sodium sulphate	*Natrum sulphuricum*	Nat. Sulph.
Silicon oxide	*Silica*	Silica

Schuessler's basic concept was as follows:

. . . the physiological fact that both the structure and vitality of the organs of the body are dependent upon certain necessary quantities and proper apportionment of its inorganic constituents. These remain after combustion of the tissues and form the ashes. The inorganic constituents are, in a very real sense, the material basis of the organs and tissues of the body, and are absolutely essential to their integrity of structure and functional activity. Any disturbance in molecular motion of these cell salts in living tissues, caused by a deficiency in the requisite amount, constitutes disease, which can be rectified and the requisite equilibrium re-established by administering the same mineral salts in small quantities . . .

SCLERA

The relatively hard external coating of the eye. It is a strong, fibrous, opaque membrane.

SCOLIOSIS

A distortion of the spinal vertebrae, either in a single curve or in an S-bend. Scoliosis can result from spinal injury or displacement of vertebrae — a condition popularly known as 'slipped disc'. It is usually treated by manipulative therapies, like chiropractic, osteopathy or physiotherapy, in conjunction with muscle-toning activities like swimming. *See also Chymopapain.*

SEA-VEGETABLES

Edible seaweeds, or algae, which feature especially in Asian and some Pacific island cuisines. Generally alkaline in content, seaweeds contain chlorine•(which assists the liver in removing toxins), potassium•(to assist the peristaltic movements of the colon), and iodine•(which is involved in the metabolism and in cleansing the blood). Sea-vegetables also contain a variety of vitamins. Brown, red and green algae are all rich in vitamins A, C, D and E,•while green and red seaweeds have comparatively higher quantities of the B•vitamins than brown varieties. Algae also have a protein content comparable to oats. Examples of sea-vegetables include hijiki, kombu, wakame, nori, arame, mekabu and dulse.

SEBUM

A fatty secretion from the sebaceous glands of the skin. Sebum lubricates the skin.

SECRETIN

A hormone produced in the small intestine, which enters the blood and causes the pancreas to secrete copious amounts of digestive juices.

SEEDS

Several types of seeds — for example, pumpkin, poppy, sesame, and caraway — represent a valuable food source. Ripe seeds of this type contain vitamins A, D, E•and B•complex, and are also a good source of unsaturated fats, protein, and the minerals calcium and phosphorus. Seeds are high in both calories and carbohydrate content, and are best taken as a snack between meals. Sunflower seeds contain up to 50 per cent protein.

SELENIUM

A mineral, the importance of which has only recently been realised. Together with vitamin E, it acts as an antioxidant which prevents the breakdown of fats to substances which can damage body tissue. It is also important in the production of sperm cells and antibodies, and in the maintenance of muscle and red blood cells. Selenium deficiency is common in farm animals and greatly reduces their rate of reproduction. It has been shown to be associated in humans with increased incidence of cancer in parts of America where the soil is lacking in this mineral, and in north-eastern China a particular type of heart disease has been linked to selenium deficiency. It has also been suggested that cataracts may be caused by a shortage of selenium. Laboratory mice fed extra selenium developed tumours 8 times less often than the controls. Recent studies have suggested that selenium can give protection against the toxic effects of mercury and other minerals which are polluting our environment.

The recommended daily dose is quite small (about 100 micrograms), and can be obtained from seafood, meat (especially liver), whole, unprocessed cereals and brewer's yeast. Too much selenium is toxic to grazing animals and probably to humans. Symptoms include fatigue, loss of hair, nails and teeth, paralysis and eventually death. Xerox machines give off selenium, but no cases of poisoning have yet been reported as the dose would have to be very high — perhaps 2000 micrograms a day.

SEMEN

The white, sticky fluid formed by the male reproductive organs and containing the fertilising spermatozoa. It discharges from the penis during sexual intercourse, impregnating the female.

SEMI-CIRCULAR CANALS

Structures in the ear, filled with fluid, which are sensitive to gravity and assist a person in attaining balance.

SEPSIS

The infection of body tissue by pathogenic bacteria.

SEPTICAEMIA

The release of bacteria into the blood, causing shock and blood poisoning.

SERINE

A non-essential amino acid important for the functioning of the lungs and the cleansing of the mucous membranes. Food sources include garlic, onion, celery, parsley, alfalfa, cucumber and apple.

SEROTONIN

An inhibitory neurotransmitter required for effective sleep. It is a precursor of the amino acid tryptophan, which is used to induce sleep, and also a treatment for aggression, hallucinations and depression.

SERUM

The residue of blood plasma after fibrin has been removed during coagulation — *see Fibrin.*

SERUM CHOLESTEROL LEVEL

Also known as the blood cholesterol level, a measure of the concentration of cholesterol in the blood serum. The range for individuals in good health is usually regarded as 80–300 mg per 100 ml, although American nutritionist Nathan Pritikin recommended a maximum of 160 and regarded 220 as the danger threshold.

SHOYU

Derived from soya beans, shoyu, or soy sauce, is a widely used condiment in the Orient.

The Chinese originally cultivated soya beans around 4000 years ago but both they, and subsequently the Japanese, discovered that it was easier to digest soya bean protein if the beans were fermented.

This process involves steaming the soya beans and roasting and 'cracking' an equal quantity of wheat. The two ingredients are then mixed and inoculated with spores of *koji* mould in an incubating room. Koji produces enzymes which convert the oils, proteins and starches in the blend to easily fermentable compounds. Shortly afterwards, the mixture is added to an equal quantity of seasalt and spring water, and the liquid is then aged for up to 3 years in cedarwood kegs. During this time the starches convert to simple sugars and these then interact with natural yeasts to produce the alcohols and esters which give rise to shoyu's distinctive aroma. The salt which is present controls the fermentation process and prevents undesirable organisms from forming in the solution.

Shoyu stimulates the secretion of digestive juices in the stomach, aids blood circulation, and strengthens the pumping of the heart. It is also one of the few vegetable sources of vitamin B12.

SIGMOID FLEXURE

That section of the large intestine which has an S-shaped curve. It is located at the higher end of the rectum.

SILICON

A mineral constituent of bones, teeth, hair, nails and skin. It plays an important part in keeping all of these healthy, in speeding nerve reactions, and in preventing the deterioration of arthritic conditions which can cause a build-up of calcium deposits round the joints. Symptoms of deficiency include exhaustion, nervous debility, cold hands and feet, hair loss and aggravation of arthritis. Good sources are lettuce, parsnips, asparagus, strawberries, sunflower seeds, celery, apricots, oats, nuts, mushrooms and tomatoes.

SINUS

A hollow cavity or passage in the body; for example, the nasal sinuses. It can also be a passage in the tissue leading to an abscess, for example, in the nose or ear.

SINUSITIS

Inflammation of the nasal sinuses leading to an accumulation of fluid.

SMOOTH MUSCLES

Those muscles in the body which are not subject to voluntary control.

SODIUM

An important mineral which works with potassium to regulate the kidneys and control most of the fluid interaction in the body, including the coagulation of blood and the maintenance of correct blood pressure. It also helps muscle contractions and is important in the lymphatic and nervous systems. Much of the sodium Western man consumes comes in the form of sodium chloride or common salt. It is well known that excessive intakes of salt can cause increased blood pressure, fluid retention and weight problems, and most modern nutritionists advise us to restrict the salt in our diets. Generally speaking, the body can obtain sufficient sodium from other foods without the addition of salt. Kelp, olives, celery, carrots, dried fruit, cheese, watercress and parsley are all rich in sodium, and if salt is desired for its taste then sea salt is preferable as it contains greater amounts of potassium and magnesium to balance the sodium.

Although more attention is given to the problems caused by excessive salt intake, it is also possible to suffer from sodium deficiency, particularly in hot climates and when strenuous physical exercise causes excessive perspiration. The symptoms are dehydration, muscle cramps, fever, heat stroke and loss of appetite. It is considered better to control these symptoms by eating foods rich in natural sodium rather than simply adding salt to the diet.

SOMATO-PSYCHIC

The influence the body can have on the mind. The term is used by Reichian and neo-Reichian therapists to describe the effects of bodywork techniques in releasing 'blocked' emotions. *See also Abreaction, Reichian therapy* (Part 2), *Psychosomatic disease.*

SORBITOL

A substance which is related to sugar and occurs naturally in several fruit species. Some authorities believe that, when taken orally, sorbitol does not increase blood sugar levels and may, for this reason, be used safely by diabetics as a sugar substitute. However, there is some controversy over the use of sorbitol by diabetics, as many authorities hold the view that it can increase blood sugar levels.

SOYA BEAN

A popular ingredient in Japanese, macrobiotic and vegetarian cooking, the soya bean is a valuable source of vegetable protein and contains all of the 8 essential amino acids in a form which can be assimilated by the body. The soya bean is free of cholesterol, has a low ratio of kilojoules to protein, and contains almost none of the indigestible saturated fats found in most animal foods. *See also Soyfoods*.

SOYFOODS

Protein-rich foods derived from soya beans. Soya bean protein contains all the essential amino acids and is thus a substitute for the protein derived from meat, eggs and dairy products. Soyfoods have no cholesterol content, are low in calories and saturated fats, and are high in vitamins and minerals. They are also easy to digest and comparatively free of chemical toxins.

Soyfoods include *soy milk* (made by grinding and cooking soaked soya beans), *soy-milk yoghurt*, *tofu* (made by curdling and pressing soy milk), *tempeh* (consisting of partially cooked soya beans which are bound together by white mould during fermentation), *miso* (fermented paste made from soya beans, rice or barley, salt and mould) and *shoyu* (a fermented soy sauce made from soya beans, wheat and salt). *Tamari* is a wheat-free form of *shoyu*.

Commercial shoyu, or soy sauce, may contain excess salt, chemicals and artificial colouring, and is not recommended. However, purer forms are available from health food shops. *See also Shoyu, Miso, Soya bean*.

SPASM

The sudden, painful, involuntary contraction of a muscle or group of muscles.

SPHINCTER

A circular muscle which contracts or expands an orifice; for example, the anal sphincter.

SPHINGOMYELIN

A phospholipid found in the brain, spinal cord, liver and kidneys. Sphingomyelin consists of phosphoric acid, choline, sphingosine and a fatty acid. It is also present in egg yolk.

Tofu, a popular form of soyfood

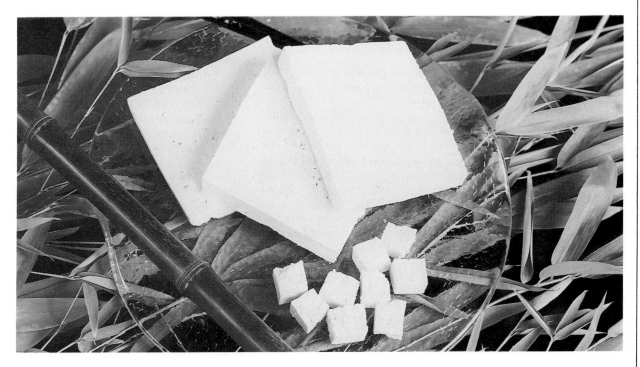

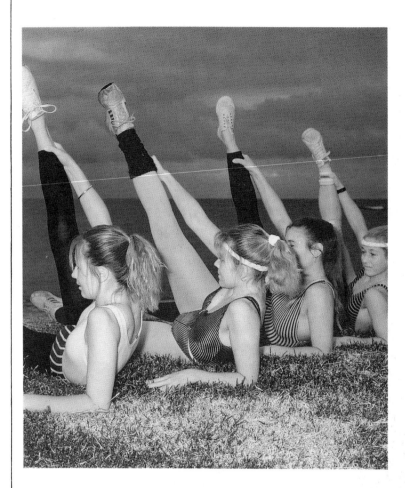

Diet affects sports performance

SPHYGMOMANOMETRY

The measurement of blood pressure. This is equivalent to the pressure in an artery at the extremities of the body. Measurement is taken by using an armband to compress the blood vessels in the left arm and placing a stethoscope over the brachial artery. A pump is utilised to produce pneumatic pressure through the cuff until the heart-beat cannot be heard through the stethoscope. The air is then released and the measurement of *systolic pressure* recorded. This represents the amount of force used by the heart to propel the blood through the arteries.

A later reading, the *diastolic pressure*, measures the tension which the arterial walls exert upon the blood. A healthy reading for a male aged 20–40 is 120 systolic:80 diastolic. Readings in females are slightly lower.

SPIRULINA

Blue-green vegetable plankton which grows in freshwater lakes in Africa and Central America, and is also harvested commercially. Spirulina consists of between 65–71 per cent protein and is claimed by some to be the world's purest source of natural protein. It contains all 8 essential amino acids, and 7 major vitamins — A, B1, B2, B6, B12, C and E.

Spirulina is not dependent on soil but grows as a result of photosynthesis — its green colour is an indicator of its high chlorophyll content. Spirulina contains as much calcium as milk, 3 times more niacin than brown rice, and 2½ times more vitamin B12 than liver. It is also especially high in vitamin A — 1 tablespoon of spirulina powder is said to be equivalent, nutritionally, to 6 carrots. It also contains all the cell-salts and enzymes required by the human body, and is only 7 per cent fat.

Despite its apparently remarkable qualities, however, spirulina is not without its detractors. According to research at the University of California, a substantial proportion of the B12 in spirulina consists of B12 vitamin analogs — constituents which are not true vitamins but which resemble them in chemical structure. It is also thought that because spirulina contains pentoses and phosphoric acid, excess consumption could lead to urinary stone formation or gout in susceptible individuals.

SPLEEN

The ductless organ located to the left of the stomach. It destroys old red-blood cells and features in the immunological system of the body.

SPONDYLITIS

Inflammation of a vertebra in the backbone.

SPORTS DIET

Many nutritionists have pointed to the connection between diet and sports performance, and several general guidelines have emerged for those actively participating in sport:

- There is no medical evidence that high protein levels improve athletic performance. Therefore substantial intake of protein in the form of steak, cheese and eggs is not recommended. However, lean meat and fish may be eaten in moderation.
- More complex carbohydrates should be consumed: including vegetables, grains and grain products. This principle has been popularised by champion tennis player Martina Navratilova, who often consumes a bowl of pasta an hour or so before an important match.
- Fibre intake should be increased.
- Artificial and salty foods, monosodium glutamate (in Chinese meals) and caffeine should all be avoided.
- Milk (especially low fat varieties) is acceptable provided it does not cause a disagreeable or allergic reaction.

SPRUE

A health complaint associated with interference to food absorption in the bowel. Sprue is accompanied by weight loss and sometimes by anaemia. It is often caused by coeliac disease, or gluten allergy.

STAPES

A stirrup-shaped bone in the middle ear, which is important for effective hearing.

STARCH

The principal food ingredient in bread, potatoes and rice. Starch is an important energy source and is made up of glucose units. It is a complex carbohydrate — *see Carbohydrates*.

STASIS

A state of stagnation or stoppage in the body.

STERNUM

The breast-bone. Pain in the region of the sternum is referred to as sternalgia.

STEROL

A solid, usually an unsaturated polycyclic alcohol, derived from plants or animals. Cholesterol is an example.

STOMATITIS

Inflamation of the mouth, tongue or gums, especially with ulcers.

STOOL

The solid waste material that passes through the anus. *See also Faeces.*

STRESSOR

Any factor resulting from changes in the environment, lifestyle or personal relationships which induces a stress-response. Stressors can be physical (temperature, radiation exposure), chemical or biological (pollutants, food additives, pesticides) or psychological (relationships with sexual partners, children, parents, work colleagues, etc.). Our ability to cope with stressors is likely to have a direct bearing on our state of health and well-being.

STROKE

The sudden rupture or clotting of a blood vessel in the brain, usually leading to unconsciousness or coma accompanied by partial paralysis. *See Hemiplegia.*

STYE

A small boil on the eyelid, resulting from infection at the root of an eyelash. Styes clear by themselves but may be aided by antiseptic eye ointments and vitamin B-complex dietary supplementation.

SUBCUTANEOUS TISSUE

Body tissue lying immediately under the skin.

SUCROSE

Another name for common sugar, a 12-carbon crystalline disaccharide. It is obtained from sugar cane, sugar beet or sorghum (a cane-like grass).

SUPPURATION

An accumulation of pus, such as in a festering ulcer.

SURROGATE

One who acts for another: for example, a surrogate mother or father who acts as a substitute for an infertile partner. This is a controversial role, fraught with legal and social difficulties.

SUTURE

The sewing up of a wound by means of silk, catgut, etc., in order to facilitate healing. The term also refers to the connection or seam between the flat bones of the skull.

SYMBIOSIS

A situation in which 2 different organisms dwell together for mutual benefit. The term is used in a popular sense for the positive interaction between 2 people.

SYMPATHETIC NERVOUS SYSTEM

The nerve system in the body which prepares it for the 'fight or flight' response in situations of potential threat or danger. The sympathetic nervous system is a branch of the autonomic nervous system, which governs involuntary responses, and includes the rapid speeding up of heart-rate, increase in blood pressure, and the rising of hairs on the skin during a state of alarm. *See also Autonomic nervous system.*

SYMPTOM

The outward indication of a given disease or disorder. Naturopaths are often inclined to disregard localised symptoms and treat the body as a whole, regarding disease as a manifestation of overall imbalance rather than the result of any invading micro-organism. Homeopaths, however, list symptoms in considerable detail and endeavour to match the pattern with the list of 'provings' established by Dr Samuel Hahnemann. *See also Naturopathy, Homeopathy* (Part 2).

SYNDROME

A group of symptoms, occurring together, which suggest the presence of a particular health condition or disease.

SYNERGY (or SYNERGISM)

The mutal action of substances which together increase each other's effectiveness.

SYNOVIA

A fluid, resembling the white of an egg, which is secreted from glands in the joints of the body.

SYNOVIAL MEMBRANES

The lining of the joints. Inflammation of one of these membranes is referred to as synovitis.

SYSTEMIC

That which affects or supplies the system or body as a whole, or a particular system of body organs.

SYSTEMIC CIRCULATION

Circulation of blood through the body vessels.

SYSTOLE

The periodic muscular contraction of the heart and arteries for the purpose of expelling blood and assisting the circulation.

SYSTOLIC PRESSURE —
see Sphygmomanometry

T

TACHOMETER

A scientific instrument for measuring the velocity of moving substances, such as running water. It can also be used to measure blood circulation.

TACHYCARDIA

A fast heartbeat. This is usually an abnormal heart condition.

T-CELLS — *see T-lymphocytes*

TECHNOLOGICAL DISEASE PATTERN

Diseases found primarily in Western industrial societies, especially the so-called 'diseases of degeneration' and stress-related illnesses. Heart disease, cancer and kidney malfunction come within this category.

TENDON

The tough, non-muscular fibrous cord attaching muscle to a bone; an example is the Achilles tendon, the tendon in the heel by which the calf muscles extend the foot.

TENOSYNOVITIS

A complaint, often confused with arthritis, caused by repeated forceful movements of the fingers, wrists, elbows and ankles at high speed. This causes painful inflammation of the tendons, leading to loss of movement in the affected limb.

Tenosynovitis occurs mainly among process and component workers, machinists, typists, and cleaners whose work is predominantly repetitive. The complaint can be prevented by re-organising work tasks so that they are more varied and do not involve lengthy periods of high-speed repetitive work.

Tenosynovitis is also known as repetitive strain injury (RSI).

TERATOGENESIS

The formation of physical defects in the foetus while it is developing in the womb. Such offspring are deformed at birth. *See also Teratoma.*

TERATOMA

An abnormal tumour consisting of many different tissues. *See also Teratogenesis.*

TESTICLES (or TESTES)

The 2 male reproductive glands within the scrotum which correspond to the ovaries in the female.

TETANY

Convulsions or muscle spasms sometimes caused by calcium deficiency, disease of the parathyroid glands or, in the case of infants, vitamin D deficiency.

A mild state of tetany is produced during rebirthing, a therapy which is characterised by a continuous breathing cycle that reduces oxygen intake to the brain. Rebirthers maintain that during the onset of tetany, subconscious traumatic memories may manifest in consciousness and that the subject can 'work through' this state to a profound catharsis, or emotional release. *See also Rebirthing* (Part 2), *Parathyroids.*

THIAMINE — *see Vitamin B1*

THORAX

The chest cavity containing the heart and lungs. It is the section of the body between the neck and abdomen. *See also Thoracic segment* (Part 2).

THREONINE

An essential amino acid important for balancing the exchange of amino acids. It is found in carrot, alfalfa, leafy green vegetables and pawpaw (papaya).

THROMBIN

A substance in the blood which causes coagulation or blood clots.

THROMBOCYTES

Platelets found in the blood which are important for the process of clotting.

THROMBOSIS

The formation of a blood clot in a vein or artery. *See also Atherosclerosis.*

THROMBUS

A blood clot occurring within a blood vessel.

THYMOSIN

A hormone which is secreted by the thyroid gland and assists the production of lymphocytes — small cells which become white blood corpuscles.

THYMUS

A small ductless gland located in the upper part of the chest. It gradually decreases in size and disappears at puberty. It nevertheless plays an important role in the immunological system, generating T-lymphocytes — *see T-lymphocytes*.

THYROID

The ductless gland located in the neck beside the trachea. It secretes hormones which help control the body's metabolism and which also affect such factors as physique and temperament. *See also Thyroxin.*

THYROXIN

A hormone secreted by the thyroid gland. Thyroxin contains a substantial amount of iodine, and a deficiency of the hormone may be responsible for such conditions as cretinism or obesity.

THYROXINE

A non-essential amino acid important for regulating metabolism and controlling the thyroid and pituitary glands. Food sources include kelp, carrot, celery, spinach, tomato and pineapple.

TIBIA

The inner bone located between the knee and ankle in the leg. It is often known as the shin bone. *See also Fibula.*

TINNITUS

A continuous ringing in the ears, often caused by catarrh or middle-ear infection. It is difficult to cure except in cases where there is a removable nerve tumour.

TISSUE, BODY — *see Body tissue*

T-LYMPHOCYTES

Cells which serve in the body as the main mechanism of cellular immunity. T-lymphocytes are produced by the thymus gland and combat viruses, bacteria, foreign cells, allergens and fungi which have invaded the body. T-lymphocytes contain a high level of vitamin C and their efficient functioning in the body is important in resisting a variety of degenerative diseases, as well as inhibiting the ageing process.

TOCOPHEROLS

A subgroup within the vitamin E group. Six years after the discovery of vitamin E in 1924, the first individual tocopherols were identified, although they do not occur singly in nature. By 1956 eight tocopherols had been isolated. They are insoluble in water, stable in acid, and are modified by heat, alkalis and light. *See Vitamin E.*

TONGUE DIAGNOSIS

A method of self-diagnosis in which characteristics of the tongue can be examined for B-vitamin deficiencies. The principal correlations are as follows:

Vitamin B1: tongue appears scarred
Vitamin B2: tongue is a purple or magenta colour
Vitamin B3: tongue is bright red and is accompanied by inflammation of the mouth and throat; the gums may be sore
Vitamin B5: tongue is enlarged and 'chunky'
Vitamin B6: there is a burning sensation in the mouth
Vitamin B12: tongue is smooth and shiny and is accompanied by sore mouth and throat, and also ulcerated lips.
Vitamin B-complex: tongue appears cracked and fissured; this indicates a serious vitamin B deficiency overall.

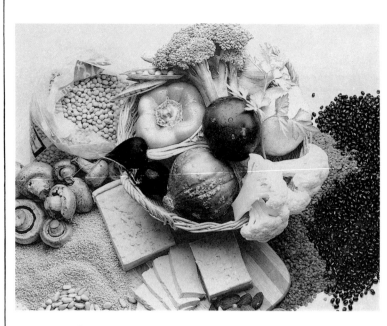

Total vegetarians eat only plant foods

TOTAL VEGETARIAN

One who abstains from eating meat, poultry, eggs, fish, dairy products and honey, and whose diet is derived solely from plants. Total vegetarians are also known as vegans — *see Veganism.*

TOXAEMIA

The presence of poisonous substances, or toxins, in the blood.

TOXICITY

A measure of degree in assessing the poisonous nature of certain substances. Toxicity is calculated as the ratio between body weight and the smallest quantity that will cause death.

TOXIN

A poison, usually of bacterial origin, capable of producing disease in the body. Some substances which are toxic in large quantities may be used as healing agents in diluted quantities because they stimulate the body's defence mechanisms. Examples are aconite and arsenic, both of which are used in minute quantities as homeopathic remedies — *see Homeopathy* (Part 2).

TRACHEA

The windpipe between the back of the throat and the lungs which is a vital organ of the respiratory system. The trachea conducts air to the lungs.

TRACHOMA

A contagious disease involving the infection of the cornea and conjunctiva of the eye. It is characterised by granulation and inflammation of the inner surface of the eye.

TRAUMA

A body injury caused by violence or aggression. It is also used to describe nervous shock and severe emotional upset.

TREMOR

An involuntary but rhythmic movement of the muscles. It is not as severe as spasm — *see Spasm.*

TRIGLYCERIDE

One of a group of edible fats and oils, a triglyceride is a fatty acid ester of the alcohol glycerol in which all 3 hydroxyl groups are joined to a fatty acid.

Trigylcerides are significant because they are associated with plaque build-up on artery walls and the possible onset of stroke or heart attack.

Normal triglyceride levels in humans range from 35 to 160 milligrams per decilitre of blood plasma. If the fats entering the system exceed the energy requirements of the body, the body adapts by producing elevated serum levels of fatty acids. These triglycerides may then be stored in the arteries, and the build-up can lead to the possibility of blockages.

Omega-3 fatty acids, found in salmon and cod-liver oil, have a unique effect on triglyceride metabolism and are recommended nutrients for people with high serum counts. Dietary fibre is also important in reducing triglyceride levels, and recommended vegetables include beans, legumes, oats and bran. High quality olive oil is also a suitable adjunct nutrient since it improves circulation. *See also Omega-3 fish oils, Fibre, dietary.*

TRYPSIN

A digestive enzyme present in the juices secreted from the pancreas. It helps to convert proteins into amino acids and has a medical application in liquefying blood clots, mucus and pus.

TRYPTOPHAN

An essential amino acid of the heterocyclic class. It is important for the generation of cells and tissues, for digestion and the eyes. Food sources include carrot, celery, fennel, brussel sprouts, spinach, alfalfa and turnips.

TUMOUR

A lump or swelling in the body tissue, which develops spontaneously. Although commonly associated with cancer, not all tumours are malignant: many are benign.

TYMPANUM

The cavity in the middle ear. The tympanic membrane is known as the eardrum, and inflammation of the middle ear is referred to as tympanitis.

TYPE A BEHAVIOUR

A behaviour pattern suggested by Californian cardiologists Dr Ray Rosenman and Dr Meyer Friedman as a correlate with the likelihood of heart disease. Type A behaviour is found in a person who is extremely competitive and aggressive, schedules more and more activities into less and less time, is in such a hurry that he or she no longer enjoys simple pleasures like the beauty of the environment, does not delegate easily, exhibits explosive speech patterns, has trouble sitting and doing nothing, and exhibits lip-clicking, head-nodding, fist-clenching and other related traits.

The Type A person may seem extremely productive in a business setting and may exude confidence, but underneath feels inferior and prone to failure.

Type A behaviour contrasts with the more relaxed style of the Type B person who can still be efficient in the work-place but is much less aggressive and rigid in style, has time for 'quality of life' pursuits and has a more peaceful manner, both professionally and at home.

TYROSINE

A non-essential amino acid of the neutral class. It is important for the development of cells, tissues and red and white corpuscles, and in the adrenal, pituitary and thyroid glands, and in the hair. Food sources include alfalfa, carrot, lettuce, asparagus, parsley, strawberries, apricots and almonds.

U

ULCER

A break in the skin or membrane, resulting in an inflamed or infected sore. Ulcers may develop in the mouth, the veins, the stomach, the duodenum and the cornea.

ULCERATIVE COLITIS

Inflammation of the colon or large intestine.

ULNA

The inner and larger of the two bones of the forearm. It is on the same side as the fifth finger.

UMBILICAL

That which relates to the umbilicus, or navel.

UMBILICAL CORD

The fibrous cord which provides the connection between the foetus and the placenta, and which is severed after birth.

UMBILICUS

The small depression or scar on the abdominal wall, which remains after the umbilical cord is severed after birth.

UNDERWEIGHT

A situation in which an individual weighs 10 per cent or more below the average weight for given height, age and sex. *See Weight-for-height ratio*.

UNSATURATED FATTY ACIDS — *see Fats*

URAEMIA

The accumulation of toxic waste substances in the blood following a malfunction of the kidneys. In a healthy person these wastes would be excreted rather than retained in the body.

URETER

One of 2 ducts in the kidney which transport urine to the bladder.

URETHRA

The duct which connects the bladder and the external orifice. Inflammation of this duct is known as urethritis.

URIC ACID

White, tasteless and odourless substance found in urine. The salts of uric acid are found in the joints of those who suffer from gout, and are a principal constituent of kidney stones.

URINARY SYSTEM

The body system consisting of the kidneys, ureters, bladder and urethra.

URINE

The fluid, normally yellowish in colour, which is secreted by the kidneys and transported through the ureters to the bladder. It is then discharged through the urethra.

UTERINE

That which relates to the uterus, or womb.

UTERUS

The womb of the female, in which the embryo develops.

UVEA

The pigmented covering of the eye. It includes the iris, ciliary body and choroid. Inflammation of the uvea is known as uveitis.

V

VAGINA

The canal which leads to the base of the uterus in the female to the external opening, or vulva. Inflammation of the vagina is known as vaginitis.

VAGUS NERVE

A cranial nerve which connects with the lungs, liver, stomach and gastrointestinal tract. Stimulation of the vagus nerve slows the heart.

VALINE

An essential amino acid important for the functioning of the corpus luteum, mammary glands and ovaries. Food sources include carrot, lettuce, celery, parsley, tomato, dandelion, green vegetables and apple.

VALVE

A membrane in a vessel of the body which allows for the flow of fluid in one direction only. Examples include the bicuspid (mitral) and tricuspid valves on the left and right side of the heart respectively.

VAS

A vessel or duct which contains blood.

VASCULAR

That which relates to the vessels or ducts which convey blood. The vascular system is the total system of blood vessels in the body.

VASOCONSTRICTOR

Any substance which causes constriction (i.e. reduction in diameter) of blood vessels in the body. *Like a boa constrictor*

VASODILATOR

Any substance which causes dilation (i.e. increase in diameter) of blood vessels in the body.

VEGANISM

A dietary practice in which no meat or animal products are consumed for strictly moral reasons. Vegans avoid any activity which flows from the killing of, or cruelty inflicted upon, animals. As a consequence the vegan diet excludes meat, fish, milk, eggs, honey, butter and other dairy foods. Vegans also avoid wearing wool or using shampoos, perfumes and soaps which have been tested on animals.

VEGETABLES

Vegetables consist primarily of carbohydrate, cellulose, fibre and water. Generally low in protein and calories, they provide vitamins, minerals and fibre, assist the digestive process, and regulate bowel activity. A person who subsists totally on vegetables is a total vegetarian. Some vegetarians eat eggs or drink milk to supplement their diet with more substantial protein and to ensure adequate vitamin B12, which is not usually found in vegetarian foods. *See Vegetarian diet, separate vegetable listings.*

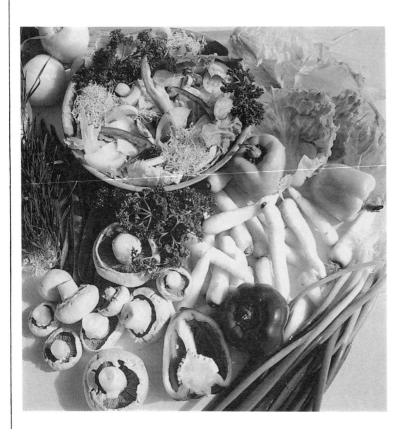

*The vegan philosophy
highlights respect for animals*

VEGETARIAN DIET

A diet in which plant foods are eaten, but fish and meat are generally excluded. Some vegetarians eat eggs and dairy products, often specifically for vitamin B12 intake, but others exclude them altogether. A vegetarian diet of the latter type resembles veganism, although the vegan philosophy is guided primarily by non-violence towards animals, whereas one can be a vegetarian strictly for nutritional rather than moral reasons. A recent Australian survey by Dr Tony Helman, comparing 50 meat-eaters (or omnivores) with 120 vegetarians of similar age, showed that vegetarians had higher levels of serum carotene, folate and vitamins B2, C and E, but lower levels of vitamin B12, B1 and ferritin. The highest vitamin levels among the vegetarians was found among those who consumed wholegrains and pulses in addition to fruit, vegetables and dairy products. Dr Helman's survey is one of several current research projects which will provide guidelines for a balanced vegetarian diet in the future. The positive aspects of a vegetarian diet include its high-fibre and low-fat content, but problems with B12 and iron deficiency remain with many 'new vegetarians' who have not paid sufficient attention to balancing their nutrient intake.

VEIN

A vessel in the body which receives blood from the capillaries and transports it toward the heart. Such blood is referred to as venous.

VENTRICLES

The two, thick muscular chambers of the heart. The left ventricle receives blood from the left atrium and pumps it through the aorta to the whole body; the right ventricle receives blood from the right atrium and pumps it to the lungs through the pulmonary vein. The latter is the only example of venous blood which is deoxygenated.

VERTEBRAE

The bony segments which make up the backbone, or spinal column in the human skeleton. There are 24 vertebrae, or movable bones, which connect at the base with the sacrum and coccyx. The vertebrae are divided into 4 groups. In descending order, the first 7 are known as the *cervical vertebrae*, which make up the neck; the next 12 are the *thoracic vertebrae*, which make up the upper and mid-back; the next 5 comprise the *lumbar vertebrae*, which support the weight of the upper half of the body, and the remaining vertebrae are the *sacral vertebrae*, extending down to the coccyx.

The vertebrae are separated by cushions of cartilage called intervertebral discs, which help prevent jarring and strain on the spine and on the paired nerves which branch out from the spinal column.

VESICAL

That which relates to the bladder.

VESICANT

Any substance which produces blisters on the body surface.

VILLI

Small, fine, hair-like projections which cover various membranes of the body. Villi are present in the small intestine, where they aid the digestive process.

VISCERA

The organs contained within the abdomen. These include the liver, gall bladder, stomach, kidney and gastrointestinal tract.

VITAMIN

From the Latin *vita*, 'life', one of several organic compounds, other than carbohydrate, protein and fat, which are present in food and essential for specialised body functions related to health and growth. Some vitamins are produced in the body, but others are not and must be obtained through normal dietary intake or supplements. *See separate vitamin listings.*

VITAMIN A

One of the first 2 vitamins to be discovered, in 1913. It is essential for the growth of new tissue and the health of the skin, the eyes, and the digestive and respiratory tracts. It is particularly important for children. Good sources are yellow/orange vegetables, especially carrot, leafy green vegetables such as lettuce and spinach, celery, tomatoes, peas, butter, cream, liver, egg yolks and cod-liver oil. Deficiency symptoms include 'night-blindness', eye infections, sensitivity to bright light, dry skin and acne, dull, falling hair, respiratory infections, ear problems and weight loss. There is strong evidence that people with inadequate supplies of vitamin A are more prone to certain types of cancer, particularly of the lung, breast, colon, oesophagus, reproductive organs and skin. Vitamin A is fat-soluble, so it can be stored in the body. Large doses can be toxic and it is usually possible to obtain an adequate supply by eating the right foods. For example, a really fresh raw carrot can supply 11 000 international units, over twice the daily requirement. However, commercially fertilised stored vegetables will develop nitrites which interfere with the body's ability to convert plant carotene to usable vitamin A, so some people may find it necessary to take a vitamin A supplement such as cod-liver oil. People who smoke need more vitamin A. RDA: 5000 IU.

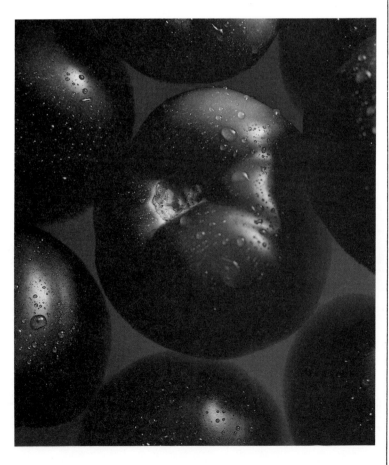

Tomatoes, a good source of vitamin A

VITAMIN ANALOG

A constituent with a chemical structure resembling a vitamin. Vitamin analogs are not true vitamins and do not necessarily act like vitamins in the human body. In some instances they may actually become antagonists to true vitamins. An example of this phenomenon is provided by spirulina, which, despite its rich range of nutrients, also contains extensive vitamin B12 analogs.

VITAMIN B1

(Thiamine, water soluble)   Vitamin B1 enables foods to be absorbed and digested, aids the appetite, promotes growth and muscle tone, inhibits pain and is connected with personal learning capacity. Deficiencies of B1 manifest as loss of appetite, muscle weakness, depression and irritability, gastric disorders, shortness of breath and slow heartbeat.

Natural sources of B1 include brewer's yeast, brown rice, fish, legumes, liver, meat, nuts, poultry, wheat germ and wholegrain cereals. Naturopaths employ B1 to treat alcoholism, anaemia, constipation, diarrhoea, diabetes, indigestion, nausea, multiple sclerosis and stress. RDA: adult, 1–1.5 mg; child, 0.5–1 mg.

VITAMIN B2

(Riboflavin, water soluble)   Vitamin B2 assists the metabolism of fat, protein and carbohydrate, increases resistance to disease, improves the quality of the skin, and aids cell respiration. Deficiencies of B2 manifest as bloodshot eyes, cracked lips, retarded growth, loss of hair, sore tongue, digestive disturbances and sensitivity to light.

Natural sources of B2 include brewer's yeast, capsicum, eggs, green leafy vegetables, legumes, milk, poultry and wholegrain cereals. Naturopaths employ B2 to treat acne, alcoholism, arthritis, baldness, cataracts, diabetes, diarrhoea, indigestion, skin disorders and stress. RDA: adult, 1.5–2 mg; child, 0.5–1 mg.

VITAMIN B3

(Niacin, water soluble) Vitamin B3 assists blood circulation, lowers blood cholesterol, aids the adrenal glands and nervous system, and helps to maintain the appetite. A B3 deficiency can cause a variety of gastrointestinal problems, including ulcers. Other symptoms may include dermatitis, fatigue, headaches, insomnia or nausea.

Natural sources of B3 include brewer's yeast, eggs, fish, legumes, liver, meat, peanuts, rice, bran, wheat germ and wholegrain cereals. Naturopaths use B3 to treat acne, arthritis, baldness, diarrhoea, halitosis, high blood pressure, leg cramps, migraines, schizophrenia, stress and tooth decay. It may also help those who are giving up smoking to recover from withdrawal symptoms. RDA: adult, 10–18 mg (depending on protein intake).

VITAMIN B5

(Pantothenic acid, water soluble) Vitamin B5 raises blood histamine levels, helps maintain healthier skin and hair, aids the liver and nervous system, and assists in the production of antibodies. Symptoms of B5 deficiency include increased susceptibility to allergies and infection, cramps, asthma, chronic fatigue, irritability and sleep disturbances. Premature greyness can also be associated with vitamin B5 deficiency.

Natural sources of B5 include beans, brewer's yeast, egg yolks, legumes, liver, oranges, peanuts, wheat germ, and wholegrain cereals.

Naturopaths use B5 to treat a variety of allergies, arthritis, baldness, cystitis, duodenal ulcers, eczema, fatigue, hypoglycaemia, indigestion, bowel problems, kidney ailments and tooth decay. RDA: 5–10 mg.

VITAMIN B6

(Pyridoxine, water soluble) Vitamin B6 helps maintain healthy teeth and gums, assists antibody formation, and is also active in DNA synthesis. It assists weight control through utilising fats and proteins. Symptoms of B6 deficiency include loss of appetite, sleepiness, convulsions, dermatitis, conjunctivitis, muscular weakness, kidney stones, and sore tongue and lips.

Natural sources of B6 include avocados, bananas, brewer's yeast, cabbage, corn oil, fish, green leafy vegetables, legumes, oranges, meat, peanuts, prunes, raisins, soya beans, walnuts, wheat germ and wholegrain cereals.

Naturopaths use B6 to treat arthritis, eczema, hypoglycaemia, muscular disorders, nausea in pregnancy, and rheumatism. RDA: 1.5–2 mg (depending on protein intake).

VITAMIN B9 — *see Folic acid*

VITAMIN B12

(Cyanocobalamin, water soluble) Vitamin B12 assists in maintaining appetite, in the biosynthesis of nucleic acids and proteins, and in the formation of red blood cells. It also helps facilitate the metabolism of fat, protein and carbohydrate, assists in the maintenance of a healthy nervous system, and counteracts cell degeneration. Symptoms of deficiency include anaemia, loss of appetite, fatigue, irritation, schizophrenia and difficulties with either walking or talking.

Natural sources of B12 include cheese, egg yolk, meat, fish, milk, kidney, liver, yeast, fermented soya beans and some sea-vegetables. Naturopaths use B12 to treat alcoholism, allergies, anaemia, arthritis, bronchial asthma, epilepsy, hepatitis, hypoglycaemia, insomnia and shingles. RDA: 0.1–0.5 mg.

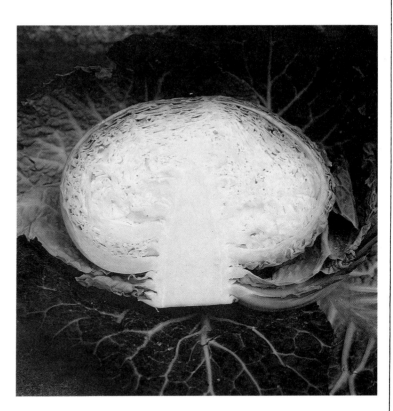

Cabbage contains vitamin B6

VITAMIN B13 — *see Orotic acid*

VITAMIN B15 — *see Pangamic acid*

VITAMIN B17 — *see Laetrile*

VITAMIN C

(Ascorbic acid, water soluble) Vitamin C is required for red blood cell formation, the healthy growth of bones and teeth, cholesterol metabolism, the healing of burns and wounds, and the building of body resistance to shock and infection. It is also an important antioxidant and helps increase iron absorption. Symptoms of deficiency include anaemia, bleeding or spongy gums, low resistance to infection, muscle degeneration, tender joints and sallow complexion.

Vitamin C occurs naturally in blackcurrants, capsicum, chilli, citrus fruits, green vegetables, pineapple, potatoes and rosehips. Naturopaths use vitamin C to treat alcoholism, allergies, atherosclerosis, arthritis, cystitis, heart disease, hepatitis, hypoglycaemia, sinusitis and tooth decay, as well as in megadoses to treat the common cold (a suggestion proposed by Dr Linus Pauling). RDA: adult, 70 mg; child, 20 mg.

VITAMIN D

(Cholecalciferol, fat soluble)   Vitamin D is required for blood clotting, heart and muscle action, the metabolism of calcium and phosphorus, tooth formation and bone growth. Symptoms of deficiency include bone deformities, cramps, dental caries, muscular weakness, and an unstable nervous condition.

Vitamin D occurs naturally in egg yolk, fish-liver oils, margarine, milk and sprouted seeds, and is also produced in the body following the action of sunlight on 7-dehydrocholesterol in the skin.

Naturopaths use vitamin D to treat acne, alcoholism, allergies, arthritis, bone fractures, conjunctivitis, cystitis, diabetes, eczema, high blood cholesterol, rickets and tooth decay. RDA: 400 IU.

Sprouts, a source of vitamin D

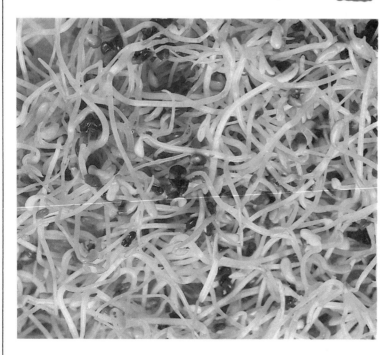

VITAMIN E

(Tocopherol, fat soluble) Vitamin E retards the ageing process, aids fertility and the circulation of the blood, helps maintain the nerves, and assists in reducing blood cholesterol. It also helps prevent the hardening of arteries. Symptoms of deficiency include dull hair, an enlarged prostate gland, muscular weakness, sterility and (in women) miscarriages.

Vitamin E occurs naturally in butter, egg yolk, fruits, nuts, vegetable oils and wheat germ. Naturopaths use vitamin E to treat arthritis, atherosclerosis, burns, baldness, cystitis, diabetes, liver problems, migraines, sinusitis and varicose veins. RDA: 12–18 IU.

VITAMIN-ENRICHED FOODS

Foods such as white flour which have much of their nutritional value removed by the refining process, but which are then 'enriched' by having vitamins and minerals added to them. It is generally considered that although white flour is nutritionally inferior to wholegrain flour, the enrichment process of adding B vitamins (thiamine, riboflavin and niacin) and iron to white flour substantially increases its food value.

VITAMIN F

A term used for a group of unsaturated fatty acids (UFA) which occur naturally in wheat-germ oil, sunflower seed oil and olive oil, as well as in some fish liver oils. Frying destroys unsaturated fats, and a diet of deep-fried foods may result in UFA deficiency — leading to psoriasis or ulcers and some types of arteriosclerosis. *See Fats.*

VITAMIN H — *see Biotin*

VITAMIN K

(Menadione, fat soluble) Vitamin K is essential for the production of prothrombin, a co-enzyme required for effective blood clotting. Symptoms of deficiency include bleeding under the skin, nosebleeds and diarrhoea.

Vitamin K occurs naturally in alfalfa, green vegetables, potatoes, kelp, eggs, bran and wheat germ. It can also be manufactured in the intestines under normal conditions. Supplements of vitamin K may be given to women in childbirth to prevent haemorrhages, to people suffering from coeliac, liver or pancreatic diseases, or to those with intestinal infections. RDA: not established.

VITAMIN SUPPLEMENT

A tablet or capsule containing a prescribed quantity of a specific vitamin which may be taken to supplement dietary deficiency. The recommended dietary allowance, or RDA, provides a guideline for daily intake. *See separate vitamin listings.*

VITILIGO

White patches of skin. Vitiligo is often caused by deficiency of PABA (para-aminobenzoic acid), which is actually a sun-blocking agent used in suntan lotions. Vitiligo can not be actually reversed, but supplementation with high potency B-complex vitamins (including PABA) will help prevent the condition from worsening.

VITREOUS HUMOUR

A clear, jelly-like substance which fills the eyeball behind the lens.

VOLUNTARY MUSCLES

Those muscles in the body which are under conscious control.

VULVA

The external opening in the female genitalia which leads into the vagina.

W

WART

A small, hard, persistent skin growth which often remains for several months or even years. Warts are caused by viral infection and may be found on the face, fingers and feet, or around the genitals or anus (in the case of venereal disease).

WATER BALANCE

The balance between intake and output of water in the body. Water is supplied to the body in food and beverages and excreted through the kidneys (in urine), the skin (in sweat), the lungs (in expired air), and from the digestive system (through faeces and saliva). Water intake should equal water output for a state of health to be maintained.

WEIGHT-FOR-HEIGHT RATIO

In many modern industrial countries, overweight and obesity are increasing problems as a result of prevalent sedentary lifestyles. Overweight and obesity increase the risk of heart disease, stroke and various other degenerative diseases, and it is clear that maintaining a healthy weight reduces one's risk of becoming sick or dying prematurely.

The following table, proposed by the National Health and Medical Research Council, is a guideline for men and women over the age of 18 years. The table lists height in centimetres on the left and the figure on the right shows body weight within the acceptable range for that height. Both the height and weight levels should be measured without shoes.

ACCEPTABLE WEIGHTS-FOR-HEIGHTS

Height (in cm, without shoes)	Body weight (in kg in light clothing, without shoes)
140	39–49
142 (4 ft 8 in)	40–50 (6 st 3 lb–7 st 9 lb)
144	41–52
146	43–53
148	44–55
150	45–56
152	46–58
154	47–59
156	49–61
158 (5 ft 2 in)	50–62 (7 st 9 lb–9 st 1 lb)
160	51–64
162	52–66
164	54–67
166	55–69
168	56–71
170	58–72
172	59–74
174 (5 ft 8½ in)	61–76 (9 st–12 st)
176	62–77
178	63–79
180	65–81
182	66–83
184	68–85
186	69–86
188 (6 ft 2 in)	71–88 (11 st–13 st 9 lb)
190	72–90

WHEAT

A widely grown grain used in the production of cereals and bread in many countries of the world. Wheat accounts for nearly 90 per cent of cereal usage and contains 5 proteins known as glutenin, gliadin, albumin, globulin and proteose. Of these, the first 2 provide around 80 per cent of the total protein which forms the gluten. Other constituents of wheat include calcium, iron, zinc, vitamin B1, vitamin B2 and folic acid. Wheat germ and wheat bran are the most nutritious wheat products and are excellent sources of dietary fibre. *See also Bread.*

WHEAT GERM

That part of the wheat kernel capable, when planted, of developing into a wheat plant. Wheat germ is one of the most nutritious parts of wholegrain wheat cereals — *see Wheat.*

WHITE BLOOD CELLS

Cells in the blood which help defend the body from invading micro-organisms. *See Lymphocyte, Macrophages.*

WHOLEFOOD

A food which is in a natural state and has, ideally, been grown in an environment free of chemicals, pesticides and weedkillers. Wholefoods include vegetables, fruit, grains, edible seeds and nuts. The refining of some wholefoods — like wheat and cane sugar — removes certain vitamins, amino acids and trace minerals, and also reduces fibre content. *See also Raw food, Vegetarian diet, Macrobiotics.*

WHOOPING COUGH

An infectious respiratory disease of the mucous membrane which lines the air passages. The condition is characterised by recurring bouts of convulsive coughing interspersed with a loud 'whoop', or drawing-in of the breath.

X

XANTHELASMA (or XANTHOMA)

A skin disease characterised by the formation of yellow patches, especially around the eyelids. It is caused by a disorder in fat metabolism leading to fatty deposits in the skin.

Y

Y CHROMOSOME

The chromosome in the genetic structure which leads an embryo to develop into a male of the species.

YEASTS

Organisms which enter the food chain primarily as a result of their association with vegetables, fruits and cereals.

Food yeasts arise as natural fermentations and are used in many ways — to leaven breads, to carbonate beer and champagne, as flavourings resulting from the formation of fruity esters and organic acids, and as nutrients in food — for they are rich in vitamins and protein.

Only a few species of yeast are used in food or in the fermentation process. The species *Saccharomyces cerevisiae* (baker's yeast, brewer's yeast) is associated with molasses, various grains and grape juice, and *Kluyveromyces marxianus* (dairy yeast) with the milk sugar derived from whey.

Yeasts contribute substantially to the protein value of fermented foods, and the food value of bread is greatly enhanced by yeast protein because it includes the essential amino acid lysine.

Nutritional forms of yeast include the following micrograms of B-complex vitamins per gram: thiamine 60–100, riboflavin 35–50, niacin 300–500, biotin 1–2, pyridoxine 25–30, pantothenic acid 70, and folic acid 13.

Yeast is not a source of vitamins A or C. However, it does contain a number of minerals, especially potassium and phosphorus, and approximately half its dried weight consists of vegetable protein.

Not all yeasts are desirable and some species are contaminants. *Candida albicans*, for example, has been identified as the cause of candidiasis, or thrush fungus. Fortunately, it is destroyed by heat — and does not occur in heat-processed foods.

YOGHURT

A dairy product noted for its regulatory effect on the digestive system and its high nutritional value. Natural yoghurt contains vitamin A, calcium, phosphorus, potassium and sodium, and also carbohydrates and protein. Yoghurt may be eaten with a variety of other foods, including wholegrain cereals, honey, fruits, salads and sprouts.

Z

ZINC

An important mineral which is an essential constituent of many enzymes involved in digestion and metabolism. Much of the zinc content in food is not absorbed, as zinc cannot be stored and used later by the body, so it is important to have a regular adequate supply in the diet. Although zinc deficiencies have been known in farm animals for many years, it is only since the 1960s that they have been recognised in humans. Symptoms include stunted growth and delayed sexual maturity, birth defects, sterility, slow healing of wounds, acne, hair loss, fatigue, aching joints, diabetes and general weakening of the immune system. Zinc deficiency is common in alcoholics. Good sources of zinc are brewer's yeast, wheat germ, unfrozen green leafy vegetables, nuts, eggs, legumes, seafood, liver, milk, sunflower seeds and mushrooms. Pregnant and lactating women need more zinc than the recommended adult dose of 15 mg a day.

ZYGOTE

The fertilised egg, or ovum, in the state just before it begins to divide and multiply.

TREATMENTS FOR COMMON HEALTH PROBLEMS

A

ACNE

This is often thought to be caused by a deficiency of vitamins A, B complex or F, or of the minerals potassium and zinc. Sufficient quantities of these vitamins and minerals are needed for healthy cell growth and development, and for the removal of unnecessary fats. It is possible to increase the quantities of these substances in the diet either by taking regular vitamin and mineral supplements in tablet form, applying them as ointments or in injections, or by eating extra amounts of certain foods. Brewer's yeast, blackstrap molasses, wheat germ and sunflower seeds are all rich in these important nutrients. Extra vitamin A can be obtained from carrots, butter, eggs and liver; vitamin B complex from wholegrain cereals; potassium from dates, raisins, peaches and bananas, and zinc from seafood, spinach and mushrooms.

RDA vitamin A: 5000–10 000 IU (adult); 1000–1500 IU (child).

RDA vitamin B complex: not established — draw on food sources such as blackstrap molasses, wheat germ or wholegrains.

RDA potassium: 0.8–1.3 g.

RDA zinc: 10–15 mg.

ALCOHOLISM

Alcoholics commonly have a vitamin B deficiency and may suffer from related symptoms like beri-beri (characterised by disorientation, faulty memory, ocular dysfunction and mental disturbance) and cirrhosis of the liver. The latter appears in around 10 per cent of all alcoholics and may be treated with supplements of vitamin B1 (thiamine). Between 80 and 100 per cent of alcoholics suffering from liver disorders are also likely to suffer from vitamin B6 deficiency. Excessive intake of alcohol interferes with the metabolism of vitamin B6 and its absorption from food in the stomach.

RDA vitamin B1: 1.0–1.5 mg.

RDA vitamin B6: 1.5–2 mg (depending on protein intake).

ALLERGIES

Hay fever, one of the most common allergic symptoms, can often be effectively controlled by taking extra vitamin C, which is a natural antihistamine. Research has also suggested that some allergy sufferers have a protein deficiency, and that they lack calcium. Extra vitamin A and F are often recommended to insure that the body's cells function normally and to reduce the likelihood of an abnormal, allergic reaction.

RDA vitamin A: 5000–10 000 IU (adult); 1000–1500 IU (child).

RDA vitamin C: 70 mg (Adelle Davis maintains that 500 mg serves as a preventive measure).

RDA vitamin F: 6 mg or 1.5% of calories (may be increased in this usage to 10% of calories).

ANAEMIA

It is well known that people whose blood contains insufficient iron tend to become anaemic. However anaemia can also be caused by insufficient quantities of vitamins B6 and B12, vitamin C or folic acid. These can be taken in tablet form or by eating extra amounts of certain foods such as liver, shellfish, spinach and wholegrains, supplemented by foods such as capsicums, parsley and citrus fruits, which are rich in vitamin C.

RDA vitamin B6: 1.0–1.5 mg.

RDA vitamin C: 70 mg (adult).

RDA vitamin B12: 0.1–0.5 mcg.

RDA folic acid: 400 mg.

ANOREXIA NERVOSA

According to two reports published in *Lancet* (11 August 1984 and 17 November 1984) it may be zinc deficiency which turns normal dieting into the behaviour pattern of starvation and emaciation which results in anorexia nervosa. Reduction of zinc intake impairs the zinc-dependent senses of taste and smell and correspondingly reduces the desire for food. Daily zinc supplementation over a period of a few months is likely to be effective against both anorexia nervosa and the related syndrome bulimia.

RDA zinc: 10–15 mg.

ARTHRITIS

This is a complaint which affects an enormous number of people in Western society, and the number of suggested remedies is almost as great. Small doses of vitamin B6 are considered by many to be the best way to control the pain of arthritis and reduce the inflammation. Vitamin B6 is plentiful in brewer's yeast, molasses, leafy green vegetables, wholegrains and meat. Another often recommended cure for arthritis is celery, which is said to be helpful because of its high silicon content. The most recent suggested cure, however, is an extract from the sea-cucumber, or bêche-de-mer, which is high in minerals and protein. Taken internally over a period of 6 weeks, the extract is said to reduce pain in 70 per cent of patients.

ASTHMA

Many people believe that patients suffering from asthma can improve their condition by changing their diet. Research by a Canadian doctor, Carl Reich, showed that many asthma sufferers improved when they took supplements of vitamins A and D in the form of cod-liver oil, as well as extra bone meal to rectify any mineral deficiencies, particularly of calcium. Other nutritionists have claimed that patients also benefit from extra vitamin B12 and F, and from supplements of manganese. Scientists in Nigeria reported decreases in the severity of asthma attacks when their patients were given 1000 mg of vitamin C daily.
RDA vitamin A: 5000–10 000 IU (adult); 1000–1500 IU (child).
RDA vitamin D: 400 IU.

ATHEROSCLEROSIS

People with high levels of cholesterol in their blood are generally considered to be more at risk, and for many years have been advised to avoid eating high cholesterol foods such as egg yolks. More recently it has been suggested that atherosclerosis may be due to deficiencies of vitamin B6 and chromium, which help to break down the fats that would otherwise be deposited on the artery walls. Increased consumption of foods such as brewer's yeast and wholegrain cereals, both rich in vitamin B6 and chromium, can be very helpful for people who are at risk of developing atherosclerosis.

RDA vitamin B6: 1.0–1.5 mg.
RDA chromium: trace elements only.

ATHLETE'S FOOT *(Tinea)*

This uncomfortable infection is usually treated by careful washing and drying and application of a medicated foot powder. Some people believe that extra vitamin A will increase the body's resistance to this infection. Vitamin A is readily available in cod-liver oil, liver, capsicums, carrots, spinach and butter.
RDA vitamin A: 5000–10 000 IU (adult); 1000–1500 IU (child).

B

BACKACHE

While back pain may often require treatment from a chiropractor, osteopath or physiotherapist, good nutrition can also help. Vitamin C helps produce collagen — the supporting tissue found between the bones — and a deficiency may have led to back weakness in the first place. RDA vitamin C: 70 mg (Dr James Greenwood of Baylor University College of Medicine, USA, recommends 500–1000 mg specifically for back pain).

BLEEDING GUMS

This condition may be caused by a deficiency of vitamin C, which can result in weak or spongy gums. Vitamin C supplementation should help to strengthen the cellular tissues.
RDA vitamin C: 70 mg.

BODY ODOUR

This may derive from a variety of factors related to disease in the body, sweat function and the excretion of toxins. Sometimes body odour results from vitamin B12 deficiency since this vitamin is involved in the efficient metabolism of fat, protein and carbohydrates, and in the health of the nervous system.
RDA vitamin B12: 0.1–0.5 mcg.

BRONCHITIS

Bronchitis — inflammation of the bronchi — often results from upper respiratory infection and may be associated with a deficiency of vitamins A and C. Both vitamins help the body to resist infection and vitamin C is particularly effective against colds — which may lead to bronchitis.

RDA vitamin A: 5000–10 000 IU (adult); 1000–1500 IU (child).

RDA vitamin C: 70 mg (adult); 20 mg (child).

BULIMIA — *see Anorexia nervosa*

C

CANCER

Cancer is a disease involving many factors but it appears that diet is a major cause of cancer — possibly even greater than the cumulative effects of smoking, X-rays and chemicals. The diet of affluent Western society includes excessive intake of saturated fat, refined carbohydrates, salt and alcohol, and reduced intake of unprocessed carbohydrate (found in cereal grains, fruit and vegetables). High fat intake increases the prospect of breast and colon cancer, while increased rates of bowel cancer appear to be associated with diets low in fibre and high in animal fats.

The ideal 'preventive' diet encompasses fresh fruit and vegetables, high-fibre foods, skinless poultry, fish, less alcohol, no cigarettes, and a reduction in the intake of fat, sugar and salt. The so-called Bristol Diet, developed by Dr Alec Forbes (former head of the Bristol Cancer Help Centre in England) allows no coffee, tea or salt, and eliminates all foods which are smoked, bottled, canned, preserved, artificially flavoured or coloured. Wholegrains are taken with every meal and 70 per cent of the diet consists of raw food. While this may seem extreme, the broad principles which emerge as the basis of a 'cancer prevention diet' are as follows:

- Eat less fat.
- Eat more fresh fruit (especially citrus) and also more fresh vegetables (especially carotene-rich and leafy green varieties like carrots, cabbage, broccoli,

spinach and brussels sprouts).
- Eat more wholegrain cereals.
- Reduce intake of salty, smoked, sugary or pickled foods.
- Reduce or eliminate intake of alcohol.

According to research at the CSIRO's Division of Human Nutrition in Adelaide, vitamin C in the diet also seems to act as a protective agent against cancer.

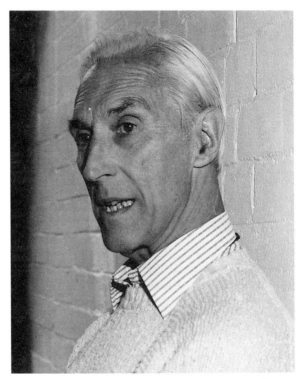

Dr Alec Forbes, who developed the Bristol Diet for cancer sufferers

CAPILLARY WALL RUPTURES

A weakness in the capillary walls may be due to a deficiency of vitamin C since this nutrient has a specific effect in maintaining the health of blood vessel walls and connective tissue.

RDA vitamin C: 70 mg (adult); 20 mg (child).

CATARACTS

Cataracts can be caused by a variety of factors, including toxaemia, inflammatory or nutritional disturbances, and continued exposure to ultraviolet rays. Opacity of the lens is often related to vitamin B2 deficiency, and supplementation of this nutrient

may help. Dr Lewis Sydenstricker of the University of Georgia Hospital, USA, treated many patients with vitamin B2 and was able to reverse the condition; treatment lasted for 9 months.
RDA vitamin B2: 1.5 mg (Dr Sydenstricker's RDA: 15 mg).

COLDS

Colds result from viral infection which affects the respiratory mucous membrane at a time of low body resistance. Vitamin C helps to protect against colds, although megadosing with this vitamin is still regarded as controversial. As a preventive measure, the standard RDA should suffice.
RDA vitamin C: 70 mg (adult); 20 mg (child).

CONSTIPATION

Characterised by sluggish action of the bowels, constipation can be prevented by increasing one's intake of foods high in fibre — especially fresh, raw fruit and vegetables — and by avoiding excessive intake of refined, sugary foods. Increased intake of unprocessed natural bran helps to soften the faeces, and in general one should eat more foods containing vitamin B complex and PABA (para-aminobenzoic acid) since these help regulate the metabolism. Foods containing these nutrients include brewer's yeast, blackstrap molasses, wholegrains and liver.

CYSTITIS

Inflammation of the bladder is more likely to arise when a person is deficient in vitamins A, B complex, C, D and E. Vitamins A and C help the body to resist infection while the other vitamins collectively help to maintain the nervous system. It is generally considered best to avoid acidic foods such as tomatoes, vinegar, rhubarb, gooseberries and spinach.
RDA vitamin A: 5000–10 000 IU (adult); 1000–1500 IU (child).
RDA vitamin B complex: not established — draw on food sources like blackstrap molasses, wheat germ or wholegrains.
RDA vitamin C: 70 mg (adult); 20 mg (child).
RDA vitamin D: 400 IU.
RDA vitamin E: 12–18 IU.

D

DERMATITIS

This condition may be caused by allergic responses and emotional stress, but can also result from deficiency of vitamin B complex. Collectively, the B vitamins assist in the healthy growth of cells, metabolism and the regulation of the nervous system. All of these relate to the skin, although vitamins B2 and B5 play a special role in the naintenance of even, healthy skin.
RDA vitamin B2: 1.5–2 mg (adult); 0.5–1 mg (child).
RDA vitamin B5: 5–10 mg.
RDA vitamin B complex: not established — draw on food sources like blackstrap molasses, wheat germ or wholegrains.

DIARRHOEA

Characterised by watery stools and frequent bowel movements, diarrhoea may simply be the result of foods that have recently been eaten which 'do not agree with the system'. However certain vitamins are related to digestive efficiency and a deficiency of these nutrients may result in diarrhoea. The vitamins are B5, D, F and K.
RDA vitamin B5: 5–10 mg.
RDA vitamin D: 400 IU.
RDA vitamin F: 6 g.
RDA vitamin K: not established — draw on food sources like green leafy vegetables, yoghurt, safflower oil or wheat germ.

E

ECZEMA

Associated with scaly, crusty skin, this form of inflammation may be psychosomatic in origin but is often due to a deficiency of vitamins B5, F and inositol — all of which relate to the metabolism and the growth of new skin cells. Infantile eczema is often caused by an allergic reaction to cow's milk and may be cured by changing to goat's milk.
RDA vitamin B5: 5–10 mg.

RDA vitamin F: 6 g.

RDA inositol: not established — draw on food sources like citrus fruits, brewer's yeast, milk, vegetables and lecithin.

F

FATIGUE

Weariness and lack of energy can, of course, be psychosomatic — a negative emotional response to a specific task or situation. However it may also result from nutritional deficiencies — specifically vitamins A and B complex and the minerals phosphorus and zinc. These nutrients assist the metabolic functioning of the body and the conversion of energy into muscular activity.

RDA vitamin A: 5000–10 000 IU (adult); 1000–1500 IU (child).

RDA vitamin B complex: not established — draw on food sources like blackstrap molasses, wheat germ or wholegrains.

RDA phosphorus: 0.6–1.2 g.

RDA zinc: 10–15 mg.

G

GALLSTONES

Gallstones form in the bladder or bile ducts as a result of the insufficient metabolism of fats. As a preventive measure, increase the intake of vegetables and fresh fruit (particularly citrus) and reduce the intake of high-cholesterol foods. Vitamin F is also beneficial because it reduces cholesterol levels and thus helps to prevent the formation of gallstones. This vitamin occurs naturally in corn, safflower, soy and sunflower seed oils and also in wheat germ.

RDA vitamin F: 6 g (or approximately 1.5% of calories).

GASTRITIS

Inflammation of the stomach can arise from overeating, infection or excess consumption of alcohol. Vitamin B complex and vitamin C help to prevent inflammation of the stomach and the latter also assists the digestive process. Small, easily digested meals should be eaten regularly, and fried, fatty or highly seasoned foods should be avoided.

RDA vitamin B complex: not established — draw on food sources like blackstrap molasses, wheat germ or wholegrains.

RDA vitamin C: 70 mg (adult); 20 mg (child).

GOITRE — *see Hypothyroidism*

H

HAEMORRHAGE

Excessive bleeding can arise either externally or internally, and may result from a lack of vitamin K, the principal role of which is to promote blood clotting. Deficiency of vitamin C will also exacerbate the effect.

RDA vitamin K: not established — draw on food sources like alfalfa, bran, eggs, green vegetables, safflower oil, yoghurt and wheat germ.

RDA vitamin C: 70 mg (adult); 20 mg (child).

HIGH BLOOD PRESSURE

High blood pressure is a risk factor for heart attacks, strokes and kidney disease. High blood pressure itself may in part be caused by eating too much salt; in modern Western society people eat 4 or 5 times more salt than is necessary. One of the solutions is to eat more rice — a food containing very little sodium but which adds 'bulk' to one's diet. Rice can be complemented by flavoursome herbs, spices and vegetables. Another approach is to eat more dairy products — thereby increasing the intake of calcium. According to Professor David McCarron of Oregon Health Sciences University, USA, people with high blood pressure have, on average, only 80 per cent of the calcium levels of healthy individuals. Calcium intake of less than 300 mg per day brings an 11–14 per cent risk of developing a systolic blood pressure of 160 mmHg or above. Low-fat cheese, milk and yoghurt are the best and cheapest sources of dietary calcium.

HYPERACTIVITY

Hyperactive children sleep only a few hours each day, are prone to eczema, asthma and respiratory problems, and may have difficulties related to speech, balance and learning. According to American nutritionist Dr Ben Feingold, such children should avoid food containing natural salicylates — almonds, apples, apricots, peaches, plums, prunes, tomatoes, tangerines, cucumbers, cherries, grapes and raisins. These can then be reintroduced one at a time to see if they cause problems. The British Hyperactive Children's Support Group (HACSG) recommends elimination of all food and drink containing synthetic colours and flavours. Glutamates, nitrites, nitrates and benzoic acid are also contraindicated.

HYPOGLYCAEMIA

Low blood-sugar levels lead to acute fatigue, irritability and weakness, and are the result of excess insulin. Vitamin B5 (pantothenic acid) is involved in the energy conversion of glucose, and hypoglycaemics sometimes lack vitamin B5 in their diet. Sufficient B5 helps to maintain stable blood-sugar levels. The diet should exclude all refined carbohydrates such as sugar, cakes, biscuits and soft drinks.
RDA vitamin B5: 5–10 mg.

HYPOTHYROIDISM (GOITRE)

Goitre is a condition in which the thyroid gland produces insufficient thyroxine. It is often associated with a deficiency of vitamin D and iodine. When there is an insufficient quantity of these nutrients a person may become lethargic and overweight. A certain amount of vitamin D is produced naturally in the body as a result of the action of sunlight, but the vitamin also occurs in egg yolk, fish-liver oils, milk

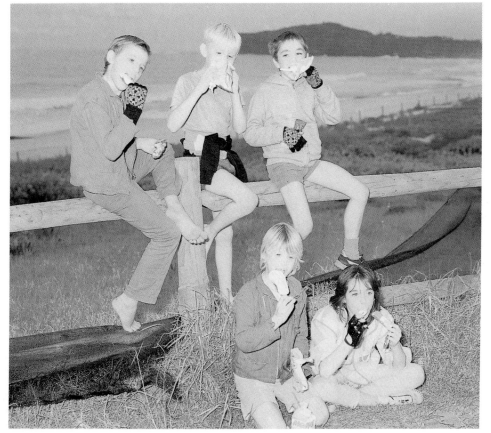

Synthetic foods may cause hyperactivity in children

and sprouted seeds. The best source of iodine is seafood or iodised salt.

RDA vitamin D: 400 IU.

RDA iodine: 100 mcg.

I

IMPOTENCE

A man's inability to achieve an erection may be the result of emotional or psychological problems, but there is a possible nutritional cause as well. Vitamin E improves male potency, possibly because of its positive effect on the blood circulation, and is regarded as an aid to fertility.

RDA vitamin E: 12–18 IU.

INFERTILITY

While infertility may be caused by a sexual malfunction or blockage, it may also be related in some instances to a deficiency of vitamin E and zinc. Vitamin E improves male potency and fertility, while zinc assists the growth and development of the sexual and reproductive organs.

RDA vitamin E: 12–18 IU.

RDA zinc: 10–15 mg.

M

MEMORY LOSS

In 1978 researchers at the National Institute of Mental Health reported that lecithin had a memory-enhancing effect. Lecithin is a primary source of choline in the diet — choline being an essential ingredient of the nerve fluid acetylcholine which helps bridge the synapses between nerve and muscle cells. It is therefore essential for the effective functioning of both the nervous system and the brain. Lecithin helps break down fatty deposits in the body,

so it is also useful in treating atherosclerosis and heart disease.

RDA lecithin: 3000 mg.

MENOPAUSE

Around 85 per cent of menopausal women experience unpleasant symptoms, including hot flushes, sweating, rheumatic aches and pains, vaginal dryness (resulting in painful sexual intercourse), depression, memory loss and other psychological or emotional problems.

While the normal treatment involves use of natural or synthetic oestrogens, there are some women who are not healthy enough to take these hormones. The herbal formulation Esten is available for women in this category, and this preparation also includes calcium, zinc and silicon in a dosage adequate to guard against osteoporosis and circulatory problems. Dr Sandra Cabot of the Women's Health Advisory Bureau in Sydney recommends the use of garlic, lecithin and vitamin E to help menopausal women overcome any potential problem with atherosclerosis. Grilled or steamed fish should also be included in the diet.

RDA vitamin E: 12–18 IU.

MIGRAINES

Migraines affect around 8 per cent of the population and a substantial percentage (around one-quarter) of all sufferers report that their migraines relate to specific foods. Chocolate is the most commonly reported offender, but other foods include cheese, citrus fruit and alcoholic drinks. Less commonly reported foods include onions, tea, coffee and seafood. Foods containing the orange-yellow colouring agent tartrazine may also precipitate migraine attacks.

Migraine sufferers aware of potential connections of this sort should avoid these foods and beverages in their diet. A healthy low-fat diet (excluding chocolate) is recommended, and the subject can test systematically whether migraine attacks appear to follow intake of cheese or alcohol. However, citrus fruits are a valuable part of the diet, supplying both nutrients and fibre, so it is unwise to exclude them unless there is a positive indication of a link with migraines.

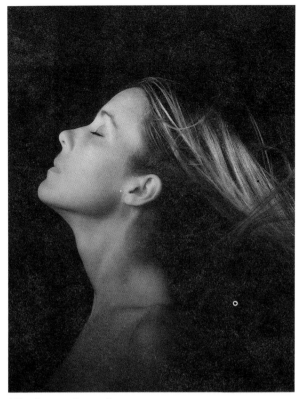

Migraines may have a dietary cause

MUSCLE CRAMPS

Muscle cramps may be caused by overexertion and fatigue, but can also result from lack of potassium since this mineral helps regulate muscle contractions and calms the nervous system. Calcium deficiency and inadequate vitamin B5 (pantothenic acid) can also cause cramps.
RDA vitamin B5: 5–10 mg.
RDA calcium: 0.4–1.3 g.
RDA potassium: 0.8–1.3 g.

N

NERVOUS TENSION

Uneasiness can often be psychosomatic in origin — the result of personal anxiety or work pressure — but it can be caused by a deficiency of vitamin B complex or vitamin C. These two nutrients facilitate the healthy functioning of the nervous system and, taken as supplements, may help to reduce nervous tension.
RDA vitamin B complex: not established — draw on food sources like blackstrap molasses, wheat germ or wholegrains.
RDA vitamin C: 70 mg (adult); 20 mg (child).

O

OBESITY

Overweight is usually caused by a combination of lethargy and overeating, but a deficiency of iodine and phosphorus can contribute to the problem. Both minerals are involved in the regulation of the metabolism and the production of energy in the body. Iodine occurs naturally in seafood and may also be taken in the form of iodised salt. Phosphorus occurs naturally in eggs, fish, poultry, milk, yoghurt and wholegrains.
RDA iodine: 100 mg.
RDA phosphorus: 0.6–1.2 g.

OSTEOPOROSIS

Eight out of 10 women are calcium deficient, and around 25 per cent of all women may develop weak and porous bones in later life. The first sign is often a broken bone or collapsed vertebra. The greatest loss of calcium occurs during the early years after menopause as a result of the lowered levels of oestrogen in the body. This corresponds to a decrease in the body's ability to incorporate calcium into bone.

As a preventive measure it is recommended that adequate calcium intake be monitored from the earlier stages of life onwards.

The RDA for children and adults is 400–800 mg, a figure which is doubled for teenagers, pregnant and lactating women. RDA for the elderly is 1000–1500 mg. One cup of milk or 35 g of cheese provide approximately 300 mg of calcium. Certain types of low-fat milk are also available with higher calcium content. High protein intake, salt, red meat and phosphorus deplete calcium levels in the body, and smoking, alcohol and coffee should also be kept to a minimum to reduce the development of osteoporosis.

Osteoporosis affects women much more markedly than men, because of hormonal differences. Men do suffer from the disease although the average man does not lose 25 per cent of his bone density until around the age of 75. By contrast 25 per cent of women aged 75 have already suffered a broken hip, wrist or crushed vertebra because of osteoporosis.

P

PHLEBITIS

Inflammation of the veins is especially common in the legs and occurs more frequently in those who are obese or who have problems with blood circulation. Vitamin E assists the circulation and may help relieve the pain caused by phlebitis.
RDA vitamin E: 12–18 IU.

PREGNANCY (Ideal Nutrition Pattern)

Additional nutrients are required during pregnancy, particularly after 20 weeks. Calcium and folate requirements double in pregnancy, and increased intake of foods rich in iron and zinc is also desirable. Milk is an ideal source of calcium, while folate occurs naturally in yeast extract, liver, bran and brussels sprouts. The best absorbed source of iron is meat, while zinc occurs in liver, kidneys, nuts and cheese.

Vegetarian pregnant women should eat additional protein and iron-rich foods (for example, peas, beans and nuts), while vegans should ideally take vitamin B12 supplements as well.
(Source: *British Medical Journal* 1985: vol. 291, pp. 263–266.)
RDA calcium (for pregnant women): 900–1300 mg.

PRE-MENSTRUAL SYNDROME (PMS)

PMS is characterised by a wide range of symptoms including irritability, anger, tension, lethargy, migraines, breast tenderness, weight gain and a feeling of being bloated. Recent medical studies con-

ducted in London and reported by the Pharmaceutical Society of Australia, indicate that vitamin B6 is effective against depression, fluid retention, irritability and breast tenderness in over half the women who suffer from pre-menstrual tension, and against headache in 80 per cent of cases. Vitamin B6 helps regulate hormonal activity in the body and it is common for a woman to become B6 deficient as additional oestrogens are produced before menstruation. The more oestrogens are released, the worse the symptoms of pre-menstrual tension become. However, taking vitamin B6 supplements, or eating foods rich in this vitamin substantially eases the problem.

The RDA for vitamin B6 in this form of supplementary treatment is 200 mg — substantially higher than the standard RDA of 1.5–2.0 mg. Foods rich in vitamin B6 include wheat germ, soya beans, peanuts, liver, yeast and citrus fruits.

PSORIASIS

This itchy skin disease can be associated with a deficiency of vitamin A — a nutrient which maintains the skin in a moist condition and helps the body to resist infection. Psoriasis can also be aggravated by a deficiency of vitamin F, which facilitates organ respiration.
RDA vitamin A: 5000–10 000 IU (adult); 1000–1500 IU (child).
RDA vitamin F: 6 g (or approximately 1.5% of calories).

R

REPETITIVE STRAIN INJURY (RSI)

RSI is characterised by constant, nagging pain in the shoulders, arms, wrists and hands, and is associated with repetitive patterns of work (for example, keying operations like typing and computer work) and jobs involving the lifting of heavy weights. A report in the *New Zealand Medical Journal* (10 June 1985) suggests that RSI may be related to subtle reactions in the body between magnesium and fluoride. Magnesium deficiency may result in nerve and muscle disorders accompanied by over-excitability, tremors, con-

vulsions or depression. Approximately 60 per cent of magnesium in the body is stored in the bones and, if the cells suffer a shortage, normally it is transported by the blood to the depleted area. However in some circumstances fluoride may react with magnesium, binding it to the bone and preventing its passage to other parts of the body. This suggests that some forms of RSI may be skeletal fluorosis. Intake of fluoride should not exceed 3 mg per day, but it is not uncommon for RSI sufferers to register higher levels than this. One way to cut fluoride intake is to use de-ionised, distilled or low-fluoride water for drinking and cooking. Increased intake of magnesium-rich foods is also recommended. Good sources include soya beans, brewer's yeast, brazil nuts, peanuts, cashews, almonds and wholewheat flour.
RDA magnesium: 0.35–0.45 g.

RHEUMATISM

Related to arthritis, rheumatism is a condition in which the joints, bones and supporting tissues become inflamed. The degenerative process of ageing is the major cause, but nutritional deficiencies of vitamins B6, C and D, as well as calcium, can aggravate the problem. Vitamin B6 helps to regulate the nervous system and vitamin C is required for the production of collagen — the basic tissue in bones. Vitamin D also promotes bone growth.
RDA vitamin B6: 1.5–2.0 mg.
RDA vitamin C: 70 mg (adult).
RDA vitamin D: 400 IU

S

SINUSITIS

Inflammation of the sinuses can be treated with antihistamines, but may be aided by vitamin A since this nutrient helps repair tissue and reduces inflammation and infection. Vitamin A occurs naturally in green vegetables like broccoli and spinach, and in reddish vegetables like raw carrots. It is also present in milk, liver and spirulina.
RDA vitamin A: 5000–10 000 IU (adult); 1000–1500 IU (child).

SKIN WOUNDS

Inadequate intake of proteins and certain specific vitamins affects the healing of skin wounds. Protein deficiency reduces and delays the rejuvenation process and inhibits the synthesis of collagen, while inadequate vitamin C prevents the formation of collagen fibrils which normally mature to produce new tissue at the location of the injury. Vitamin B5 (pantothenic acid) is also important in treating skin wounds, burns, nipple fissures, nappy rash and skin ulcers.
RDA vitamin C: 70 mg (adult); 20 mg (child).
RDA vitamin B5: 5–10 mg.

STROKE — *see Atherosclerosis*

T

TONSILLITIS

Inflammation of the throat area can be caused by infection, by environmental pollutants in the air, or by overusing one's voice. Vitamin C serves as a preventive and can also help minimise the risk that more acute infection might follow the sore throat.
RDA vitamin C: 70 mg (adult); 20 mg (child).

V

VARICOSE VEINS

Varicose veins may result from poor circulation, but can also arise as a consequence of vitamin F deficiency. The principal role of this vitamin is to facilitate efficient blood flow by preventing hardening of the arteries and regulating blood pressure.
RDA vitamin F: 6 g (or approximately 1.5% of calories).

BIBLIOGRAPHY

Selected sources for further reading

GENERAL

BERKELEY HOLISTIC HEALTH CENTRE. *The Holistic Health Handbook.* And/Or Press, Berkeley, California, 1978.

CARLSON, R. J. *The Frontiers of Science and Medicine.* Regnery, Chicago, 1975.

EAGLE, R. *Alternative Medicine.* Futura, London, 1978.

FADIMAN, J., AND FRAGER, R. *Personality and Personal Growth.* Harper & Row, New York, 1976.

FULDER, S. *The Handbook of Complementary Medicine.* Hodder & Stoughton, London, 1984.

GROSSINGER, R. *Planet Medicine.* Doubleday, New York, 1980.

HALL, D. *The Natural Health Book.* Nelson, Melbourne, 1974.

HILL, A. *A Visual Encyclopaedia of Unconventional Medicine.* Crown, New York, 1979.

HORNE, R. *The New Health Revolution.* Happy Landings Publications, Sydney, 1983.

HULKE, M. *The Encyclopaedia of Alternative Medicine and Self-Help.* Rider, London, 1978.

KRIPPNER, S., AND VILLOLDO, A. *The Realms of Healing.* Celestial Arts, Millbrae, California, 1976.

LAW, D. *A Guide to Alternative Medicine.* Turnstone, London, 1974.

REGUSH, N. M. *Frontiers of Healing.* Avon, New York, 1977.

SHEPHARD, B. D., AND SHEPHARD, C. A. *The Complete Guide to Women's Health.* New American Library, New York, 1985.

STANWAY, A. *Alternative Medicine.* Rigby, Adelaide, 1979.

STANWAY, A. (ed). *The Natural Family Doctor.* Century, London, 1987.

ACUPUNCTURE

ACADEMY OF TRADITIONAL CHINESE MEDICINE. *An Outline of Chinese Acupuncture.* Foreign Language Press, Peking, 1975.

CROIZIER, R. C. *Traditional Medicine in Modern China.* Harvard University Press, Cambridge, Massachusetts, 1968.

DUKE, M. *Acupuncture.* Harcourt Brace Jovanovich, New York, 1977.

LOW, R. *The Acupuncture Atlas and Reference Book.* Thorsons, Wellingborough, 1985.

MACDONALD, A. *Acupuncture.* Allen & Unwin, London, 1982.

MANN, F. *Acupuncture, the Ancient Chinese Art of Healing.* Heinemann, London, 1962.

MANN, F. *The Meridians of Acupuncture.* Heinemann, London, 1964.

MANN, F. *Treatment of Disease by Acupuncture.* Heinemann, London, 1967.

SEASON, S. M. WONG. *The Basic Knowledge of Acupuncture and Moxibustion.* Commercial Press, Hong Kong, 1975.

STIEFVATER, E. W. *What is Acupuncture?* Health Science Press, Sussex, 1962.

TAI, D. *Acupuncture & Moxibustion.* Gower Medical Publishing, London, 1987.

ALEXANDER TECHNIQUE

ALEXANDER, F. M. *Alexander Technique.* Thames and Hudson, London, 1974.

BARKER, S. *The Alexander Technique.* Bantam, New York, 1978.

BARLOW, W. *The Alexander Technique.* Random House, New York, 1973.

BYLES, M. B. *Stand Straight Without Strain.* Fowler, Essex, 1978.

MAISEL, E. *The Resurrection of the Body.* University Books, New York, 1969.

AROMATHERAPY

LAUTIE, R., AND PASSEBECQ, A. *Aromatherapy.* Thorsons, Northamptonshire, 1979.

MAURY, M. *The Secret of Life and Youth.* Macdonald, London, 1964.

RYMAN, D. *The Aromatherapy Handbook.* Century, London, 1984.

TISSERAND, R. B. *The Art of Aromatherapy.* C. W. Daniel, London, 1977.

ASTROLOGY

CULPEPER, N. *Astrological Judgment of Disease.* American Foundation of Astrologers, Tempe, USA, nd.

GARRISON, O. *Medical Astrology.* Warner, New York, 1971.

GAUQUELIN, M. *The Cosmic Clocks.* Peter Owen, London, 1967.

GAUQUELIN, M. *Cosmic Influences on Human Intelligence.* Futura, London, 1974.

GEDDES, S. *Astrology and Health.* Aquarian Press/Thorsons, Wellingborough, 1981.

JANSKY, R. *Modern Medical Astrology.* Astro-Analytics Publications, Van Nuys, California, 1974.

RUDYAR, D. *An Astrological Mandala.* Random House, New York, 1973.

AURAS

BAGNALL, O. *The Origin and Properties of the Human Aura.* University Books, New York, 1969.

LEADBEATER, C. W., AND BESANT, A. *Man, Visible and Invisible.* Theosophical Society, Adyar, Madras, 1974.

LEADBEATER, C. W., AND BESANT, A. *Thought Forms.* Theosophical Society, London, 1971.

KILNER, J. W. *The Aura.* Weiser, New York, 1973.

BATES METHOD

CORBETT, M. *Help Yourself to Better Sight.* Wilshire, Los Angeles, 1949.

HUXLEY, A. *The Art of Seeing.* Montana Books, Washington, 1975.

BIOENERGY

JOHNSON, L. *Bioenergetics.* Espiritu, Houston, 1974.

Lowen, A. *Bioenergetics.* Viking, New York, 1975.
Lowen, A. *The Way to Vibrant Health.* Harper & Row, New York, 1977.

Biofeedback
Blundell, G., and Cade, C. M. *Self Awareness and E.S.R.* Audio Publications, London, nd.
Cade, C. M., and Coxhead, N. *The Awakened Mind.* Wildwood House, London, 1979.
Green, E. and A. *Beyond Biofeedback.* Delacorte, New York, 1977.
Karlins, M., and Andrews, L. M. *Biofeedback.* Garnstone Press, London, 1973.

Biorhythms
Gittelson, B. *Biorhythm.* Warner, New York, 1977.

Chiropractic
Cannon, W. B. *The Wisdom of the Body.* Norton, New York, 1939.
Dintenfass, J. *Chiropractic: A Modern Way to Health.* Pyramid, New York, 1977.
Hassard, G. H., and Redd, C. L. *Elongation Treatment of Low Back Pain.* C. Thomas, Springfield, USA, 1959.
Jause, Houser and Wells. *Chiropractic Principles and Technique.* National College of Chiropractic, Lombard, Illinois, 1947.
Sordoni, A. J. *Chiropractic in Industry.* American Chiropractic Association, Des Moines, Iowa, 1962.

Colour therapy
Anderson, M. *Colour Healing.* Weiser, New York, 1975.
Birren, F. *Colour Psychology and Therapy.* University Books, New York, 1961.
Clark, L. *Colour Therapy.* Devon-Adair, Old Greenwich, USA, 1975.
Leadbeater, C. W., and Besant, A. *Man Visible and Invisible.* Theosophical Society, Adyar, Madras, 1974.

Diet and health
Altman, N. *Eating for Life.* Theosophical Publishing House, Illinois, 1973.
Atkinson, R. F. *Your Lifestyle — Health & Nutrition.* Doubleday, Sydney, 1984.
Cilento, Lady. *Nutrition of the Child.* Blackmores, Sydney, 1980.
Davies, S., and Stewart, A. *Nutritional Medicine.* Pan Books, London, 1987.
Lesser, M. *Nutrition and Vitamin Therapy.* Grove Press, New York, 1980.
Lewis, C. (ed). *Growing Up With Good Food.* Allen & Unwin, London, 1982.
Phillips, D. *Guide Book to Nutritional Factors in Edible Foods.* Pythagorean Press, Sydney, 1977.
Sattilaro, A. J. *Living Well Naturally.* Houghton Mifflin, Boston, 1984.
Steele, M. *The Warburton Programme.* Methuen, Sydney, 1985.
Stone, I. *The Healing Factor: Vitamin C Against Disease.* Grosset and Dunlap, New York, 1972.

Wahlqvist, M., and Collins, L. *Australian Kitchen Nutrition.* Sun Books/Macmillan, Melbourne, 1984.
Williams, R. *Nutrition Against Disease.* Bantam, New York, 1971.
Yudkin, J. *Encyclopedia of Nutrition.* Viking, New York and London, 1985.

Encounter therapy
Howard, J. *Please Touch.* McGraw-Hill, New York, 1970.
Rogers, C. *Carl Rogers on Encounter Groups.* Harper & Row, New York, 1970.
Schutz, W. *Here Comes Everybody.* Harper & Row, New York, 1971.

Fasting
Bragg, P. *The Miracle of Fasting.* Health Science, Santa Ana, California, nd.
Cott, A. *Fasting: The Ultimate Diet.* Bantam, New York, 1975.
Phillips. D. 'Fasting Can Save Your Life' *in N. Drury, Frontiers of Consciousness.* Greenhouse Press, Melbourne, 1975.
Shelton, H. *Fasting Can Save Your Life.* Natural Hygiene Press, Chicago, 1964.

Flower remedies of Dr Bach
Bach, E., and Wheeler, F. J. *The Bach Flower Remedies.* Keats, New Canaan, Connecticut, 1977.
Chancellor, P. *Handbook of the Bach Flower Remedies.* C. W. Daniel, London, 1971.
Drury, N. and S. *Healing Oils and Essences.* Harper & Row, Sydney, 1987.
Scheffer, M. *Bach Flower Therapy.* Thorsons, Wellingborough, 1986.
Vlamis, G. *Flowers to the Rescue.* Thorsons, Wellingborough, 1986.

Gestalt therapy
Naranjo, C. *The Techniques of Gestalt Therapy.* SAT Press, Berkeley, 1973.
Perls, F. *The Gestalt Approach.* Science and Behaviour Books, Ben Lomond, California, 1973.
Perls, F. *Gestalt Therapy Verbatim.* Real People Press, Lafayette, California, 1969.
Perls, F. *In and Out of the Garbage Pail.* Real People Press, Lafayette, California, 1969.

Herbalism
Bethel, M. *The Healing Power of Herbs.* Wilshire, Los Angeles, 1974.
Culpeper, N. *Culpeper's Herbal Remedies.* Wilshire, Los Angeles, 1973.
Grieve, M. *A Modern Herbal.* Dover, New York, 1971.
Griggs, B. *The Home Herbal.* Hale, London, 1986.
Hall, D. *Herb Tea Book.* Pythagorean Press, Sydney, 1980.
Hall, D. *The Book of Herbs.* Angus & Robertson, Sydney, 1972.
Hylton, W. *The Rodale Herb Book.* Rodale, Emmaus, USA, 1974.

KLOSS, J. *Back to Eden*. Woodbridge, Santa Barbara, 1972.

LAW, D. *The Concise Herbal Encyclopaedia*. St Martins Press, New York, 1973.

LEVY, J. *Common Herbs for Natural Health*. Schocken, New York, 1974.

LOEWENFELD, C., AND BACK, P. *The Complete Book of Herbs and Spices*. David and Charles, London, 1974; A. H. Reed, Sydney, 1974.

LUST, J. *The Herb Book*. Bantam, New York, 1974.

ROSE, J. *Herbs and Things*. Grosset and Dunlap, New York, 1974.

HOMEOPATHY

CAMPBELL, A. *The Two Faces of Homeopathy*. Hale, London, 1984.

COULTER, H. L. *Homeopathic Medicine*. Formur, St Louis, 1972.

GIBSON, D. M. *First Aid Homeopathy in Accidents and Ailments*. British Homeopathic Association, London, 1975.

HAHNEMANN, S. *The Chronic Diseases*. Jain Publishers, New Delhi, 1898.

HAHNEMANN, S. *The Organon of Medicine*. Hermes Press, Boulder, Colorado, 1977.

ROSS, A. C. GORDON. *Homeopathy*. Thorsons, Northamptonshire, 1976.

SHARMA, C. H. *A Manual of Homeopathy and Natural Medicine*. Dutton, New York, 1976.

VITHOULKAS, G. *Homeopathy: Medicine of the New Man*. Formur, St Louis, 1975.

VITHOULKAS, G. *The Science of Homeopathy*. Grove, New York, 1980.

HYPNOTHERAPY

FRENCH, N. *Successful Hypnotherapy*. Thorsons, Wellingborough, 1984.

MEARES, A. *A System of Medical Hypnosis*. W. B. Saunders, Philadelphia, 1960.

RHODES, R. H. *Therapy Through Hypnosis*. Wilshire, Los Angeles, 1975.

SPIEGEL, H., AND D. *Trance and Treatment*. Basic Books, New York, 1978.

VAN PELT, S. J. *Hypnotism and the Power Within*. Skeffington, London, nd.

WAXMAN, D. *Hypnosis*. Allen & Unwin, London, 1981.

IRIDOLOGY

HALL, D. *Iridology*. Nelson, Melbourne, 1980.

JENSEN, B. *The Science and Practice of Iridology*. Jensen's Nutritional and Health Products, Solana Beach, California, 1974.

KRIEGE, T. *Fundamental Basis of Irisdiagnosis*. Fowler, Essex, 1969.

LINDLAHR, H. *Irisdiagnosis and other Diagnostic Methods*. Health Research Press, Mokelume Hill, California, nd.

KIRLIAN DIAGNOSIS

DAVIS, M., AND LANE, E. *Rainbows of Life*. Harper & Row, New York, 1978.

KRIPPNER, S., AND RUBIN, D. *The Kirlian Aura*. Anchor/Doubleday, New York, 1974.

MOSS, T. *The Body Electric*. J. P. Tarcher, Los Angeles, 1979.

MACROBIOTICS

ABEHSERA, M. *Cooking For Life*. Avon, New York, 1972.

KUSHI, M. *The Book of Macrobiotics*. Japan Publications, Tokyo and New York, 1976.

OHSAWA, L. *The Art of Just Cooking*. Autumn Press, California, 1974.

MASSAGE

INKELES, G. *The New Massage*. Unwin, London, 1987.

INKELES, G., AND TODRIS, M. *The Art of Sensual Massage*. Unwin, London, 1977.

MEDITATION

ABDULLAH, S. 'Meditation: Achieving Internal Balance' in E. Goldwag, *Inner Balance*. Prentice-Hall, New Jersey, 1979.

COURT, S. *The Meditator's Manual*. Aquarian Press/Thorsons, Wellingborough, 1984.

DASS, B. R. 'Relative Realities' in R. Walsh and F. Vaughan, *Beyond Ego*. J. P. Tarcher, Los Angeles, 1980.

DRURY, N. (ed). *Inner Health*. Harper & Row, Sydney, 1985.

GOLEMAN, D. 'A Map for Inner Space' in R. Walsh *op. cit.*

GRIFFITH, F. 'Meditation Research' in J. White, *Frontiers of Consciousness*. Avon, New York, 1975.

JOHNSTON, W. *Silent Music: The Science of Meditation*. Collins, London, 1974.

KIEFER, D. 'Meditation and Biofeedback' in J. White, *The Highest State of Consciousness*. Anchor/Doubleday, New York, 1972.

NARANJO, C. *The One Quest*. Wildwood House, London, 1972.

RUSSELL, P. *The TM Technique*. Routledge and Kegan Paul, London, 1977.

WALSH, R. N. 'Meditation Research' in R. Walsh and F. Vaughan, *Beyond Ego*. J. P. Tarcher, Los Angeles, 1980.

MUSIC (NEW AGE)

HALPERN, S. *Sound Health*. Harper & Row, San Francisco, 1985.

WATSON, A., AND DRURY, N. *Healing Music*. Prism Press, Dorset, 1987.

NATURAL BIRTH AND BIRTH CONTROL

BILLINGS, E., AND WESTMORE, A. *The Billings Method*. Ann O'Donovan, Melbourne, 1980; Random House, New York, 1981.

DRAKE, K. AND J. *Natural Birth Control*. Thorsons, Wellingborough, 1984.

EWY, D. *Preparation for Childbirth*. New American Library, New York, 1976.

HAZELL, L. *Commonsense Childbirth*. Berkley, New York, 1976.

KITZINGER, S. *The Experience of Childbirth*. Viking, New York, 1972.

THOMPSON, J. *Healthy Pregnancy the Yoga Way*. Doubleday, New York, 1977.

NATUROPATHY

BENJAMIN, H. *Everybody's Guide to Nature Cure*. Thorsons, Northamptonshire, 1961.

BERKELEY HOLISTIC HEALTH CENTRE. *The Holistic Health Handbook*. And/Or Press, Berkeley, California, 1978.

HALL, D. *The Natural Health Book*. Nelson, Melbourne, 1974.

HALL, D. *What's Wrong With You?* Nelson, Melbourne, 1984.

TURNER, R. N. *Naturopathic Medicine*. Thorsons, Wellingborough, 1984.

NEGATIVE IONS

SOYKA, F., AND EDMONDS, A. *The Ion Effect*. Bantam, New York, 1977.

KRUEGER, A. P. 'Are Negative Ions Good For You?', *New Scientist* (UK), 14 June, 1973.

OSTEOPATHY

HOAG, J. M. *et al. Osteopathic Medicine*. McGraw Hill, New York, 1969.

STODDARD, A. *Manual of Osteopathic Practice*. Hutchinson, London, 1969.

STODDARD, A. *Manual of Osteopathic Technique*. Hutchinson, London, 1962.

PAST LIFE THERAPY

HAGON, M. *Journey Within*. Iona Sanctuary, Sydney, 1981.

NETHERTON, M., AND SHIFFRIN, N. *Past Lives Therapy*. Compendium, Melbourne, 1978.

RAMSTER, P. *The Truth About Reincarnation*. Rigby, Adelaide, 1980.

STEVENSON, I. *The Evidence for Survival from Claimed Memories of Former Incarnations*. Privately published, Tadworth, Surrey, 1961.

STEVENSON, I. *Twenty Cases Suggestive of Reincarnation*. American Society for Psychical Research, New York, 1966; reissued by University of Virginia Press.

WAMBACH, H. *Reliving Past Lives*. Harper & Row, New York, 1978.

POLARITY THERAPY

GORDON, R. *Your Healing Hands: The Polarity Experience*. Unity Press, Santa Cruz, 1978.

STONE, R. *Energy: The Vital Principle in the Healing Art*. Privately published, Chicago, 1948.

STONE, R. *Health Building*. Pannetier, Orange, California, 1978.

PRIMAL THERAPY

JANOV, A. *The Primal Revolution*. Abacus, London, 1975.

JANOV, A. *The Primal Scream*. Abacus, London, 1973.

JANOV, A. *Prisoners of Pain*. Anchor/Doubleday, New York, 1980.

JANOV, A., AND HOLDEN, E. *Primal Man: The New Consciousness*. T. Y. Crowell, New York, 1975.

PSIONIC MEDICINE

REYNER, L., AND V. *Psionic Medicine*. Routledge and Kegan Paul, London, 1974.

PSYCHIC SURGERY

DOWNS, C. 'My Meeting with Benji' in *Simply Living*. Vol. I, No. 2, Sydney, 1976.

FULLER, J. G. *Arigo — Surgeon of the Rusty Knife*. Panther, London, 1977.

KRIPPNER, S., AND VILLOLDO, A. *The Realms of Healing*. Celestial Arts, Millbrae, California, 1976.

PLAYFAIR, G. L. *The Indefinite Boundary*. Panther, London, 1977.

PLAYFAIR, G. L. *The Unknown Power*. Panther, London, 1975.

PSYCHOMETRY

HAGON, M. *Journey Within*. Iona Sanctuary, Sydney, 1981.

PSYCHOSOMATIC HEALING

CARLSON, R. J. *Frontiers of Science and Medicine*. Regnery, Chicago, 1975.

PYRAMID ENERGY

RIXON, G. *Discover Pyramid Power*. Pythagorean Press, Sydney, 1981.

RADIESTHESIA

BENHAM, W., AND WILLIAMSON, J. *Handbook of the Aura Biometer*. Society of Metaphysicians, London, 1968.

REYNER, L., AND V. *Psionic Medicine*. Routledge and Kegan Paul, London, 1974.

WETHERED, V. D. *An Introduction to Medical Radiesthesia and Radionics*. C. W. Daniel, London, 1974.

RADIONICS

RUSSELL, E. *Report on Radionics*. Spearman, London, 1973.

RUSSELL, E. 'Radionics — Science of the Future' in J. White and S. Krippner, *Future Science*. Anchor/Doubleday, New York, 1977.

TANSLEY, D. V. *Radionics and the Subtle Anatomy of Man*. Health Science Press, Bradford, Devon, 1972.

REFLEXOLOGY

BERGSON, A., AND TUCHAK, V. *Zone Therapy*. Pinnacle, New York, 1975.

INGHAM, E. D. *Stories The Feet Have Told Me*. Ingham, Rochester, NY, 1951.

KAYE, A., AND MATCHAN, D. C. *Reflexology for Good Health*. Wilshire, Los Angeles, 1978.

REICHIAN THERAPY

BOADELLA, D. *Wilhelm Reich — the Evolution of his Work*. Vision Press, London, 1973.

LUTON, L. 'Reichian and Neo-Reichian Therapy' in N. Drury (ed.), *The Bodywork Book*. Harper & Row, Sydney, 1985.

MANN, W. E. *Orgone, Reich and Eros*. Simon and Schuster, New York, 1973.

ROLFING

PIERCE, R. 'Rolfing' in Berkeley Holistic Health Centre, *The Holistic Health Handbook*. And/Or Press, Berkeley, 1978.

SEXUAL THERAPY

BUTTON, J. *Making Love Work.* Turnstone Press/Thorsons, Wellingborough, 1985.

CRENSHAW, T. L. *Your Guide to Better Sex.* Rigby, Adelaide, 1985.

KAPLAN, H. S. *The Illustrated Manual of Sex Therapy.* Granada, London, 1981.

LIDELL, L. *The Sensual Body.* Unwin, London, 1987.

MASTERS, W. H., AND JOHNSON, V. E. *Human Sexual Response.* Little Brown, Boston, 1966.

MASTERS, W. H., AND JOHNSON, V. E. *Human Sexual Inadequacy.* Little Brown, Boston, 1970.

MASTERS, W. H., AND JOHNSON, V. E. *Homosexuality in Perspective.* Little Brown, Boston, 1979.

PIETROPINTO, A., AND SIMENAUER, J. *Beyond the Male Myth.* Times Books, New York, 1977; Harper & Row, Sydney, 1979.

SZASZ, T. *Sex By Prescription.* Anchor/Doubleday, New York, 1980.

SHAMANIC HEALING

DRURY, N. *The Shaman and the Magician.* Routledge and Kegan Paul, London, 1982.

ELIADE, M. *Shamanism.* Princeton University Press, New Jersey, 1964.

FURST, P. T. *Flesh of the Gods.* Allen and Unwin, London, 1972.

HARNER, M. *Hallucinogens and Shamanism.* Oxford University Press, New York, 1973.

HARNER, M. *The Way of the Shaman.* Harper & Row, San Francisco, 1980.

RIOS, M. DE. *Visionary Vine.* Chandler, San Francisco, 1972.

SHIATSU AND ACUPRESSURE

BLATE, M. *The Natural Healer's Acupressure Handbook.* Routledge & Kegan Paul, London, 1978.

EWALD, H. *Acupressure Techniques.* Thorsons, Wellingborough, 1984.

HOUSTON, F. M. *The Healing Benefits of Acupressure.* Thorsons, Northamptonshire, 1958.

MASUNAGA, S., AND OHASHI, W. *Zen Shiatsu.* Japan Publications, Tokyo, 1977.

OHASHI, W. *Do-It-Yourself Shiatsu.* Mandala/ Unwin, London, 1977.

WARREN, F. Z. *Freedom From Pain Through Acupressure.* Frederick Fell, New York, 1976.

YAMAMOTO, S. *Barefoot Shiatsu.* Japan Publications, Tokyo, 1979.

SPIRITUAL HEALING

EDWARDS, H. *The Healing Intelligence.* Hawthorn, New York, 1965.

EDWARDS, H. *The Power of Spiritual Healing.* Herbert Jenkins, London, 1963.

HAMMOND, S. *We Are All Healers.* Turnstone, London, 1973.

WORRALL, A. AND O. *The Gift of Healing.* Rider, London, 1969.

TAI CHI CH'UAN

HORWITZ, T., AND KIMMELMAN, S. *Tai Chi Ch'uan.* Rider, London, 1979.

HUANG, A. C. *Embrace Tiger, Return to Mountain.* Bantam, New York, 1978.

KHOR, G. *Tai Chi.* Boobooks, Sydney, 1981.

LIANG, T. T. *Tai Chi Ch'uan for Health and Self-Defence.* Redwing, Boston, 1974.

MAISEL, E. *Tai Chi for Health.* Dell, New York, 1963.

TONING

KEYES, L. E. *Toning: The Creative Power of the Voice.* De Vorss, Santa Monica, 1973.

YOGA

CHAUDHURI, H. 'Yoga Psychology' in C. Tart, *Transpersonal Psychologies.* Harper & Row, New York, 1975.

ELIADE, M. *Yoga, Immortality and Freedom.* Princeton University Press, New Jersey, 1969.

KRISHNA, G. *Kundalini.* Robinson and Watkins, London, 1971.

MUMFORD, J. *Psychsomatic Yoga.* Aquarian Press, Northamptonshire, 1979.

PICTURE CREDITS

All photographs, tables and illustrations in this book appear courtesy of *Nature & Health* magazine except for the following, which are gratefully acknowledged:

page 113 — Anne O'Donovan Ltd, Melbourne; pages 114, 115, 116 (upper), 137, 146, 149, 153, 156, 157, 158, 160, 193, 226, 270 — the collection of Nevill and Susan Drury; page 135 — Dorothy Hall; pages 141, 147 — East-West Centre, Sydney; page 152 — K. Benveniste/ Doubleday, New York; page 165 — Trager Institute; and page 255 — Irene Lorbergs.